9
自我保健

	中文	英文
主　编	张文高	徐象才
副主编	尹常健	李　磊　黄嘉陵
编　者	欧阳兵	王正忠　孙祥燮
		张　苏　雷希濂
审　校		约翰·布莱克

MAINTAINING YOUR HEALTH

	English	Chinese
Chief Editor	Xu Xiangcai	Zhang Wengao
Deputy Chief Editors	Li Lei Huang Jialing	Yin Changjian
Editors	Wang Zhengzhong Sun Xiangxie Zhang Su Lei Xilian	Ouyang Bing
Reviser	John · R · Black	

The Leading Commission of Compilation and Translation
编译领导委员会

Honorary Director 名誉主任委员	Hu Ximing 胡熙明		
Honorary Deputy Directors 名誉副主任委员	Zhang Qiwen 张奇文	Wang Lei 王镭	
Director 主任委员	Zou Jilong 邹积隆		
Deputy Director 副主任委员	Wei Jiwu 隗继武		
Members 委员 (以姓氏笔划为序)	Wan Deguang 万德光	Wang Yongyan 王永炎	Wang Maoze 王懋泽
	Wei Guikang 韦贵康	Cong Chunyu 丛春雨	Liu Zhongben 刘中本
	Sun Guojie 孙国杰	Yan Shiyun 严世芸	Qiu Dewen 邱德文
	Shang Chichang 尚炽昌	Xiang Ping 项平	Zhao Yisen 赵以森
	Gao Jinliang 高金亮	Cheng Yichun 程益春	Ge Linyi 葛琳仪
	Cai Jianqian 蔡剑前	Zhai Weimin 瞿维敏	
Advisers 顾问	Dong Jianhua 董建华	Huang Xiaokai 黄孝楷	Geng Jianting 耿鉴庭
	Zhou Fengwu 周凤梧	Zhou Ciqing 周次清	Chen Keji 陈可冀

The Commission of Compilation and Translation
编译委员会

Director 主任委员	Xu Xiangcai 徐象才

Deputy Directors 副主任委员	Zhang Zhigang 张志刚	Zhang Wengao 张文高	Jiang Zhaojun 姜兆俊
	Qi Xiuheng 亓秀恒	Xuan Jiasheng 宣家声	Sun Xiangxie 孙祥燮
Members 委员 (以姓氏笔划为序)	Yu Wenping 于文平	Wang Zhengzhong 王正忠	Wang Chenying 王陈应
	Wang Guocai 王国才	Fang Tingyu 方廷钰	Fang Xuwu 方续武
	Tian Jingzhen 田景振	Bi Yongsheng 毕永升	Liu Yutan 刘玉檀
	Liu Chengcai 刘承才	Liu Jiaqi 刘家起	Liu Xiaojuan 刘晓娟
	Zhu Zhongbao 朱忠宝	Zhu Zhenduo 朱振铎	Xun Jianying 寻建英
	Li Lei 李磊	Li Zhulan 李竹兰	Xin Shoupu 辛宁璞
	Shao Nianfang 邵念方	Chen Shaomin 陈绍民	Zou Jilong 邹积隆
	Lu Shengnian 陆胜年	Zhou Xing 周行	Zhou Ciqing 周次清
	Zhang Sufang 张素芳	Yang Chongfeng 杨崇峰	Zhao Chunxiu 赵纯修
	Yu Changzheng 俞昌正	Hu Zunda 胡遵达	Xu Heying 须鹤瑛
	Yuan Jiurong 袁久荣	Huang Naijian 黄乃健	Huang Kuiming 黄奎铭
	Huang Jialing 黄嘉陵	Cao Yixun 曹贻训	Lei Xilian 雷希濂
	Cai Huasong 蔡华松	Cai Jianqian 蔡剑前	

Preface

I am delighted to learn that THE ENGLISH-CHINESE ENCYCLOPEDIA OF PRACTICAL TRADITIONAL CHINESE MEDICINE will soon come into the world.

TCM has experienced many vicissitudes of times but has remained evergreen. It has made great contributions not only to the power and prosperity of our Chinese nation but to the enrichment and improvement of world medicine. Unfortunately, differences in nations, states and languages have slowed down its spreading and flowing outside China. At present, however, an upsurge in learning, researching and applying Traditional Chinese Medicine (TCM) is unfolding. In order to maximize the effect of this upsurge and to lead TCM, one of the brilliant cultural heritages of the Chinese nation, to the world for it to expand and bring benefit to the people of all nations, Mr. Xu Xiangcai called intellectuals of noble aspirations and high intelligence together from Shandong and many other provinces in China and took charge of the work of both compilation and translation of THE ENGLISH-CHINESE ENCYCLOPEDIA OF PRACTICAL TRADITIONAL CHINESE MEDICINE. With great pleasure, the medical staff both at home and abroad will hail the appearance of this encyclopedia.

I believe that the day when the world's medicine is fully

developed will be the day when TCM has spread throughout the world.

I am pleased to give it my preface.

Prof. Dr. Hu Ximing
 Deputy Minister of the Ministry of Public Health of the People's Republic of China,
 Director General of the State Administrative Bureau of Traditional Chinese Medicine and Pharmacology,
 President of the World Federation of Acupuncture —Moxibustion Societies,
 Member of China Association of Science & Technology,
 Deputy President of All—China Association of Traditional Chinese Medicine,
 President of China Acupuncture & Moxibustion Society.

December, 1989

Preface

The Chinese nation has been through a long, arduous course of struggling against diseases and has developed its own traditional medicine—Traditional Chinese Medicine and Pharmacology (TCMP). TCMP has a unique, comprehensive, scientific system including both theories and clinical practice. Some thousand years since ito—beginnings, not only has it been well preserved but also continuously developed. It has special advantages, such as remarkable curative effects and few side effects. Hence it is an effective means by which people prevent and treat diseases and keep themselves strong and healthy.

All achievements attained by any nation in the development of medicine are the public wealth of all mankind. They should not be confined within a single country. What is more, the need to set them free to flow throughout the world as quickly and precisely as possible is greater than that of any other kind of science. During my more than thirty years of being engaged in Traditional Chinese Medicine(TCM), I have been looking forward to the day when TCMP will have spread all over the world and made its contributions to the elimination of diseases of all mankind. However it is to be deeply regretted that the pace of TCMP in extending outside China has been unsatisfactory due to the major difficulties in expressing its concepts in foreign languages.

Mr. Xu Xiangcai, a teacher of Shandong College of TCM, has sponsored and taken charge of the work of compilation and translation of The English-Chinese Encyclopedia of Practical Traditional Chinese Medicine—an extensive series. This work is a great project, a large-scale scientific research, a courageous effort and a novel creation. I deeply esteem Mr. Xu Xiangcai and his compilers and translators, who have been working day and night for such a long time, for their hard labor and for their firm and indomitable will displayed in overcoming one difficulty after another, and for their great success achieved in this way. As a leader in the circles of TCM, I am duty-bound to do my best to support them.

I believe this encyclopedia will be certain to find its position both in the history of Chinese medicine and in the history of world science and technology.

Mr. Zhang Qiwen
Member of the Standing Committee of
All-China Association of TCM,
Deputy Head of the Health Department
of Shandong Province.
March, 1990

Publisher's Preface

Traditional Chinese Medicine(TCM) is one of China's great cultural heritages. Since the founding of the People's Republic of China in 1949, guided by the farsighted TCM policy of the Chinese Communist Party and the Chinese government, the treasure house of the theories of TCM has been continuously explored and the plentiful literature researched and compiled. As a result, great success has been achieved. Today there has appeared a world-wide upsurge in the studying and researching of TCM. To promote even more vigorous development of this trend in order that TCM may better serve all mankind, efforts are required to further it throughout the world. To bring this about, the language barriers must be overcome as soon as possible in order that TCM can be accurately expressed in foreign languages.

Thus the compilation and translation of a series of English–Chinese books of basic knowledge of TCM has become of great urgency to serve the needs of medical and educational circles both inside and outside China.

In recent years, at the request of the health departments, satisfactory achievements have been made in researching the expression of TCM in English. Based on the investigation into the history and current state of the research work mentioned above, the English–Chinese Encyclopedia of Practical TCM has been published to meet the needs of extending the knowledge of TCM around the world.

The encyclopedia consists of twenty-one volumes, each dealing with a particular branch of TCM. In the process of compilation, the distinguishing features of TCM have been given close attention and great efforts have been made to ensure that the content is scientific, practical, comprehensive and concise. The chief writers of the Chinese manuscripts include professors or associate professors with at least twenty years of practical clinical and / or teaching experience in TCM. The Chinese manuscript of each volume has been checked and approved by a specialist of the relevant branch of TCM. The team of the translators and revisers of the English versions consists of TCM specialists with a good command of English professional medical translators, and teachers of English from TCM colleges or universities. At a symposium to standardize the English versions, scholars from twenty-two colleges or universities, research institutes of TCM or other health institutes probed the question of how to express TCM in English more comprehensively, systematically and accurately, and discussed and deliberated in detail the English versions of some volumes in order to upgrade the English versions of the whole series. The English version of each volume has been re-examined and then given a final checking.

Obviously this encyclopedia will provide extensive reading material of TCM English for senior students in colleges of TCM in China and will also greatly benefit foreigners studying TCM.

The assiduous efforts of compiling and translating this encyclopedia have been supported by the responsible leaders of the State Education Commission of the People's Republic of China, the State Administrative Bureau of TCM and Pharmacy, and the Education Commission and Health Department of Shandong

Province. Under the direction of the Higher Education Department of the State Education Commission, the leading board of compilation and translation of this encyclopedia was set up. The leaders of many colleges of TCM and pharmaceutical factories of TCM have also given assistance.

We hope that this encyclopedia will bring about a good effect on enhancing the teaching of TCM English at the colleges of TCM in China, on cultivating skills in medical circles in exchanging ideas of TCM with patients in English, and on giving an impetus to the study of TCM outside China.

Higher Education Press
March, 1990

Foreword

The English–Chinese Encyclopedia of Practical Traditional Chinese Medicine is an extensive series of twenty–one volumes. Based on the fundamental theories of traditional Chinese medicine(TCM) and with emphasis on the clinical practice of TCM, it is a semi–advanced English–Chinese academic works which is quite comprehensive, systematic, concise, practical and easy to read. It caters mainly to the following readers: senior students of colleges of TCM, young and middle–aged teachers of colleges of TCM, young and middle–aged physicians of hospitals of TCM, personnel of scientific research institutions of TCM, teachers giving correspondence courses in TCM to foreigners, TCM personnel going abroad in the capacity of lecturers or physicians, those trained in Western medicine but wishing to study TCM, and foreigners coming to China to learn TCM or to take refresher courses in TCM.

Because Traditional Chinese Medicine and Pharmacology is unique to our Chinese nation, putting TCM into English has been the crux of the compilation and translation of this encyclopedia. Owing to the fact that no one can be proficient both in the theories of Traditional Chinese Medicine and Pharmacology and the clinical practice of every branch of TCM, as well as in English, to ensure that the English versions express accurately the inherent meanings of TCM, collective translation measures have been taken. That is, teachers of English familiar with TCM, professional medical translators, teachers or physicians of TCM and even teachers of palaeography with a strong command of English were all invited together to co-translate the Chinese manuscripts and, then, to co-deliberate and discuss the English versions. Finally English-speaking foreigners studying TCM or teaching English in China were asked to polish the English versions. In this way, the skills of the above translators and foreigners were merged to ensure the quality of the English versions. However, even using this method, the uncertainty that the English versions will be wholly accepted still remains. As for the Chinese manuscripts, they do reflect the essence, and give a general picture, of traditional Chinese medicine and pharmacology. It is not asserted, though, that they are perfect, I whole-heartedly look forward to any criticisms or opinions from readers in order to make improvements to future editions.

More than 200 people have taken part in the activities of compiling, translating and revising this encyclopedia. They come from twenty-eight institutions in all parts of China. Among these institutions, there are fifteen colleges of TCM:Shandong, Beijing, Shanghai, Tianjin, Nanjing, Zhejiang, Anhui, Henan, Hubei, Guangxi, Guiyang, Gansu, Chengdu, Shanxi and Changchun, and scientific research centers of TCM such as China Academy of TCM and Shandong Scientific Research Institute of TCM.

The Education Commission of Shandong province has included the compilation and translation of this encyclopedia in its scientific research projects and allocated funds accordingly. The Health Department of Shandong Province has also given financial aid together with a number of pharmaceutical factories of TCM. The subsidization from Jinan Pharmaceutical Factory of

TCM provided the impetus for the work of compilation and translation to get under way.

The success of compiling and translating this encyclopedia is not only the fruit of the collective labor of all the compilers, translators and revisers but also the result of the support of the responsible leaders of the relevant leading institutions. As the encyclopedia is going to be published, I express my heartfelt thanks to all the compilers. translators and revisers for their sincere cooperation, and to the specialists, professors, leaders at all levels and pharmaceutical factories of TCM for their warm support.

It is my most profound wish that the publication of this encyclopedia will take its role in cultivating talented persons of TCM having a very good command of TCM English and in extending, rapidly, comprehensive knowledge of TCM to all corners of the globe.

    Chief Editor Xu Xiangcai
           Shandong College of TCM
              March, 1990

Contents

Notes ··· 1
1 Principles of Health Care in TCM ····································· 1
  1.1 Mental Health Care ··· 1
    1.1.1 Being Open—minded and Optimistic ··································· 3
    1.1.2 Keeping a Clear Mind and Reducing Desire ······················· 7
    1.1.3 Controlling Joy and Anger ·· 10
    1.1.4 Abstaining from Too Much Worry ······································ 13
    1.1.5 Refraining from Grief, Sorrow and Misery ························ 15
    1.1.6 Avoiding Terror and Fear ·· 16
  1.2 Dietetic Health Care ·· 17
    1.2.1 Choosing a Simple and Light Diet ·· 18
    1.2.2 Seasoning Food with the Five Tastes Properly ················· 21
    1.2.3 Dining at Regular Times and Controlling the Intake ········ 24
    1.2.4 Regulating Cold and Heat of Food ······································ 28
    1.2.5 Following Proper Methods of Cleanliness ························· 29
    1.2.6 Following Some Instructions in Diet ··································· 30
  1.3 Regular—life Health Care ·· 41
    1.3.1 Leading a Regular Life ·· 42
    1.3.2 Following a Correct Way of Sleeping ·································· 43
    1.3.3 Adjusting One's Clothing According to Climate ················ 48
    1.3.4 Paying Attention of Hygiene ··· 50
  1.4 Balance between Work and Rest for Health Care ······· 54
    1.4.1 Avoiding Overwork ··· 54
    1.4.2 Avoiding Irritability ··· 57

1.4.3	Regulating Sexual Life	59
1.4.4	Avoiding Excessive Leisure	64

1.5 Health Care by Sports ... 66
    1.5.1 Participating in Physical Labour ... 67
    1.5.2 Taking Part in Physical Training ... 68
    1.5.3 Brief Introduction to Common Exercises ... 68

1.6 Health Care by Conforming to Nature ... 70
    1.6.1 Conforming to the Four Seasons ... 71
    1.6.2 Adjusting the Environment ... 77

2 Practical Chinese Materia Medica for Health Care ... 83
2.1 Commonly Used Chinese Material Medicines for Health Care ... 83
2.1.1 *Qi* Tonics ... 83
1. Ren Shen
2. Xi Yang Shen
3. Tai Zi Shen
4. Ci Wu Jia
5. Dang Shen
6. Huang Qi
7. Bai Zhu
8. Gan Cao
9. Shan Yao
10. Huang Jing
11. Da Zao
12. Yi Tang
13. Feng Mi

2.1.2 Blood Tonics ... 93
1. E Jiao
2. Dang Gui
3. Shu Di Huang
4. He Shou Wu
5. Bai Shao
6. Long Yan Rou
7. Sang Shen

2.1.3 Yang Tonics ... 98
1. Lu Rong
2. Ge Jie
3. Ba Ji Tian
4. Du Zhong
5. Dong Chong Xia Cao
6. Zi He Che

    7. *Tu Si Zi*   8. *Hu Tao Ren*

    9. *Yang Qi Shi*   10. *Bu Gu Zhi*

    11. *Yin Yang Huo*

2.1.4 Yin Tonics ······ 105

    1. *Sha Shen*   2. *Tian Dong*

    3. *Shi Hu*   4. *Mai Dong*

    5. *Yu Zhu*   6. *Bai He*

    7. *Gou Qi Zi*   8. *Nü Zhen Zi*

    9. *Hei Zhi Ma*   10. *Bie*

    11. *Yin Er*

2.1.5 Other Chinese Medicines for Health Care ······ 113

    1. *Suan Zao Ren*   2. *Shan Zha*

    3. *Lian Zi*   4. *Ling Zhi*

    5. *Fu Ling*   6. *Yi Yi Ren*

    7. *Qian Shi*   8. *Xiang Gu*

    9. *Mu Er*   10. *Ju Hua*

    11. *Dan Shen*   12. *San Qi*

    13. *Tian Ma*   14. *Hua Fen*

2.2 Commonly Used Chinese Patent Medicines for Health Care ······ 122

2.2.1 Patent Medicines for Tonifying *Qi* ······ 122

    1. *Bu Zhong Yi Qi Wan*   2. *Shen Ling Bai Zhu Wan*

    3. *Si Jun Zi Wan*   4. *Shi Quan Da Bu Wan*

    5. *Liang Shen Jing*   6. *Ren Shen Feng Wang Jiang*

    7. *Bei Jing Feng Wang Jing*   8. *Yan Nian Yi Shou Jing*

    9. *Wu Jia Shen Chong Ji*   10. *Da Li Shi Bu Ye*

    11. *Ren Shen VitC Zi Bu Pian*   12. *Qing Chun Bao*

    13. *Wan Nian Chun Zi Bu Jiang*

2.2.2 Patent Medicines for Nourishing Blood ······ 132

1. *Ba Zhen Wan*　　　　2. *Fu Fang E Jiao Jiang*
3. *Kang Bao*　　　　　4. *Shen Qi Wang Jiang Yang Xue Jing*
5. *Ren Shen Shou Wu Jing*　6. *E Jiao Zi Bu Jing*
7. *Liang Yi Chong Ji*　　8. *Yi Shou Zi Bu Jiang*
9. *Bu Xue Ning Shen Pian*　10. *Shen Gui Zao Zhi*

2.2.3　Patent Medicines for Supporting *Yang* ·················· 138
1. *Jin Kui Shen Qi Wan*　　2. *Hai Long Ge Jie Jing*
3. *Nan Bao*　　　　　　4. *Shen Rong Bian Wan*
5. *Yang Chun Yao*　　　6. *Yi Shen Tang Jiang*
7. *Shen Rong Da Bu Wan*　8. *Chu Feng Jing*
9. *Hai Ma Bu Shen Wan*　10. *Mei Hua Lu Rong Xue*
11. *Hai Shen Wan*

2.2.4　Patent Medicines for Nourishing *Yin* ·················· 148
1. *Liu Wei Di Huang Wan*　2. *Ren Shen Gu Ben Wan*
3. *Jian Nao Chong Ji*　　4. *Shen Qi Feng Huang Jiang*
5. *Zi Yin Bai Bu Wan*　　6. *Kang Fu Wan*
7. *Qing Gong Shou Tao Wan*

2.2.5　Other Patent Medicines for Health Care ·················· 154
1. *Ling Zhi Pian*　　　　2. *Yi Nao Fu Jian Wan*
3. *Nao Ling Su*　　　　4. *You Kang Ping*
5. *An Shen Bu Xin Wan*　6. *Yi Chun Bao Kou Fu Ye*
7. *Ling Zhi Qiang Ti Pian*　8. *Dan Qi Pian*
9. *Nü Bao*　　　　　　10. *Geng Nian An*

2.3　Chinese Medicated Liquor for Health Care ·················· 161
2.3.1　Health-care Effects of Chinese Medicated Liquor ········· 163
1. Regulating *Yin* and *Yang*　2. Invigorating *Qi* and blood
3. Tonifying the five *Zang*　4. Eliminating illness and expelling evils
5. Prolonging life

2.3.2　Mechanism of Chinese Medicated Liquor ·················· 165

2. 3. 3　Characteristics of Health Care with Chinese Medicated Liquor ················· 168
　1. Liquor Helps Potentiate Medicines
　2. Wide Endications and Easy Preparation
　3. Stable Effect and Convenient Administration
2. 3. 4　Indications of Chinese Medicated Liquor for Health Care ················· 169
　1. Indications of Medicated Liquor for Replenishing *Qi*
　2. Indications of Medicated Liquor for Nourishing blood
　3. Indications of Medicated Liquor for Nourishing *Yin*
　4. Indications of Medicated Liquor for Reinforcing *Yang*
　5. Indications of Medicated Liquor for Tonifying the Five *Zang* Organs
　6. Indications of Medicated Liquor for Prolonging Life
　7. Indications of Medicated Liquor for Preventing Diseases and Building up health
2. 3. 5　Preparation of Medicated Liquor ················· 171
2. 3. 6　Cautions for Taking Medicated Liquor ················· 174
2. 3. 7　Commonly Used Medicated Liquor ················· 177
　1. Medicated Liquor for Tonifying *Qi* ················· 177
　　Ren Shen Jiu　　Shen Qi Yi Qi Jiu　　San Sheng Jiu　　Huang Qi Sheng Mai Jiu　　Chang Sheng Gu Ben Jiu
　2. Medicated Liquor for Nourishing Blood ················· 181
　　E Jiao Jiu　　Long Yan Sang Shen Jiu　　Gui Yuan Jiu　　Yuan Rou Bu Xie Jiu　　Jiao Ai Jiu
　3. Medicated Liquor for Nourishing *Yin* ················· 186
　　Nü Zhen Zi Jiu　　Er Dong Jiu　　Yin Er Xiang Gu Jiu　　Gou Qi Yao Jiu　　Yang Shen Gu Ben Jiu　　Chun Shou Jiu　　Gu Jing Jiu
　4. Medicated Liquor for Supporting *Yang* ················· 192
　　Xian Ling Pi Jiu　　Ge Jie Jiu　　Lu Rong Jiu　　Fu Fang Lu

   Rong Chong   *Cao Jiu*   *Yang Shen Er Xian Jiu*   *San Bian Bu Jiu*   *Dong Bei San Bao Jiu*   *Qiong Jiang*

  5. Medicated Liquor for Tonifying both *Qi* and Blood ·················· 199

   Qi Gui Shuang Bu Jiu   *Ba Zhen Jiu*   *Shi Quan Da Bu Jiu*

  6. Medicated Liquor for Tonifying *Yin* and *Yang* ·················· 201

   Chong Cao Jiu   *Er Xian Jiu*   *Zi Yin Bai Bu Yao Jiu*

  7. Medicated Liquor for Tonifying the Five-*Zang* ·················· 205

   Fu Ling Jiu   *Shen Xian Yao Jiu Wan*   *Yang Xin An Shen Jiu*   *Shen Ge Chong Cao Jiu*   *Fu Fang Hai Ma Jiu*   *Shou Wu Qi Ju Jiu*   *Bu Xue Shun Qi Yao Jiu*

  8. Medicated Liquor for Prolonging Life ·················· 210

   Bai Sui Jiu   *Yan Shou Jiu Xian Jiu*   *Liao Bai Ji Yan Shou Jiu*   *Jing Shen Yao Jiu*

  9. Medicated Liquor for Preventing Diseases ·················· 215

   Ju Zha Yi Xin Jiu   *Jian Xin Ling Jiu*   *Tu Su Jiu*   *Du Huo Ji Sheng Jiu*   *Shen Rong Jiu*

2.4   Soft Extract for Health Care ·················· 221

2.4.1   Soft Extract for Invigorating *Qi* ·················· 226

  1. *Ren Shen Gao*   2. *Dai Shen Gao*

  3. *Yi Qi Kai Wei Gao*

2.4.2   Soft Extract for Nourishing the Blood ·················· 228

  1. *Sang Shen Gao*   2. *Qi Yuan Gao*

  3. *Shou Wu Bu Xue Gao*   4. *Dang Gui Bu Xue Gao*

2.4.3   Soft Extract for Nourishing *Yin* ·················· 231

  1. *Er Dong Gao*   2. *Er Zhi Gao*

  3. *Yang Yin Gao*

2.4.4   Soft Extract for Supporting *Yang* ·················· 233

  1. *Suo Yang Gao*   2. *Cong Rong Er Xian Gao*

  3. *Ge Jie Dang Shen Gao*

2.4.5 Soft Extract for Tonifying Both *Qi* and Blood 235
 1. *Liang Yi Gao*   2. *Shi Quan Da Bu Gao*
 3. *Yang Shen Shuang Bu Gao*

2.4.6 Soft Extract for Tonifying the Five-*Zang* Organs............ 238
 1. *Gou Qi Gao*   2. *Cang Zhu Gao*
 3. *Fu Ling Gao*   4. *Run Fei Gao*

2.4.7 Other Soft Extract for Tonifying the Body and Prolonging Life 242
 1. *Qiong Yu Gao*   2. *Yi Shou Yang Zhen Gao*
 3. *He Che Gao*   4. *Gui Lu Er Xian Gao*
 5. *Hong Yu Gao*   6. *Jia Jian Fu Yuan He Zhong Gao*
 7. *Jia Jian Fu Yuan Yi Yin Gao*

2.4.8 Soft Extract for Health Care Used to Prevent and Treat Diseases 250
 1. *Ju Hua Yan Ling Gao*   2. *Ming Mu Yan Ling Gao*
 3. *Jia Zhu Li Li Gao*   4. *Li Yan Gao*
 5. *Shou Wu Ju Zha Gao*   6. *Yi Qi Huo Xue Gao*
 7. *Lao Guan Cao Gao*

2.5 Chinese Herbal Tea for Health Care 256
 2.5.1 Herbal Tea for Invigorating *Qi* and Enriching Blood 259
  1. *Shen Qi Dai Cha Yin*   2. *Wu Bao Cha Tang*
  3. *Guan Yin Mian Cha*   4. *Wu Xiang Nai Cha*
  5. *Zhu Dong Dai Cha Yin*   6. *Sang Long Dai Cha Yin*
  7. *Yi Qi Sheng Jin Dai Cha Yin* 8. *Bu Xue He Wei Dai Cha Yin*

 2.5.2 Herbal Tea for Nourishing *Yin* and Supporting *Yang* 265
  1. *Yu Shi Dai Cha Yin*   2. *Er Shen Er Dong Dai Cha Yin*
  3. *Shen Ling Dai Chan Yin*   4. *Xian Ling Pi Cha*
  5. *Fu Fang Du Zhong Cha*   6. *Xin Er Xian Dai Cha Yin*
  7. *Fu Fang Gou Qi Cha*

2.5.3 Herbal Tea for Regulating the Function of the Spleen and Stomach to Promote Digestion 269

1. He Wei Dai Cha Yin
2. Er Shen Dai Cha Yin
3. Wu Xian Dai Cha Yin
4. Gan Lu Cha

2.5.4 Herbal Tea for Tranquilizing the Mind 272

1. An Shen Dai Cha Yin
2. Yuan Rou Er Ren Cha
3. Qing Xin Dai Cha Yin

2.5.5 Herbal Tea for Preventing and Treating Common Diseases 273

1. Ju Zha Dai Cha Yin
2. Shou Wu Jue Ming Cha
3. Fu Fang Yu Mi Xu Cha
4. Jian Fei Dai Cha Yin
5. Xiao Fei Jian Shen Cha
6. Fu Fang Luo Bu Ma Cha
7. Huang Yu Shi Dai Cha Yin
8. He Pei Fang Shu Cha
9. Wen Zhong Cha
10. Jian Wei Cha
11. Qing Jie Cha

2.6 Medicated Gruel for Health Care 278

1. Ren Shen Zhou
2. Bu Xu Zheng Qi Zhou
3. Da Zao Zhou
4. Shen Ling Zhou
5. Shan Yao Zhou
6. Bai Bian Dou Zhou
7. Huang Qi Zhou
8. Luo Hua Sheng Zhou
9. Zhu Yu Er Bao Zhou
10. Nuo Mi E Jiao Zhou
11. Long Yan Rou Zhou
12. Xian Ren Zhou
13. Ru Zhou
14. Hai Shen Zhou
15. Sang Shen Zhou
16. Ji Zhi Zhou
17. Tu Si Zi Zhou
18. Cong Rong Yang Rou Zhou
19. Hu Tao Zhou
20. Li Zhi Zhou
21. Li Zi Zhou
22. Que Er Yao Zhou
23. Lu Jiao Jiao Zhou
24. Gou Qi Yang Shen Zhou
25. Shan Yu Rou Zhou
26. Yu Zhu Zhou

  27. *Tian Men Dong Zhou* 28. *Sha Shen Zhou*

  29. *Bai He Fen Zhou*   30. *Lian Zi Fen Zhou*

  31. *Suan Zao Ren Zhou* 32. *Shan Zha Zhou*

  33. *Yi Yi Ren Zhou*

 2. 7 Medicated Cake for Health Care ·············· 310

  1. *Yang Chun Bai Xue Gao* 2. *Mi Chuan Er Xian Gao*

  3. *Jiu Xian Wang Dao Gao* 4. *Ba Xian Bai Yun Gao*

  5. *Ba Xian Zao Chao Gao* 6. *Ba Zhen Gao*

  7. *Jian Pi Yang Xin Gao* 8. *He Zhong Xiao Shi Gao*

 2. 8 Medicated Pancake for Health Care ············ 322

  1. *Tian Dong Bing Zi*   2. *Huang Jing Bing*

  3. *Zhuang Yang Nuan Xia Yao Bing* 4. *Qi Yi Bing*

  5. *Yi Pi Bing*   6. *Yi Shou Bing*

  7. *Jiu Xian Bao Jian Bing*

 2. 9 Externally-applied Plaster for Health Care ········· 332

  1. *Yang Xin Gao*   2. *Xin Shen Shuang Bu Gao*

  3. *Zhuan Yi Yuan Qi Gao* 4. *Yong Quan Gao*

  5. *Si Yin Bai Bing Gao*   6. *Bao Yuan Gu Ben Gao*

  7. *Yu Lin Gu Ben Gao*   8. *Yi Shou Bi Tian Gao*

 2. 10 Medicated Pillows for Health Care ············ 352

  1. *Qi Huang Pai Gao Xiao Bao Jian Yao Zhen* 2. *Shen Zhen Fang*

  3. *Bao Sheng Yao Lu Yao Zhen Fang* 4. *Ding Gong Xian Zhen*

  5. *Gao Xue Ya Bing Yao Zhen*   6. *Bao Jian Yao Zhen*

  7. *Jian Kang Chang Shou Yao Zhen* 8. *Jing Zhui Bing Yao Zhen*

  9. *Xiao Er Bi Yuan Yao Zhen*   10. *Li Shizhen Yao Zhen*

  11. *Shen Nong Pai Bao Jian Yao Zhen* 12. *Yi Shou Yao Zhen*

3 Health Care Independent of Medicines ············ 373

 3. 1 Acupuncture and Moxibustion for Health Care ········ 373

  3. 1. 1 The Effects of Acupuncture and Moxibustion in

· 9 ·

    Health Care ··· 374
 3. 1. 2 Mechanism of Acupuncture and Moxibustion for
    Health Care ··· 377
 3. 1. 3 Commonly Selected Acupoints in Health Care ················ 378
   1. Zusanli(ST36)   2. Shenque(RN8)
   3. Zhongji(RN3)   4. Guanyuan(RN4)
   5. Qihai(RN6)   6. Shenshu(BL23)
   7. Mingmen(DU4)   8. Sanyinjiao(SP6)
   9. Zhongwan(RN12) 10. Tianshu(ST25)
   11. Quchi(LI11)   12. Neiguan(PC6)
   13. Shenmen(HI7)   14. Dazhui(GB14)
   15. Feishu(BL13)   16. Xinshu(BL15)
   17. Ganshu(BL18)   18. Pishu(BL20)
   19. Weishu(BL21)   20. Huantiao(GB30)
   21. Yongquan(KI1) 22. Baihui(DU20)
   23. Danzhong(RN17)
 3. 1. 4 Acupuncture and Moxibustion for Health Care ············· 392
   1. Acupuncture for Health Care ··································· 392
   2. Moxibustion for Health Care ··································· 395
   3. Selection and Compatibility of Points in Acupuncture and
    Moxibustion for Health Care ································· 400
   4. Cautions in Acupuncture and Moxibustion for Health Care ········ 402
 3. 1. 5 Magnetotherapy for Health Care ······························ 404
3. 2 *Qigong* Exercises for Health Care ································· 405
 3. 2. 1 Ways of Exercising ·· 407
   1. Regulation of Posture 2. Regulation of Mental Activities
   3. Regulation of Respiration
 3. 2. 2 Types of *Qigong* Exercises ····································· 415
   1. *Songjing Gong*   2. *Neiyang Gong*

3. *Qiangzhuang Gong*

    3. 2. 3 Principles in Doing *Qigong* Exercises ················ 420

  3. 3 TCM Massage for Health Care·················· 421

    3. 3. 1 Classification and Manipulation ················ 423

    3. 3. 2 Self—massage for Health Care ················ 429

    3. 3. 3 Indications and Contraindications ················ 434

The English—Chinese Encyclopedia of Practical TCM (Booklist) ··· (628)

Notes

MAINTAINING YOUR HEALTH is the ninth volume of The English-Chinese Encyclopedia of Practical Traditional Chinese Medicine(TCM).

This volume consists of three chapters:Principles of Health Care in TCM, Practical Chinese Materia Medica for Health Care and Health Care Independent of Medicines, introducing the methods of mental health care, dietetic health care, regular-life health care, balancing work and rest for health care, health care by sports, and health care **by** conforming to nature;56 commonly used Chinese material medicines for health care, 51 commonly used Chinese patent medicines for health care, 47 commonly used medicated liquor for health care, 34 soft extract for health care, 33 Chinese herbal tea for health care, 33 medicated gruel for health care, 8 medicated cake for health care, 7 medicated pancake for health care, 8 externally-applying plaster for health care, and 12 medicated pillows for health care;acupuncture and moxibustion for health care, *Qigong* exercises for health care and TCM massage for health care;all suitable for self-application.

The Chinese manuscript was compiled by combining plenty of relevant information from a great many medical books with the author's own experience and knowledge, checked and approved by the famous specialist Prof. Chen Keji, and translated into English by translators, including Miss Feng Xiuping, Jiang Wenying, Huang Qingxian, etc. , from quite a few colleges all over China. To generalize the first draft of the English version, another seven translators and revisers, including Liu Qiang, Cao Huilai, John Black, etc. , were called in to work uninterruptedly together for one more year. They readjusted and re-translated part of the version, re-examined, re-corrected, refreshed, re-copied and re-typewrote the whole version, and at last produced the present version. Prof. Qi Xiuheng, Wang Zhengzhong, etc. once endeavoured to help check the first draft of English version.

In the English version, the names of Chinese Materia Medica are expressed with both Chinese spelling and Latin words. The Chinese spelling words are all monosyllabified and italicized for the foreign readers's convenience. The Latin words are capitalized to show the difference from English ones. Nearly all the Latin names of Chinese Materia Medica are from The Pharmacopoeia of The People's Republic of China published in 1990. The locations and numbers of acupoints are all from The Location of Acupoints—State Standard of the People's Republic of China published in 1990.

The Editors

1 Principles of Health Care in TCM

The principles of health care in TCM have been gradually developed and perfected through our forefathers' prolonged pratice of the techniques and methods of health care. The book *Nei Jing* generalizes the ways of health care into the following principles:"The techniques and methods should be based on the theory of *Yin* and *Yang* and should conform to the natural law; one should keep an orderly life with proper and controlled diet and avoid overwork; pathogenic wind and other ill factors should be prevented at all times;the essential *Qi* will result from a state of serenity and empty-mindedness, and one will be kept from diseases if he has a sound mind. Highly appreciated and advocated by experts of past ages in health care, these principles have been followed by people keeping themselves in good health. And it is just under the guidance of these principles that the content and methods of health care have been gradually developed and perfected.

1.1 Mental Health Care

In TCM, great attention has always been paid to the close relationship between mental activities and health. Its established theory of "integrating spirit with body" holds that both together make up an organic unity: to strengthen the spirit, one must strengthen the body, and to strengthen the body, one must strengthen the spirit, putting stress on the guiding position of regulation of the spirit in health care. TCM also holds that essence (*Jing*), vital energy (*Qi*), and spirit (*Shen*), are three treasures of one's life, granting longevity as well as resistance to diseases if they are conserved and cultivated. One can be healthy and free from illnesses only when he cultivates essence, uses *Qi* sparingly and takes good care of his spirit, so that he will be full of vigour with every organ performing its proper function. An imbalance of spirit, on the other hand, may result in various illnesses or even early death through exhaustion and loss of the body's essential *Qi*. This is what is meant by saying that "Failure to keep a sound mind may weaken resistance and invite attacks by pathogenic factors." and "Those who keep a sound mind will survive, and those who don't will die; those who gain a sound mind will live and those who don't will perish." Therefore, it is imperative, for the sake of preventing diseases and promoting longevity, to keep a sound mind. Man has seven emotions and six desires. But the seven emotions, i.e. joy, anger, melancholy, anxiety, grief, fear and terror, will cause, when excessive, disorder of the functions of *Zang* and *Fu*, which will lead to the reverse disorder of *Qi* and blood together with resultant pathological changes, bringing about great harm to human body. As is stated in the book *Nei Jing*, "It is known that all diseases arise from the upset of *Qi*: Anger pushes the *Qi* up, joy makes the *Qi* slacken, grief disperses the *Qi*, fear brings the *Qi* down... terror confuses the *Qi*... and anxiety causes the *Qi* to stagnate; and that anger harms the liver, joy the heart, anxiety the spleen, grief the lungs and fear the kidney." In short, loss of balance in mind and *Qi* will greatly affect one's health.

Mental health care has always been highly valued and applied as a major means of maintaining health and achieving longevity. It serves as a means of building up the body, strengthening resistance against disease, prolonging life through conscious adjustment, avoiding excessive stimulation of emotions, and keeping a sound mind and good mental balance. TCM works and documents on health care handed down from various historical periods have a great many discussions on mental health care and on effective and practical ways of building up by achieving a mental balance, which still guide the modern mental health care.

1.1.1 Being Open-minded and Optimistic

As the proverb goes, "Optimism will help you forget sorrow." An optimistic, stable mood and good mental balance will calm the vital energy and spirit, aid the circulation of blood and *Qi*, and improve health. The ancient book *Guan Zi* states, "The quality of one's life depends on maintaining a positive happy state of mind. Anxiety and anger lead to confusion of mind. There can be no mental balance when anxiety, grief, joy and anger exist. Thus desire should be subdued, and disorder be checked. Happiness and luck will arrive on their own if there is no such disturbance of mind." The book *Nei Jing* also points out that one should strive for tranquility and happiness, remaining free from anger, resentment and troubled thoughts. It indicates that by avoiding angry moods and a troubled state of mind and by cultivating tranquility, optimism and happiness, one will obtain longevity with a sound body which will not be easily degenerated and with a sound mind which will not be easily distracted. The book *Huai Nan Zi* advocates "happiness and cheerfulness", which is said to be a part of human nature. The book *Zun Sheng Ba Jian* also maintains that to tranquilize the mind one should have a happy mood. These statements indicate that good health is always based on happy and tranquil moods. To keep a happy mood, one must have a noble spirit, high ideals, an expanded outlook, a sanguine and lively disposition and an open and broad mind. While dealing with daily affairs and people, one must not be disposed to feeling extremely depressed from personal losses. As is said in the book *Ji Zhong San Ji,* "Cultivate a good temperament for the sake of mind;tranquilize the mind for the sake of life;avoid emotional extremes and adopt a care—free attitude. "If one can achieve such equanimity, he will be safe from unnecessary worries and enjoy an undisturbed mind and a sound body.

Also, to keep a happy state of mind, one should be able to tackle a problem in a composed manner. As the book *Shou Shi Qing Bian* says, "Don't worry about a problem before it has actually manifested don't worry too much after it has existed, and don't cling to what has already passed; instead; one should adopt a detached attitude towards its coming or going, leaving it alone and checking all emotions as anger, fear, desire, joy and anxiety. That is the way to health and longevity. "

Happiness lies in contentment, which is important not only for physical and mental health, but also in keeping a happy mood. The book *Dao De Jing* says, "There is no sin greater than discontent, and no error greater than covetousness. " Therefore, knowing what contentment is means constant satisfaction. The book *Zun Sheng Ba Jian* maintains, "Contentment will bring neither abuse nor danger. " Both statements express the idea that lasting happiness can be achieved only through contentment. In our actual life, most anxieties and worries result from going after and covetting fame, a higher status and material comfort. In face of such desires, one should always keep this in mind:"There are many others who have less than I. " In so doing, it will be easier for one to refrain from excessive desire and competition, to remain content with what one has, and to be cheerful and open-minded, so that anxiety will be expelled, tranquility of soul obtained, and the mind maintained in an optimistic and stable state.

The self-cultivation of one's sense of morality is another important method to maintain optimism, to which the ancients paid great attention. They professed, "The kind will enjoy longevity. " The kind here mean all those who have a well-developed sense of morality. The cultivation of morality involves devoted attention. The methods discoursed upon by the ancients, such as moderating desires, remaining content, and being tolerant, kind and courteous are all essential for that purpose. They also believed:"A person of great morality is sure to obtain longevity. " The reason why such a person lives a long life lies in the fact that he is "apt to cultivate the great-Qi", being broad-minded, and strong-willed as well as having great ideals and aims;meanwhile, those who respect others will receive respect from others, and those who are content will enjoy lasting happiness... all of these factors, together with tolerance and avoidance of anxiety, contribute to a balanced mind and a cheerful mood.

One guarantee of maintaining an optimistic frame of mind is to continuously enrich one's life by cultivating a great variety of interests and hobbies, such as reading, meeting friends, travelling, fishing, playing chess, practising calligraphy, painting, reciting poetry, singing, playing musical instruments, watering flowers, growing bamboo, etc. There are many discussions handed down from the ancients, maintaining that such activities can bring on cheerful mood and refine one's sensibility. The book *Yi Qing Xiao Lu* says, "One should always enjoy simple pleasures such as sunshine in winter or shade in summer, beautiful scenes on a bright day, walking cheerfully with a stick, watching fish in a pond, listening to birds singing in the woods, drinking a cup of wine or playing a stringed musical instrumnet." What is meant by this quotation is that one should relax the mind, choose and cultivate one's own hobbies and increase continually one's interest in life so that comfortable feelings, a stability of mind and cheerfulness will result, all of which contribute to good health and longevity.

In short, open—mindedness and optimism are important principles in regulating the mind and in health care. As it has been explained in the book *Nei Jing*, "That is why the saints did not concern themselves with purposeful actions. They cultivated tranquility and developed emptiness of mind. Their way of health care brought about a substantial longevity." This points out that those competent at health care will not do anything they feel reluctant to do, remaining free from whimsical and improper thoughts, keeping a cheerful and happy mood, cherishing a rich variety of interest, leading a tranquil and undisturbed life, maintaining a mind which is relaxed, happy, open and optimistic... this contributes to longevity.

1.1.2 Keeping a Clear Mind and Reducing Desire

Experts in health care of various historical periods of China have always attached great importance to clarification of mind and desirelessness, believing this to be an important point in regulating mind and prolonging life. The book *Li Lun Yao Ji* also says, "Health care lies in reducing desire."

Selfishness and desire exist in the mind; therefore, if they become extreme, the spirit and *Qi* will be disturbed, and, peace and tranquility of mind damaged. Thus, Lao Zi, the founder of *Daoism,* especially emphasized the maintenance of a clear mind and reduction of desire, advocating "the simple and plain life with least selfishness and desire". The book *Nei Jing* also regards a tranquil mind with least desire as a way to ensure longevity. Ge Hong, a famous physician and world known alchemist in the Jin Dynasty, stressed that to adjust one's mind requires "purify, modesty, freedon from desire and anxiety, maintenance of essence of life, and simple living with no indulgence in material comforts". The book *Zun Sheng Yao Zhi* states, "... Man has three treasures... essence, vital energy and spirit. People apt at health care will not spend them lavishly, but will keep hold of spirit, essence and *Qi* by reducing desire, refraining from talkativeness and avoiding anxiety respectively." This emphasizes that good health can be achieved through reduction of desire and elimination of improper thoughts, thus resulting in adjustment of *Qi* and blood, preservation of a peaceful mind, clarification and tranquilization of spirit and *Qi* in the interior, and resistance to harm from pathogenic factors. To the same effect, the book *Lei Xiu Yao Jue* holds, "To cultivate the mind, one must resist selfish thoughts." and the book *Hong Lu Dian Xue* stresses, "Long persistence in maintaining a clear mind and reducing desire will keep all diseases away."

For that purpose, the following three points are to be followed:

1. Controlling the mind with the understanding that selfishness and excessive desire are harmful to health

The book *Yang Sheng Lun* maintains, One should cultivate an empty and tranquil mind in which there is no place for selfishness and excessive desire to take root. He should avoid the pursuit of fame and power, knowing that they harm one's virtue. It is better that excessive desire not arise at all than that it be suppressed after it has emerged. In the same light, one should eliminate desire for wealth and possessions, knowing that it injures one's nature, rather than check the greediness for them after its emergence. Once excessive desire has emerged, it will be beyond suppression; and once greed has occurred, suppression may make it even greater; in such a case, no effect of tranquilizing the mind can be obtained. "The book *Yi Xue Ru Men* has this, "If one does not see the law of life and fails to grasp the essence, then even if he closes his eyes all day long, his mind is full of self-concern and he is only outwardly quiet but inwardly active. But if he realizes that there is a regulating law governing his life, he will do everything according to the law of nature without greed, haste and haughtiness, thus resisting illness and achieving longevity. "The upshot of this is that to control the mind with reason helps to eliminate selfish, improper thoughts and the mind is naturally tranquilized." All the above suggests that selfish and excessive thoughts are easy to eliminate and the mind is easy to calm by understanding why and how.

2. Eliminating six dangers and taking a correct attitude towards personal gains and losses

The book *Tai Shang Lao Jun Yang Sheng Jue* says, "Those good at health care will first try to eliminate six dangers before they can maintain life and achieve longevity. Then what are the things they must do? They are as follows: First, care little about fame and position; second, refrain from indulgence in entertainment and sexual life; third, discount riches; fourth, abstain from greed for food; fifth, get rid of haughtiness; sixth, eliminate jealousy." If the six dangers are not eliminated, the mind will be filled with various anxieties, and cannot remain tranquil.

3. Avoiding excessive stimulation of the eyes and ears

Of the five sense organs, the eyes and ears are two important ones with which the mind receives outside stimulation. Their functions are governed and controlled by the mind. If the eye and ear are protected from unhealthy stimulations. the vital energy and the mind will not be disturbed. Failing this, the case will be quite different. Lao Zi believed that "the maintenance of a tranquil mind" can be managed through "the effect not to see the desired objects". The ancient philosopher Zhuang Zi also held the view of keeping stimulation away from the eyes and ears, saying: "Without looking and listening, the mind will preserve its peace and the body will thereupon be in good condition." Such a proper attempt to refrain from watching and listening in order to decrease the unhealthy stimulation from the exterior to the mind can, though passive and seemingly impractical, succeed and be beneficial to health. To the same effect, the book *Qian Jin Yi Fang* has this to say, "What is important in health care for the aged is that they should not listen to anything improper, nor talk about anything improper, nor have any desire improper. These requirements are quite essential for their benefit." It is true that no one will not watch with his eyes nor listen with his ears, but the key point is that he should not see and listen improperly lest the mind and vital energy be disturbed.

Moreover, in order to control one's personal desire, the ancients came up with some specific measures, such as cultivating a clean conscience, acquiring knowledge of what is to be respected and what is to be distanced, developing the ability to be resolute and to detect errors and redress them, etc. These measures have positive significance in suppressing desire and calming the mind.

1.1.3 Controlling Joy and Anger

Everybody experiences joy and anger, but too much of either is harmful. The book *Ling Shu* says, "Those overjoyed have their minds distracted rather than preserved..., those extremely enraged have their minds confused rather than calmed." Therefore, many of the ancients upheld the measure of preserving a sound mind and vital energy by controlling joy and anger. The book *Nei Jing* lists the controlling of joy and anger as one of the most important measures in health care. The book *Peng Zu She Sheng Yang Xing Lun* says, "Excessive joy or anger makes it impossible for the spirit to be in its proper position." This indicates that too much joy or anger will disturb the mind, causing the vital energy to be scattered, dispersed and upset rather than preserved and calm. The book *Ling Shu* has this to say, "Unchecked joy and anger will injure the viscera, and then illness will arise from the consumption of *Yin*." This indicates that uncontrolled joy and anger may also injure one's viscera and the balance of *Yin* and *Yang* and hence cause various diseases.

1. Suppressing Joy

Joy itself is a sort of cheerful mood, but raptures and overjoy will bring harm to health. That's why the ancients said, "Overjoy weakens *Qi*." and, also, "Overjoy injures the heart." In our daily life, if we cannot calmly deal with unexpected joys and delight, and hence become over-excited, beyond the mental and physical capacity, diseases are liable to occur. The story of Fan Jin, who went mad from over-excitedness after succeeding in passing the provincial service examination, is just a case in point. Over-excitement may cause heart disease and hypertension to become serious, so serious as to endanger life. The book *Yang Sheng Yan Ming Lu* says, "Too much joy causes the mind to be exposed, and too much delight confuses it." Therefore, excessive emotional excitement should be avoided. One should regard calmly the events in one's life, judging any matter in an objective and rational way, so that strong and transitory emotions are avoided in favour of long-lasting happiness, in which stability and harmony of the mind are achieved.

2. Controlling Anger

Among the seven emotions, anger is the most harmful, as anger diverts *Qi* and injures the liver. That is why it is regarded as the first to be avoided. The book *Hong Lu Dian Xue* points out, "Anger and rage should be avoided, as what is important in *Qi* is its confluency rather than diversion; with the confluency of *Qi* all channels will be regulated, while diversion of *Qi* will disturb the harmony of the human body." The book *She Sheng San Yao* says, "When one flies into rage, the *Qi* becomes tough, diverted, disordered and dispersed rather than gentle, fluent, stable and consistent." This points out the danger. The book *She Sheng Yao Lu* says, "Intense anger injures the eyes and dims the sight. Too much anger will disturb all the channels, wither the hair and weaken the tendons. Those who get angry easily tend to exhaust their spirit; their illness is hard to cure, and their *Qi* drains away with each passing day; hence, they will not be able to enjoy longevity." This indicates that anger is also one of the major causes of accelerating ageing and geriatric diseases. Intense anger may even cause syndromes of serious and fatal illness, as the book *Nei Jing* says, "Fierce anger causes the exhaustion of *Qi*, leading to the accumulation of blood in the head and to fainting." in reality, there are indeed cases of fainting or shock due to fierce anger, which may even endanger life.

Since anger is such a great harm, to maintain health, one must refrain from it or check it, reducing stimulation of the mind and preventing excessive emotional fluctuations. Thus, one must first strengthen the training of temper and cultivate the mind. In one's behaviour and treatment of everyday affairs, one should keep the mind calm and controlled;following what Sun Simiao, a famous physican in the Tang Dynasty, advocated:"I say little while others talk a lot; I remain tranquil while others get entangled in affairs; I keep my temper while others lose it; I refrain from feeling troubled by my staying away from improper affairs, and I do not follow vulgar custom, so as to reach the state of empty-mindedness." Cao Tingdong, an eminent figure in the Qing Dynasty, said:"When one encounters something really offensive, he/she should automatically realize that health is, by comparison, much more important, and then, with a change of mind, the anger would soon vanish. " This indicates that one should quieten down even if he / she really had some reason for being angry because, compared with the value of his health, the trouble should be regarded as trivial, and by diverting the thought, he can disperse the anger.

In fact, it is not that one can always completely avoid stimulation of emotions, but that the effect of such stimulation should be reduced or softened, just as Sun Simiao held, "No one can be free from troubled thoughts, but they should be dispelled." When one gets angry, he should make timely effort to comfort himself and dispel his worried thoughts so as to minimize their ill effects on health.

The ancients advocated "tolerance and forbearance", and regarded them as a person's virtues, which are, in effect, important measures for checking anger. The book *Yang Lao Feng Qin Shu* says, "Being invincible in fighting is not so preferable as tolerance, ten thousand words or reactions are not comparable to reticence." In this attitude, or better still, by keeping such a state of mind where even suffering from utter wrong cannot make him angry, and by controlling himself while respecting others, and by holding fast to the beneficial but avoiding the harmful... with all this he will naturally be able to check anger, keep the body and mind from being disturbed, and will thus achieve longevity.

1.1.4 Abstaining from Too Much Worry

Worry is one of the activities of the spirit. Everybody has something to think of or to worry about, but less worry will ease the spirit while too much anxiety will hurt the spirit and shorten life. The book *Ling Shu* also says, "Too much anxiety injures the spirit. "The book *Peng Zu She Sheng Yang Xing Lun* says, "Hard and continuous worry will lead to destruction of the spirit." The book *Wan Shou Dan Shu* says, "The heart houses the spirit, and therefore, when the heart is not disturbed, the spirit will be tranquil, but when the heart is agitated, the spirit will become exhausted. Since the spirit is the master of the limbs, a sound spirit, which can naturally be fostered through worrying less, desiring less, eliminating disturbing ideas and hence resisting all encroachment, will bring about a sound body, which in turn will bring about longevity. This is essential in health care." The book *Yang Shen Fu Yu* compares the relationship between worry and spirit to the one between fire and oil. The more one worries, the less his spirit becomes; just as the more the fire burns, the drier the oil will go. This shows that worry has to be controlled. Likewise, the book *Lei Xiu Yao Jue* advocates "nurturing one's spirit through reducing anxiety and worry". The book *Qian Jin Yao Fang* states, "One could also achieve longevity by restraining from the thought of clothing and food, music and sex, victory and defeat, right and wrong, gain and loss, honour and indignity, etc., thus preventing the mind from being worried and the body from being extremely exhausted." Here worrying less and refraining from anxiety should be interpreted as avoiding excessive and improper anxiety and worry.

Excessive anxiety and worry are detrimental to health. In real life, man can not be released from anxiety and worry, but he can reduce them to a minimum, especially in the case of personal gains or losses, fame or position, money or material comforts, etc., which one should not constantly worry about lest psychological balance should be lost and health affected. For that we must be open-minded, taking a realistic attitude and a practical way in analysing and dealing with affairs, refraining from groundless pursuit but starting from reality as the basis. When anxiety is found difficult to release, attention may be diverted to other things, putting anxiety aside for the time being until, as time passes by, it is readily solved.

1.1.5 Refraining from Grief, Sorrow and Misery

The great ancient poet Su Dongpo in the Song Dynasty said, "Man has his grief and happiness just as the moon has its different phases: dark and bright, full and crescent." The road of one's life can not be safe from sorrow, grief and misery, whose influence on health has always been carefully noted by ancient people. The book *Huai Nan Zi* has this to say, "Too much sorrow and misery lead to illness." and "Those in grief cannot fall asleep in bed, nor get pleasure even from their best food, nor enjoy music and dance." This demonstrates the fact that grief and sorrow not only have great effect on the mind but also cause illness. The book *Nei Jing* says, "Grief and anxiety are harmful to man." As the book *She Sheng Yao Lu* puts it: "Too much grief and sorrow impair uterine collaterals, and too much Yang–Qi existing in the interior causes pain in the epigastrium." Also the book *Ling Shu* says, "The Qi of those grieved and worried is blocked and its movement checked.", besides, "One's heart–Qi begins to decline when he reaches the age of sixty, and he will be more liable to suffer from anxiety and grief." Thus, too much anxiety and grief injure the heart–Qi and, consequently, the health. The same view can be also found in two other books: the book *Peng Zu She*

Sheng Yang Xing Lun and the book *Yang Sheng Yan Ming Lu*.

So, the conclusion is that anxiety and grief do great harm to one's health. On the other hand, one can hardly avoid them in one's life. This grim fact requires a means of subduing and eliminating them. One should first of all cultivate the character of open-mindedness, optimism and broad-mindedness so as to "refrain from attachment to material gains and from grief over one's personal loss. He should also have a strong will to overcome sentimentality. Besides, nothing in the world can, in terms of pleasure, be compared with valuable friendship, which can replace regret and hatred, and heal the old wounds of the mind. Such fine things as sincere help, consolation and encouragement, all filled with friendship, are magic weapons for eliminating grief and anxiety. With one's life free from anxiety and grief, he will find food tasty, sleep restful, life tranquil and recreation enjoyable, and his mental tranquility will thus be regained, with the bad effects of grief and anxiety eliminated thereupon.

1.1.6 Avoiding Terror and Fear

Terror and fear, at whatever degree, are abnormal mental activities.

Although they both have the sense of 'dread', there is some difference between them: Terror means panic, which is mainly caused by outside factors such as sudden stimulation, thus terror disperses and disorders the spirit and *Qi*, whereas, fear means apprehensions, which is mainly caused by inner factors and is actually inner dread and uneasiness. Fear depresses the spirit and impairs *Qi*. The book *Nei Jing* maintains, "Fear depresses *Qi*.", while "Terror disorders *Qi*.". Terror and fear not only harm one's spirit and health, cause disorder of *Qi*, hinder normal physiological function, but may also cause congenital diseases for one's descendants. The book *Nei Jing* also says, "Some people are born with congenital diseases. What are these diseases called? How do people contract them?As Qi Bo, one of the greatest founders of TCM, explained, they are called embryopathia, which are contracted in the embryo when the mother experiences a great fright that causes the *Qi* to stay up in confusion and thus plants epilepsy in the infant. This indicates that such epilepsy is closely related to terror experienced by the mother during pregnancy, and that terror is a great threat to health care and aristogenesis, and should therefore be avoided as much as possible. Those who have a weak personality should not travel alone at night or walk alone through thick forests, mountains, or other deserted places. In addition, attention should be paid to the training of one's will in favour of freedom from unnecessary panic and of maintaining mental peace and tranquility.

1.2 Dietetic Health Care

Food provides nutrients for the maintenance of body function and growth; it is a basic guarantee of health and longevity. Traditional Chinese medicine has, through long health care, developed systematic theories and come up with a series of principles and methods which have contributed a great deal to the health and longevity of the Chinese people. As early as in the Zhou Dynasty, there were officials called "diet doctors" responsible for medical treatment through proper diet. During the Wei, Jin, Northern and Southern Dynasties, there was a book entitled *Shi Jing*(The Classic on Diet) which systematically defines the nourishing functions of food. Sun Simiao, writer of the *Qian Jin Yao Fang*, held the view that the medical treatment function of diet must never be neglected, saying, "Proper food can beat back pathogenic factors, tranquilize *Zang* and *Fu*,inspire the mind and strengthen blood and *Qi*."The book *Yang Sheng Lu* puts forward two ways of health care:first to keep a sound mind by cultivating one's character, and second, to keep fit through proper diet, with the latter as the basis. This indicates that the ancients has long since realized the importance of proper diet to health and longevity. Later, in the Song Dynasty, dietetic health care was developed into a branch of science; and since the Ming and Qing Dynasties, works concerning this branch have appeared one after another, with theories and methods increasingly perfected, drawing general and universal attention.

Dietetic health care plays an important part in longevity; the study of it covers a wide field and rich content; many of the theories and methods concerned are highly scientific and of great value, and are therefore well worth following.

1.2.1 Choosing a Simple and Light Diet

Simple and light diets had always been advocated by ancient Chinese experts in health care, who believed that simple and light diets can prevent diseases, strengthen the body and prolong life, whereas, long consumption of heavy, greasy and sweet food has the disadvantage of producing heat, phlegm and dampness, which is harmful to health and tends to cause illness. The book *Nei Jing* says, "Heavy and greasy food causes a change that may result in serious illness." The book *Lü Shi Chun Qiu* states, "One must refrain from fatty meat and quality wine which are dubbed intestine-corroding food." The book *Han Fei Zi* says, "Tasty food, excellent wine and fatty pork are pleasing to the tongue but damaging to the body." Zhu Danxi, a noted physician from 1281 to 1358, pointed out, "Various diseases may arise from one's indulgence in enjoying food." All these statements help to show the fact that such heavy food is dangerous to health. In his book *Yang Sheng Lun*, Ji Kang made a comparison between the different diets of southen people and northen people, whose life spans were also different: "In north China, people there are habitually frugal, with only pickled vegetables and soybean sauce as their dishes, but they suffer less from illness and live longer than those in the south, although the latter live in rich areas where all kinds of savoury food from both land and sea are available."

It is because heavy food harms the body that experts in health care have always upheld simple and light food. Sun Simiao said, "One should cut down on quality food and delicacies, and rely mainly on economical food." The same statement can also be found in another medical book *Yi Xue Xin Wu*. Likewise, the book *Bao Yang Shuo* stresses, "Contentment with simple and light food which will benefit the *Zang* (visera) is essential. This applies to both the old and the young." The book *Lü Shi Chun Qiu* points out, "One should refrain from heavy, spicy food and strong wine."and, "Too much heavy food will cause the stomach to be overloaded, and hence the blocking of *Qi*. Thus, how can longevity be achieved?" Sun Simiao maintained that the diet for the old should mainly consists of non-heavy, light-salted food;barley, wheat and non-glutinous rice are preferable. He also pointed out that those paying attention to health care should usually take less meat but more rice. The same view was held by

Zhu Danxi in his book *Ru Dan Lun*.

    The above mentioned simple and light food refers in effect to grain and vegetables, whose action of resisting diseases and benefitting health was discovered through long practice by the ancient people. Modern research has proved that too much intake of fat in the body may cause the accumulation of fat clinging to blood vessels, promoting arteriosclerosis which will most probably cause hypertension and coronary heart disease. These diseases are often the main cause of death among old people. It is, therefore, quite necessary to control the intake of animal fat and high cholesterol food. It manifests that emphasis by TCM on vegetarian diet has its scientific basis. Besides, according to statistics, in all those regions famous in the world for the longevity of their inhabitants, most people there take vegetables, grains, melons and fruit as their main food.

    Apart from vegetarian diet, the ancients also advocated mild tasting food, food being referred to mainly in terms of tastes. Tastes, especially saltiness, should not be too strong and the intake of salt should be strictly controlled. the book *Nei Jing* states, "Too much salt will enlarge bones but shrink muscles, exhaust *Qi* and, in particular, depress the heart—*Qi*." The book *Lao Lao Heng Yan* says, "Dishes cannot be prepared without salt, but its amount must be controlled, and the taste of saltiness must be mild so that food may keep its natural flavour and quality." and, "Blood congeals and dries when it meets with salt." Chen Jiru, the author of the book *Yang Sheng Fu Yu*, presented from his own experience the fact that there was much evidence which proved that much intake of salt injured the body whereas food with mild taste prolonged life. He was of the opinion that people living in the palace mostly lived a short life partly because of their food which was too salty and whose other tastes were too strong. On the other hand, he took for examples three elderly people who, all their lives, had rarely taken salt, and mainly consumed mild-tasting food, and yet who still enjoyed excellent health at the age of over eighty. Sun Simiao also held the view that less salty food promotes longevity. Modern researches have discovered that many diseases such as hypertension, arterioclerosis, cardiac infarction, cirrhosis, apoplexy and kidney diseases are all connected, to some extent, with over intake of salt. Some foreign scholars have also stated that hypertension is actually the result of salt intoxication. The diseases mentioned ablve are all detrimental to health. Therefore, the observation in TCM that mild-tasting food helps to prolong life is in accordance with the truth, Everybody who hopes to enjoy good health and longevity must follow this principle.

1.2.2 Seasoning Food with the Five Tastes Properly

Food with "five tastes" is the source of *Qi* and blood and of their interpromotion. Proper adjustment of food and tastes will result in the promotion of *Qi* and blood, and in the maintenance of good health;whereas, if blood and tastes are not properly coordinated, harm will be done to *Qi* and blood, and one's life span will be cut down. The book *Nei Jing* states repeatedly that one must have a "fixed diet" and "arrange the five tastes carefully", pointing out that careful mixture of the five tastes will strengthen the bones, make the tendons flexible, promote the circulation of blood and *Qi*, keep the skin and muscles in good condition, and thus enhance the bones and tendons. Following this principle, one will achieve longevity.

The so-called five tastes are: sour, sweet, bitter, acrid and saltiness. They are the main tastes of food. Adjustment of food and tastes is an important principle in TCM and, in terms of its content and significance, there is a difference between its wide sense and its narrow one. In the wide sense, it means rational adjustment of diet, while in the narrow sense, it means the adjustment of five tastes.

1. Adjusting Food Rationally

The ancients had long since realized that different food contains different nutrients and that only through an all-round and rational adjustment of different food can the body gain different kinds of nutrients to satisfy the needs of various physiological functions. As the book *Nei Jing* points out, grains, fruits, meat and vegetables contain the integral nutrition, and a diet should consist mainly of grains, meat, fruits and vegetables, all of which have the action of strengthening essence and *Qi*, and hence are indispensable to the human body. Grains should be the staple food, because it contains rich carbohydrate, supplying the human body with the necessary heat and energy. Fruits, meat of domestic animals and vegetables are secondary food. Fruits and vegetables provide various vitamins, fibers and microelements, which are also indispensable in metabolism and other life activities. Domestic animals such as pigs, cattle, sheep and chickens provide the human body with necessary proteins, fat and amino acid. Protein is a major material for forming tissue cells, fat provides heat while amino acid is even more necessary for metabolism. This diet itself with various kinds of food rationally matched in accordance with the Chinese diet tradition is just as much as a scientific cookery book can suggest. Meanwhile, such a diet is beneficial to health also because it prevents food bias. Thus anyone who wants to enjoy good health and longevity should accept it.

2. Adjusting the Five Tastes Rationally

Each food is different from others in terms of taste. The five major tastes are sour, sweet, bitter, acrid and saltiness. They have different actions and effects and should be carefully adjusted to keep them from being too strong and to avoid bias towards one or any other of the tastes. Excess or bias in tastes is detrimental to health and should be guarded against. The book *Nei Jing* points out that excessive sour harms the liver—*Qi* and exhausts the spleen—*Qi*; too much salt enlarges bones, shrinks muscles and suppressed the heart—*Qi*; the excess sweet causes excessiveness of the heart—*Qi*, blue face, and the loss of balance of the kidney—*Qi*; excessive bitter leads to weakness of the spleen—*Qi* and fullness of the stomach—*Qi*; while excessive acrid brings about relaxation and debility of tendons and vessels and, consequently, causes the depression of spirit. This indicates that bias towards a particular taste will hurt the *Zang* and *Fu* organs, causing diseases, because each of the five tastes links with a particular channel. The book *Nei Jing* also says, " After the five tastes have entered the stomach, each goes first to its favourite organ—the sour to the liver, the bitter to the heart, the sweet to the spleen, the acrid to the lungs and the salty to the kidney. "As a rule, a long practice of diet with tastes properly matched will strengthen *Qi*, otherwise, *Qi* will be impaired and trouble will ensue.

Excessive tastes will not only do invisible harm to the respective *Zang* and *Fu* organs, but also cause visible pathologic changes. As the book *Nei Jing* has put it, consumption of too much salt will thicken blood in the vessels and give rise to change of skin colour, too much bitter will dry the skin and reduce hair, too much acrid will tighten tendons and weaken fingers and toes, too much sour will cause a person to grow fatter, and too much sweet will make the bones ache and the hair fall out. This accounts for the fact that the ancients had repeatedly stressed the importance of keeping the five tastes in the right proportion. The same principle was also mentioned by Zhang Zihe, a well-known ancient doctor.

To keep the five tastes in regulation, we must, firstly, select food according to the principle of arranging tastes in the right proportion and, secondly, regulate the tastes by means of cookery, thus making full use of their mutual checking and promoting functions. This will prevent nourishment diminishing and therefore benefit the health.

1.2.3 Dining at Regular Times and Controlling the Intake

Dining at regular times and controlling the intake is an important part of traditional Chinese medical health care. The so-called 'regular time' means dining at comparatively fixed time, while intake control means the rational control of amount, so that there is no excessive hunger or fullness, and no excessive eating or drinking.

1. Keeping Regular Dining Hour

The book *Lü Shi Chun Qiu* says, "One is sure to be safe from diseases if he keeps regular dining hours.", pointing out the importance of having meals on time as early as over 2000 years ago. The book *Shang Shu* also has the same statement, asserting that keeping regular dining hours is an essential measure for maintaining good health. It is an important principle in diet regulation keeping the time interval between meals neither too short nor too long. The dining habit of three meals a day, with an interval of 5 hours in between, which has long since been practised by the Chinese is quite rational and scientific, as it takes at least four or five hours to digest most ordinary foods. Therefore, the suitable dining hours are: breakdast around seven o'clock, lunch around twelve o'clock and supper around six o'clock. Such a time-table of meals is beneficial to health, as it not only makes the various nutrients meet the needs of the body, but also suits the arrangement of one's daily life, such as work and study.

Keeping correct dining hour has another aspect, i. e. to dine according to whether one feels hungry or thirsty. As the book *Qian Jin Yao Fang* puts it, those good at health care dine when they feel hungry and drink when thirsty. The book *Zun Sheng Ba Jian* holds the same view that one should not eat until he feels hungry, and not drink until very thirsty, and in either case no haste should be involved. But it stresses that one should not form the habit of eating and drinking only when excessively hungry or thirsty. Hunger and thirst may be felt at different times, for example, intense movement, overwork or work on night shift may all make an individual feel hungry and thirsty at a time outside the ordinary time-table for meals, and consequently, some people may have a night meal. This is, of course, a rational regulation of dining time.

2. Controlling the Amount of Intake

Rational diet principle requires not only correct timing, but the controlling of intake as well, to suit the needs of the body.

The general principle of food intake is "neither too much nor too little", as traditional Chinese medicine holds the view that being too full or too hungry is harmful to health. The book *Nei Jing* says, "Taking no food for half a day will decline the *Qi*, and a whole day exhaust the *Qi*." but "Eating twice as much as enough will injure the spleen and the stomach." The book *Dong Wei Jing* states that hunger injures the spleen, but eating too much harms the *Qi* because the spleen depends on food, and hunger will cause insufficiency of spleen due to lack of supply; furthermore, as *Qi* travels through the spleen, the stuffiness of spleen due to overeating will cause the *Qi* to stagnate. Thus, one eats when hungry in order to aid the spleen but tries to avoid overfilling the spleen for the sake of supplying the *Qi*. Sun Simiao held that it is advisable to eat more meals a day in lesser amount instead of having fewer meals in larger amount, and that one should try to be in a semi-hungry and semi-full state. This principle of being neither too full nor too hungry is quite beneficial to health. As to the amount of food for each of the three meals daily, the Chinese ancients believed it should be different. The book *Nei Jing* says, "*Yang Qi* is strong at noon but declines at sunset, so it is advisable to have a big breakfast, but one should eat less after noon and even less in the evening." Later, a principle was developed under the guidance of that theory and through long practice in life: quality food for breakfast, enough quantity for lunch and less quantity for supper.

The Chinese ancient experts in health care believed that control of intake is of great importance, especially to old people, and that less intake may result in longevity. The book *Bo Wu Zhi* says, "Less intake benefits the heart, while too much intake hurts the heart and reduces one's life." The book *Lao Lao Heng Yan* maintains that relatively small intake benefits the health as it helps the spleen to function well, turning food into essential body fluid, whereas, too much intake hurts the spleen, even if the food is easy to digest. The book *Dong Gu Zhui Yan* points out, "Those overeating will suffer from five bad results: first, frequent bowel movement;second, frequent urination; third, disturbance of sleep; fourth, a body too fat to be able to exercise; fifth, poor digestion." The book *Shou Shi Bao Yuan* draws a good conclusion in terms of amount of intake: eat food only to half one's capacity and drink wine to only one third.

The principle of less intake developed by the ancients agrees with dietary physiological reality and is of great scientific value. Modern medicine has proved that constant excessive intake of food overburdens the stomach and intestines, causes insufficient supply of digestive fluid and, hence, indigestion; besides, it will concentrate too much blood in the stomach and intestines. Thus major organs like the heart and brain will have a short supply of blood, and this in turn causes lassitude and mental exhaustion. Those with coronary disease may develop angina pectoris. Moreover, it may lead to obesity due to accumulation of fat, which may a give rise to hypertension, coronary disease, diabetes, cholelithiasis and so on. Many scholars maintain that long and constant full—loading of the stomach causes early deterioration of health and shortens one's life, and should be consciously avoided, especially in the case of old people whose physiological functions of various kinds, including the digestive function, are declining.

1.2.4 Regulating Cold and Heat of Food

Regulating cold and heat of the food one takes is an important aspect of diet regulation practised by the ancients. The book *Zhou Li* states that food should be warm like the weather in spring, soup shoud be hot like the weather in summer, food pickled in soy sauce should be cool like the weather in autumn, and drinks should be cold like the weather in winter, indicating that the character of cold or heat varies with different foods and that it needs proper regulating. What should be emphasized is that the above mentioned regulating principle does conform to practical necessity, and it is still being observed even to the present.

Also, the ancients had a clear understanding about the danger of food either too cold or too hot for the *Zang—Fu* organs and for one's health in general. The book *Nei Jing* and some other medical classics also point out the above danger, saying that food which is too cold or too hot harms *Fu* organs, and that hot food hurts the bones while cold food the lungs, and that food should not be so hot as to scald the lips or so cold as to hurt the teeth, and that food excessively hot and cold should not enter the stomach lest it should disorder the proper functions of the stomach and spleen.

Meanwhile, some people maintained that one's diet should consist mainly of warm food. This view is held by the book *Qian Jin Yao Fang* and the book *Shou Shi Bao Yuan*. The latter says, "In whichever season, food should always be warm, especially in summer when *Yin* is stored internally." The book *Zun Sheng Ba Jian* even advocates that food should never be eaten cold or raw. These statements sound somewhat exaggerated, but there is something in them since what is underlined is warm food rather than hot food.

Modern medicine shows that frequent intake of hot food damages the mucous membrance in the mouth and esophagus and generates correponding diseases, while too much intake of cold or raw food is apt to impair the digestive function of the stomach and spleen and to cause gastrointestinal diseases. Therefore, the regulating of cold and hot food is of great significance as regards the maintenance of health and should be carfully observed.

1.2.5 Following Proper Methods of Cleanliness

The ancient paid great attention to the role played by cleanliness in health care, maintaining that dirty and spoiled food must never be eaten. The book *Lun Yu,* written by disciples of Confucius during the Warring States Period, 476 B. C—221 B. C, says, "Rotten fish, decaying meat and food with hideous colour or smell must not be eaten." The book *Jin Gui Yao Lüe* holds a similar view and even especially points out what kind of meat, fish or fruit cannot be eaten, saying: "The meat and fish which dogs will not eat and birds will not peck should not be eaten", "Meat with red spots should not be eaten", "Squashed food kept for many days is, if eaten, harmful to health." and "Fruit fallen to ground and bitten by worms or ants should never be eaten". These statements show that our ancients guarded closely against unclean food. The noted physcian Zhang Zhongjing further observed that animals that have died of illnesses might be toxic and should not be eaten.

Clinically, many diseases of the digestive tract such as dysentery and intestinal parasitosis are mostly caused by dirty and unclean food. Although the ancients were not yet aware of those pathogenic organisms, they had already recognized the danger of unclean food to health. Their observations enriched the theory and practice of hygiene in diet, and , therefore, has some realistic guiding significance.

1.2.6 Following Some Instructions in Diet

In dietetics there are some principles to be advocated and some practices to be advoided. The Chinese ancients summarized their rich experience. The book *Yang Sheng Lu* points out that one should eat a bit earlier rather than a bit later, slowly rather than fast; the amount should be small rather than large; and the food should be warm but not hot, soft rather than hard and salty but of not too much salt. This demonstrates that the ancients had, in terms of diet, principles and advice in many respects, such as proper time, rate, amount, taste, property of food, and the cold-heat factor. These principles conform with the reality of diet and will naturally benefit one's health if they are followed.

The book *Qian Jin Yi Fang* says, "Without the knowledge of correct diet, one cannot enjoy good health. "It should go without saying that a knowledge of what is right or wrong in diet has great significance and an important role in health care. Instructions in diet are very rich in content and cover a wide range. Broadly speaking, almost all the discussions on diet in TCM are within the scope of dietetic instructions. But they have their specific content and significance, which may roughly be divided into two parts: instructions in methods of dining and in choosing proper beverage.

1. Methods of Dining

Method of dining centers on the question of what should be followed and what should be avoided. In terms of time, there are instructions concerning methods to be adopted at the time of dining and those after dining.

(1) Do's and Don'ts during Eating

A. Dining with Concentration of Mind

The ancients held the view that one should concentrate his mind when dining rather than allow oneself to be distracted by thinking, talking, reading, etc. , because such things affect the taste and hamper the digestion as well as assimilation of food. As the book *Lun Yu* puts it, "Refrain from talking while dining or after going to bed. "The book *Qian Jin Yao Fang* also says that one should not talk loudly when eating, especially when hungry. All this stresses concentration of mind in dining.

B. Dining in a Relaxed and Cheerful Mood rather than in Anger or Resentment

A good mood in dining helps digestion and assimilation whereas anxiety, depression and anger are harmful to health. The book *Qian Jin Yao Fang* has this to say, "One must abstain from anxiety when dining. If he dines in great anger, his spirit will be shocked and he will be troubled by dreams in sleep. " The book *Da Sheng Yao Lu* also says, "One mustn't eat immediately after anger, nor must he lose his temper right after a meal. He must not eat at such moments as those of anger, deep speculation or fear, and he must not eat when drowsy or sleepy, lest the food should stay halfway in the stomach. " This statement points out clearly the danger of dining in unsuitable moods. Moreover, the ancients also believed, " The stomach tends to favour tranquility and cheerfulness while the spleen favours music. ", implying that music is of great benefit to the digestion and assimilation of food. The book *Shou Shi Bao Yuan* also states, "The spleen is fond of music. It starts to move and 'grind' food at the rhythm of music." To the same effect, the Taoists also had such statements in their works. It has been indicated that soft and gently music, or even a cosy and tidy environment, serves as a benign stimulation that may regulate the digestive function through the central nervous system, whereas, noise, messy environment and bad smell may affect one's mood and, consequently, one's digestion and health.

C. Chewing the Food Thoroughly and Taking It Gradually

Thorough chewing and gradual ingesting both help digestion and assimilation, as the book *Qian Jin Yao Fang* puts it, "One must chew his food thoroughly when eating.", and "... raw food should not be swallowed.". Other medical works like the book *Yang Bing Yong Yan* and the book *Yi Shu* have statements to the same effect. They stress thorough chewing and gradual ingestion as an important link in diet, which should not be neglected.

(2) Do's and Don'ts after a Meal

Health care after a meal was always emphasized by the ancients, who had accumulated rich experience. Some statements and discussions concerned are reasonable and practical with general significance and considerable scientific value.

A. Walking Slowly rather than Hastily

A walk after dining aids digestion, as is pointed out in the book *Qian Jin Yao Fang*, "One should take a walk after a meal, which will help digestion and prevent various diseases."The book

Yang Xing Yan Ming Lu has this to say, "According to principles of health care, one should not lie down immediately after having a big meal or keep sitting all day, because this will result in damage to one's life." The book *Lao Lao Heng Yan* also states, "Since the food stays in the stomach after a meal, it is necessary to walk a distance of a few hundred steps with the intent of helping circulate the *Qi* and the essence of food, and of letting the stomach massage itself to aid digestion... Thus elderly people in ancient times always took a walk after a meal as a care-free pastime."

The ancients were opposed to the practice of fast walk and intense movement after a meal, regarding it as a great harm to health, as is stated in the book *Shou Shi Bao Yuan*, "One should not walk fast, nor ride a horse, nor go to high or dangerous places lest the *Zang* and *Fu* organs should be injured due to excessive fullness of *Qi*."

B. Rubbing the Stomach rather than Lying Down

Rubbing the stomach after meal will assist digestion, as is advocated in the book *Qian Jin Yao Fang*, "After taking a meal or a snack, one should help digest it by rubbing the stomach with warm hands and by walking outdoors a few dozen paces." and "If one rubs his stomach, walks one or two hundred paces slowly without getting out of breath and then returns to lie in bed awake with the limbs stretched, the *Qi* will quieten down in a few moments." The book *Shou Shi Bao Yuan* states, "Rubbing the stomach a few hundred times, exhaling a few hundred breaths with eyes looking up to the sky and walking slowly a few hundred paces are all within the scope of benefitting digestion." all these statements lead to the conclusion that rubbing the stomach after a meal is essential to the digestion of food.

To lie down immediately after a meal is injurious to health, as it holds back the food in the stomach, unfavourable for digestion. It is a practice opposed by the ancients, as is stated in the book *Qian Jin Yi Fang*, "To sleep right after a meal will result in various diseases."

2. Choosing Proper Beverages and Taking Them in a Proper Way

This is an important part of dietetic health care. The main beverages popular in China are tea and wine. The quantity of intake, the way and the time for taking them are related to health, and hence are observed closely.

(1) Discussion on Tea Drinking

China is the native land of tea. As early as in the fourth century B. C., tea was already used as a drink in China where tea-bushes were first discovered and tea-leaves were first cultivated. In many ancient books such as the book *Shi Jing*, the book *Er Ya* and the book *Shen Nong Shi Jing*, descriptions and records about tea can be found. The first book in the world specially treating the subject of tea was written by Lu Yu in the Tang Dynasty(618—905). The benefit of tea to health has long been highly valued. It is not only a popular drink among the Chinese but is enjoyed by more and more people internationally as one of the three main drinks in the world, the other two being coffee and cocoa. Its beneficial role in health care and medical treatment was recognized by the ancients long ago. The book *Shen Nong Ben Cao Jing* states, "With a bitter taste, tea aids one's mind, combats listlessness, invigorates one's body, reduces one's weight and improves one's eye sight." The book *Ben Cao Gang Mu* says,

"The main medical action of tea lies in its effect on cough with dyspnea and in dispelling phlegm accumulation." The book *Yang Sheng Sui Bi* states, "If drunk after a meal, tea may counteract the bad effect of heavy food." The book *Cha Pu* maintains, "Tea drinking can quench one's thirst, assist digestion, dispel phlegm, reduce sleepiness, clear the urethra, strengthen one's eye sight, aid one's mind and expel one's feeling of anxiety or weariness and the effect of heavy food. With so many advantages, tea drinking is indeed a daily necessity to man." These statements show clearly the varied actions and effects of tea.

Modern research in medicine proves that, apart from cellulose, colloid and chlorophyl, tea contains various alkaloids, vitamins, flavonoids, tannin, ergosterol, volatile oil, certain amounts of hydrochloric acid, thiamine, folacin, protein and minerals. Therefore it has the action of refreshing the brain, getting rid of fatigue, improving memory, preventing dental caries, improving eye sight, lowering blood-lipid, preventing hypertension, acting as diuretic against calculi and supplementing nutrition. It can even reduce the effect of radioactivity. All these indicate that proper tea-drinking is beneficial to health.

Although tea-drinking has so many advantages, it may also bring some detriment to health if drunk excessively or improperly.

A. Drinking Tea in Appropriate Amount

The ancients realized the detriment of excess tea-drinking long ago, as is recorded in the book *Sun Zhen Ren Wei Sheng Ge Zhu Shi*, "Although tea has the effect of clearing away the heart fire and bettering the eye sight..., it has many disadvantages, and should not be drunk excessively in any season of the year, especially in the case of those people who suffer from insomnia and those who are thin and weak; for, lacking in fat and body fluid, how could they sustain the exhausting effect of tea? In moments of hunger and exhaustion or after sexual intercourse one should strictly refrain from drinking tea, especially cold tea. " The book *Shou Yang Cong Shu* says, "Tea should be drunk hot and in small quantity. Long practice of improper tea-drinking, reduces fat in the body, causes cold of deficiency type in the lower-*Jiao*. Drinking tea in hunger is particularly improper, as it causes insomnia." Modern mendicine also holds that excessive drinking of strong tea will cause overstimulation; accelerate palpitation; lead to precipitant urination, insomnia and over-hydration; increase the burden on both the heart and kidney owing to the increased amount of water in the body; and effect the deficiency of vitamin B as well.

B. Refraining from Drinking Tea Right before or after a Meal

The suitable time for drinking tea is during breaks by day when one is taking a rest rather than just before or after a meal, since tea contains tannin which will combine with proteins in food to synthesize albutannin. And this may make food hard to digest, cause the contraction of membrane in the digestive canal, affect appetite, digestion and assimilation, or even lead to constipation. As Li Shizhen, a famous physician in the Ming Dynasty, put it, "Tea has a bitter and cool taste, long practice of improper tea drinking may result in abdominal distention and loss of appetite." The book *Bai Yao Yuan Quan* states, "The middle-*Jiao* is itself full of dampness;over-drinking of tea will add to dampness and is bound to injure the spleen and cause the fullness in the middle—*Jiao.*" These statements indicate that too much intake of tea or drinking it in improper times will affect the digestive function of the stomach and spleen.

C. Refraining from Drinking Tea before Going to Bed

Since tea contains such elements as caffeine, theocin and theobromin which have stimulating properties, it should not be taken just before sleep lest it should affect sleep and rest through stimulation and frequent urination. A similar view can be found in some ancient books such as *Bo Wu Zhi* and *Tong Jun Lu*.

Furthermore, tea-drinking is not suitable for parturients or people suffering from hypertension, cardiac diseases, habitual constipation and neurosism. It also should be noted that tea-drinking should not be accompanied by certain food, such as leeks.

(2) Guidance in Liquor-drinking

Liquor has a long history in China. The book *Nei Jing* contains a chapter specially devoted to discussions on liquor, which was made from grain. With continuous creative efforts made by working people in various historical periods, the variety of liquor has been continually increasing and liquor has become an important drink for many people.

Traditional Chinese medicine holds that liquor has the action of promoting blood circulation through the vessels, potentiating a medicine, increasing one's appetite, dispelling fatigue and invigorating one's spirit. It can be used for the prevention of diseases and for achieving longevity as well. The number of the varieties of medicated liquor produced in the past historical periods is estimated at several hundred. The book *Qian Jin Yao Fang* says, "Drinking two or three doses of medicated liquor in winter until spring begins——a practice which, if it is observed all one's life, will prevent all diseases. ", confirming the positive action of liquor in health care. Li Shizhen, a great physician and naturalist in the Ming Dynasty, said, "Liquor is a heavenly drink. Taken in small quantities, it warms up the blood, improves the circulation of *Qi,* invigorates the spirit, resists cold, dissolves anxiety and raises one's interest in life. "Chen Cangqi, a noted physician, said, "... It facilitates the circulation of blood through the vessels, strengthens the stomach and intestines, moistens the skin and scatters dampness. "Scientific researches indicate that drinking a little liquor each day can strengthen one's body, prevent angiocardiopathy as well as raise one's appetite. The property of liquor varies with different kinds. Generally, spirits (Chinese white liquor) is thought to have the action of resisting cold and used for soaking medicinal material; rice wine is often used as a guiding drug; yellow rice or millet wine can improve blood circulation and suppress pain; grape wine can strengthen the heart and aid the spirit; beer is rich in nutrition and capable of nourishing the stomach and helping digestion; as to various medicated liquors, they can prevent or cure many kinds of diseases.

Although the amount and way of drinking vary with the particular constitution of individuals, there is a general principle for liquor-drinking: drink in small quantity and choose mild liquor rather than drink different kinds of liquor at a time or in an abandoned manner. The book *Yang Sheng Yao Lu* quoted from Ruan Janzhi, a noted physician, that "Drinking mild liquor from a small cup over a chat is not only good entertainment to one's friends but also beneficial to one's health. "To the same effect, the book *Qing Ji Lu* points out, "Different liquor should not be drunk together, otherwise even those good at drinking would get drunk."

It is believed that, with regard to drinking, attention should be paid to what is called the "three proper" : proper quantity, proper time and proper mood. It has been proved through practice that by following these principles, liquor-drinking will prove enjoyable and beneficial to health, but if one's practice is contrary to these principles, liquor-drinking will be detrimental to one's body and mind.

A. Proper Amount

No kind of liquor should be drunk to excess, or in a abandoned, manner or it may harm one's health and cause diseases or even death. This fact had long been known by the ancients. The book *Yang Sheng Yao Lu* says, "Liquor may benefit the drinker but it may also ruin his health. When drunk in proper amount, it will regulate the channels and vessels, drive out pathogenic factors and resist cold. But when drunk to excess over a long period, it will weaken one's constitution, and impair one's mind. Thus one must be careful in drinking and keep it under control. " The book *Ben Cao Gang Mu* has this to say, "Should a person abandon himself to alcoholic drinks and always get drunk, he would, in mild cases, behave in an abnormal manner, or, in serious cases, damage his health and ruin his life. The harm as such is indeed beyond description. " and " Excessive alcoholic drinking may cause sudden death. "The book *Yin Shan Zheng Yao* holds exactly the same view.

Modern researches have proved that alcohol, or ethanol, is the essential element of liquor. In some spirits, the percentage of alcohol is as high as 40−60%. Alcohol does great harm to health, and too much intake of it will lead to acute or chronic alcoholism. The state of being drunk occurs when the concentration of alcohol in the blood reaches 0.05–0.2%, and death will result from acute alcoholic poisoning when it reaches 0.4%. Constant alcoholic incitation may cause chronic gastritis and hence malnutrition, Long practice of alcoholic drinking also causes cirrhosis of the liver and fatty liver owing to the fact that alcohol is decomposed in the liver. The disease incidence among the alcoholics is eight times as high as that among non-alcoholics. In addition, chronic alcoholism may result in various other diseases such as cardiac diseases and cerebrovascular accidents, directly affecting one's health.

B. Proper Time

It is imperative that one should not drink when hungry. The book *Yang Sheng Sui Bi* states, "It was always after taking some food that the ancients drank their liquor." Drinking liquor on an empty stomach is most detrimental, since stomach and intestines will assimilate 60% of it in an hour, and 90% in one and a half hours with only 10% excreted out of the body through urination, perspiration and exhalation. If the amount of alcohol contained in the contents of the stomach is greater than 0.5% of those, it will become harmful.

Nor should one drink before going to bed. Wang Ying, a noted physician, was opposed to alcoholic drinking before sleeping at night, as he put it, "If one goes to sleep after getting drunk, his heart and eyes will be injured through overabundance of heat ... and the resulting stagnated dampness will give rise to skin and other external diseases; it increases fire and incites sexual desire, leading to various diseases." There are certain truths in this statement.

C. Proper Mood

By mood is meant here the state of one's mind and some other conditions. Liquor must not be drunk when one is in improper moods, such as anxiety, worry or anger. Some people are in the habit of suppressing anger with alcoholic drinking, but in fact it is a bad habit, as a famous Chinese saying describes, "To suppress anxiety with liquor will only add to the anxiety. " Although alcoholic drinking may cause the drinker to have a temporary feeling of comfort, it will make him become more depressed as if he had lost something. To drink liquor at such moments is most likely to cause drunkeness, harming the body and one should, therefore, take great pains to refrain from such practice.

Furthermore, one should also abstain from liquor drinking under some special circumstances such as the moment before having sex. In such a moment, if pregnancy should result, the alcohol would cause harm to the fetus, seriously affecting its growth.

Moreover, patients suffering from fever, liver trouble, gallbladder disease, angiocardiopathy, cerebrovascular disease, kidney trouble and serious enterogastric diseases, etc. should also abstain from alcoholic drinking lest the diseases worsen.

1.3 Regular-life Health Care

Traditional Chinese medicine has always attached great importance to an orderly life for maintaining good health, and has treated this as an important component of the science of health care. The book *Qian Jin Yao Fang* says, "Those good at health preservation follow a regular discipline for harmonious life, as well as a suitable time-table for going to bed and rising, which varies with different seasons. "And the book *Shou Qin Yang Lao Xin Shu* also has the same statement. Both books indicate that regularity in one's life and work is essential for preserving health both physically and mentally, and for achieving longevity. An orderly life involves many aspects, including regular hours for sleeping and resing, correct way of sleeping, proper clothing and personal hygiene, the principles of which are rational, the ways correct, and therefore are worth following.

1.3.1 Leading a Regular Life

This principle was specially underlined by the Chinese ancients, as can be seen in the book *Nei Jing* which regards keeping regularity in one's daily life as an important measure for achieving longevity. The ancient experts in health care were of the opinion that whether one could enjoy health or not depended largely on whether or not his/her daily life was rationally arranged. The book *Shang Shu* has this to say: "The channels and vessels will be affected if there is no regularity in one's life and no restraint in using one's energy." Other medical classics such as the book *Shou Shi Mi Dian* and the book *Yang Sheng Yao Lun* also stress that, to achieve health and longevity, one should take pains to arrange one's daily life properly, be restrained in one's hobbies and preserve one's vital energy. No one will enjoy longevity if he doesn't observe these principles and leads an irregular life.

What is most important in keeping regular hours for bed and rise is to adjust to the change of seasons, because the natural climate and environment vary with seasons and different times of the day while man's physiological functions also change with the changes of the outside world; as the book *Nei Jing* puts it, "All living things, even their birth and death, depend on the law governing the change of seasons and the relation between *Yin* and *Yang*. Those who go against the law will incur disasters and those submitting themselves to it will keep diseases away." The book also raises a principle concerning health preservation: "to cultivate *Yang* in spring and summer, and to cultivate *Yin* in autumn and winter." Meanwhile it puts forward a time-table for daily life based on the change of seasons: in spring, "late to bed and early to rise, followed by a leisurely walk around the courtyard", in summer, "late to bed and early rise, with no drowsy feeling in the day time," in autumn, "early to bed and early to rise, as a rooster", and in winter, "early to bed and late to rise, lying in bed until sunrise." Moreover one's daily activities should be adjusted to different times of a day, because, as the book *Nei Jing* states, "*Qi* begins to grow in the morning, and the *Yang-Qi* culminates at noon and weakens at sunset, and its entrance is closed." This statement clearly indicates that the increase and decrease of *Yin* and *Yang* varies with the different times of the day, to which one should adapt his daily activities. The ancients' practice of "beginning one's activities at sunrise and stopping to rest at sunset" is, so to speak, a kind of time-table showing their regular hour for daily activities

1.3.2 Following a Correct Way of Sleeping

Since sleeping is not only a major means of dispelling fatigue and restoring one's energy, but also an important process of regulating various physiological functions and stablizing the balance of the nervous system, the ancients paid great attention to the proper way of sleeping, believing that it is closely connected with health and longevity. An ancient poem says, "Were I to meet with the Huashan Immortal, I'd ask him for no divine medicine but his way of sleeping." Traditional Chinese medicine has, by using the theory of *Yin* and *Yang*, established the truth that sleeping is a necessity for balancing *Yin* and *Yang*, and for continuing life process, as is stated in the book *Ling Shu*, "One falls asleep when the *Yang-Qi* has run out and the *Yin-Qi* is abundant, whereas one awakes when the condition is reversed.

1. Pre-sleep Adjustment

(1) Keeping a peaceful Mind and a Calm Mood

Unrestrained joy, anger, grief and anxiety are all capable of affecting one's mind and disturbing one's sleep. The book *Shui Jue* states, "As far as sleep is concerned, one should keep regular hours, and try to let his / her mind sleep before the eyes do." Only by making the mind sleep first can the eyes fall asleep afterwards. One can not go to sleep, or may even suffer from insomnia if he / she is full of worry and anxiety. It is, therefore, necessary to eliminate, before sleep, various thoughts and calm down the mind and spirit. The book *Yan Shou Yao Yan* says, "It will be much easier to go to sleep if one, before going to bed, washes his feet in hot water, drives away all anxiety, thinks only of the pleasant things in life, or reads some serene and comforting poems so as to broaden the mind and tranquilize the spirit." It has been proved through practice that washing feet in hot water before going to bed does help calm the mind and enable one to enjoy a better sleep.

(2) Controlling the Intake of Food before Sleep

The practice of "sleeping right after eating one's fill" is detrimental to health, which was recognized long ago by the Chinese ancients who emphasized that "One should refrain from eating one's fill late at night, nor should he go to sleep right after that." The book *Nei Jing* states, "When there is discomfort in the stomach, sleep will not be peaceful." If one eats his fill before sleep, it will add to the burden of one's stomach and intestines, and this in turn will affect sleep and harm one's health. In addition, one should, before going to bed, abstain from taking such things as strong tea, cigarettes, wine, coffee, etc., because they also affect sleep.

(3) Doing a Suitable Amount of Exercise

A suitable amount of exercise before bedding down can help stabilize one's mood as well as relax one's limbs and torso. The book *Zi Yan Yin Shu* maintains, "It is advisable to walk a thousand steps around the room before going to bed every night ...When you walk, you exercise your body and you cease to think. So there is something in the statement that enough movement leads to a peaceful mind ... A thousand-pace walk before sleep is just the technique of seeking peace through movement." This indicates that proper exercise helps one sleep better through relaxing the mind and stabilizing the mood. But intense exercise before sleep is not advisable.

(4) Trying to Induce Oneself into the State of Quietness

The ancient experts in health care developed a number of techniques of inducing the state of quietness for those who toss and turn in bed, failing to fall asleep. For instance, the book *Lao Lao Heng Yan* says, "There are two kinds of techniques for inducing oneself into sleep, which are called respectively the controlled and the uncontrolled. The former includes such methods as concentrating one's mind on the crown, counting silently the number of breaths or contemplating the point of *Dantian*, so that the mind may have a place to stay rather than wander about, which will help one fall asleep. The latter is to allow one's mind to travel to distant places in situations where oneself is not involved, which can also bring one gradually into the state of drowsiness." The method of counting numbers silently to help fall asleep adopted by some people nowadays is, in effect, the application of the above—mentioned technique.

2. Principles to Be Followed during Sleep

(1) Adopting a Proper Sleeping Posture

A sleeping posture has a direct influence upon sleep. The Chinese ancients advocated the posture of lying on one's right flank with the body relaxed and the legs slightly bent. The book *Xiu Ling Yao Zhi* says "sleeping on one's right flank, stretching out when waking up". The book *Hua Shan Shi Er Shui Gong Zong Jue* gives similar instructions. The book *Lao Lao Heng Yan* states, "One should sleep on the right flank, not the left flank, to soothe the spleen and to regulate the circulation of *Qi*..., with the body bent like a bow." These instructions of the ancients concerning sleeping postures have been proved to be quite rational. The posture of lying on one's stomach or on one's back is not advisable.

(2) Avoiding Exposure to Wind during Sleeping

Wind is the number one cause of various diseases. One is liable to be attacked by wind—cold pathogens when one is sleeping soundly. Therefore, one should not sleep in the open air, nor ask other people to fan him, for although he may thus enjoy a temporary pleasure, the pathogenic wind is, in such case, most likely to enter the striae of the skin, muscles and viscera, causing serious effects. The book *Qian Jin Yao Fang* says, "Sleeping in the open air induces stagnation of food in the stomach, and within a month will cause any such person to be ill, whether he / she be young or old." The book *Sun Zhen Ren Wei Sheng Ge* says, "When sitting or lying, one must see to it that the wind is not blowing at the back of the head, for it harms one's health."

(3) Sleeping not too near a Fire

The book *Suo Sui Lu* points out, "One should not sleep with his head near a fire or it may injure the brain." Sleeping near a stove, it is most likely that the pathogenic fire may cause diseases, and besides, one is liable to catch cold when getting up at night.

(4) Sleeping with the Head not Wrapped or the Nose not Covered

The book *Shou Qin Yang Lao Xin Shu* contains an account describing how three elderly men achieved longevity, stressing, "It is imperative not to wrap one's head during sleep at night." As is generally believed, wrapping one's head in sleep hinders breathing and, with impure air inhaled, harms the health.

(5) Making Bedding Warm and Pillow Comfortable

The book *Dao Lin Yang Sheng Lun* says, "Make the bed warm and comfortable before sleep." It is necessary before sleep to make sure that the bed is well arranged, firm and stable, the bedding is made warm and comfortable, the pillow soft and springy and at its proper height. In some circumstances it is preferable to select a suitable kind of medical-herb-padded pillow, which is capable of preventing and curing diseases as well as comfortable. The book *Lao Lao Heng Yan* points out, as regards the height of the pillow, "It should be at the same height as one's shoulder when sleeping on one's flank, and one should feel equally comfortable when sleeping on one's back." It has manifested that these requirements are scientific. Sun Simiao, a noted physician, also stressed the necessity of "soft pillow and adequately warm bedding." These principles they advocated are practical and worth following.

3. Health Care after Waking up

Great attention was paid to health care after waking up by the ancients, who developed many means in this field. As the book *Lao Lao Heng Yan* puts it, "When waking up, one should turn and twist lest the lower body should be numb, or the waist and flank ache or the limbs twing." The book *Zun Sheng Ba Jian* suggests techniques such as tapping the teeth, doing breathing exercise, ingesting saliva and doing massage. The author believed them to be the methods easy to apply in general practice and capable of strengthening the body.

1.3.3 Adjusting One's Clothing According to Climate

Clothing is an outer expression of one's material and spiritual life as well as a means of preserving warmth and preventing diseases. The close relation between health and clothing was known long ago to the ancients, who emphasized that clothing should vary with the climate and be comfortable to wear.

1. Making One's Clothing Suitable and Comfortable

It was believed by the ancients that it was not the glamour of clothing that matters but the fitness for wearing, as is stated in the book *Lao Lao Heng Yan*, "Food and clothing are two essentials in health care. One's desire for food should be confined to the simple and non-heavy while his clothing should be comfortable to wear. This requirement is, so to speak, a wonderful medicine in health preserving." and "The size of clothes should agree with the shape of the wearer individual ... while their thickness or layers the particular season." These statements indicate that what the ancients emphasized in clothing was its cosiness and its value for practical use rather than its glamorous appearance. The general principle to be adopted in selecting clothes is to see to it that they are light, soft, big enough, cosy, simply-designed and convenient to wear. Moreover, the underwear should, preferably, be made of cotton material.

2. Changing Clothes according to Climate

The year has its differences between seasons while the day the differences between night and daytime; the clothes one wears should, accordingly, increase or decrease with the change of seasons and climate. The book *Sun Zhen Ren Wei Sheng Ge* has this to say, " In spring time clothes should be thick enough as the weather is still cold; in summer days clothes should be changed frequently as the weather is hot and sweat is profuse; in autumn when weather becomes colder, clothes should be added before diseases arise and medicine is called for ." The book *She Sheng Xiao Xi Lun* says, "Since the temperature is not yet stable in lunar January and February, alternating between cold and warm, the clothes that one wears should not be reduced abruptly; and elderly people, whose *Qi* is relatively weak, whose bones are far from strong, and whose resistance to illness is declining, should have more extra clothes at hand for wear, for in their case cold wind is more likely to injure the striae of their skin, muscles and viscera. During the three months of winter the heaven and earth are closing ..., adding of clothes should begin only when it is cold enough and the increase must be gradual and not abrupt. "This is because, in spring time, although the weather gets warmer, the temperature still fluctuates, tending to attract pathogenic factors, and thus the clothes one wears must not be reduced suddenly; whereas, when winter comes, the pathogenic dryness of the autumn still persists although the weather gets cold, and therefore, the clothes and bedding should not be thickened abruptly. A similar view was also held by Tao Hongjing, a notable physician in the Epoch of Division between the Northen and the Southen Dynasties.

As was stated by Sun Simiao, one will benefit a great deal both in health preservation and in preventing diseases if he follows the law of nature, to which he should adjust his food, clothing, sleeping and housing.

1. 3. 4 Paying Attention to Hygiene

The ancients had always pain much attention to personal hygiene, believing that only through hygiene will it be possible to achieve prevention of illness and good health. On such techniques as mouth-rinsing, tooth-brushing, bathing, face-washing, foot-washing and tooth-tapping, they have handed down a lot of detailed instructions, many of which are quite scientific and still have practical, guiding significance even up to now.

1. Mouth-rinsing and Tooth-brushing

Ancient experts in health care were aware long ago that oral hygiene is important for preventing stomatosis. They maintained that one should rinse his mouth after a meal and brush his teeth each night. The book *Qian Jin Yao Fang* says, " The mouth should be rinsed several times after a meal so that the mouth and teeth will not smell." The book *Lao Lao Heng Yan* states, "The remains of food clinging to the tooth-gaps after a meal are most detrimental to the teeth; if they are of sweet food, it will be all the more necessary to rinse the mouth. Those people we often find who lose their teeth before old age are victims of sweet food remaining between teeth, causing, as a result, the decaying of teeth." There were, too, quite a few experts in health care who upheld the practice of rinsing the mouth before sleep, as is stated in the book *Suo Sui Lu*, "Rinsing the mouth at night is better than in the morning." The book *Lao Lao Heng Yan* also contains the same statements to the same effect.

Tooth brushing is one of the ancient inventions of the Chinese. As early as in the Song Dynasty (A.D. 960-1278) tooth powder and tooth brushes were already used. The book *Tai Ping Sheng Hui Fang* records ways of producing tooth paste. In the Yuan Dynasty (A.D. 1206-1333), Hu Sihui, a noted physician, recorded in his book *Yin Shan Zheng Yao*, "Brushing teeth with salt in the morning can prevent odontopathy." The book *Jin Dan Quan Shu* states rightly, "Most people today clean their teeth in the morning, but this has wrongly been inverted. Teeth should be brushed at night instead, for the remains of food held in between the teeth will be cleared away in time to keep them from decaying. Some wise people are found to have their teeth white, firm and free from decay until they are old just because they have persisted in brushing teeth each night."And the book *Wei Sheng Bao Jian* advocates tooth-brushing both in the morning and at night, a rational practice which is popular even today.

2. **Points for Attention on Bathing**

The cleanliness of the body is a necessity for health—preserving. Bathing, including washing the hair and the body, was practised long ago in China. Some classical works such as the book *Chu Ci*, the book *Shi Ji* and the book *Meng Zi* have all mentioned the practice of bathing by the Chinese ancients, indicating that they had the tradition of taking care of personal hygiene. The book *Lun Yu* advocates bathing in cold water and has a description of a group of people, including several children, taking a bath in the River of *Yi* in late spring.

In terms of water temperature, the book *Lao Lao Heng Yan* has this to say, "The water for bathing should not be too hot, its temperature should be agreeable to the body." Also, it recommends 'dry bath' and 'medical bath', saying, "By 'dry bath' is meant the method of rubbing one's hands on the stomach before sleeping at night ... Bathing in special decoction from wolfberry is called 'medical bath', which helps one resist diseases and ageing. Even if it does not achieve that effect in some circumstances, it never does the least harm to the health." When taking a bath in spring and autumn, one should, as the book holds, "put a large basin with hot water filled to half the capacity and with a tent covering it. Moreover, one should put on warm enough clothes as soon as bathing is over, for if one feels somewhat chilly after a bath, he / she is likely to catch cold." The book *She Sheng Xiao Xi Lun* states, "During winter, the *Yang—Qi* stays inside while the *Yin—Qi* outside, thus it is not advisable for old people to bath in winter, for they usually suffer from the disorder of heat in the upper body and cold in the lower." The book *Qian Jin Yao Fang* maintains that it is not advisable to bathe too frequently. Modern medicine also holds that elderly people needn't bathe so often, because their sebaceous glands are shrinking, and frequent baths may cause dryness of skin and itching. For them, 'dry bathing' or rubbing the body with a dry towel is preferable. As regards the frequency of baths, the book *Tai Ding Yang Sheng Zhu Lun* says, "Taking a bath every ten days is recommendable except in summer. Frequent baths only make a person feel seemingly comfortable and regulated, but inwardly his / her essential *Qi* is dispersed and dissipated." In addition, the book *Lao Lao Heng Yan* states, "One should not take a bath when hungry." and "Wind must be avoided when one is taking a bath." These requirements are quite scientific with practical value of reference.

3. **Hygiene of Hands and Feet**

Hands directly contact the outside world most frequently, but are the least protected; they are most vulnerable to contamination of various kinds. The hygiene of hands is closely related with the health of a person. Apart from regular washing of hands and keeping them clean, one should also cut one's finger nails regularly, as the book *Yang Sheng Shu* puts it, "Finger-nails are the ends of tendons; if they are not cut regularly, the tendons will not be easy to renew." The book *Yan Shou Yao Yan* recommends, "It is advisable to wash one's feet in hot water before sleep." This will help stablize one's mind and promote sleep. As an old saying goes, "A basin of hot water before sleep will keep the medicine away.", indicating vividly the benefit of washing the feet, esp. right before sleep. It is indeed a practice worth observing persistently.

In addition, the ancients have handed down some analects specially treating methods of health preserving, such as tapping teeth and ingesting saliva, these analects still have their value for practical application up to the present.

1.4 Balance between Work and Rest for Health Care

Work here implies "tiredness", while rest means leisure, ease and comfort. Man has to work and struggle against nature in order to survive. In doing so, however, one must do his work within the limits of his tolerance. And he needs proper rest to relieve the tension from work. That is called striking a proper balance between work and rest. Traditional Chinese medicine has invariably insisted that the balance has great beneficial effect on health. Moderate work or rest is advocated rather than excessive hard work or too much rest. Experts through the ages in health care have maintained that imbalance between work and rest was a great taboo. The book *Yang Xing Yan Ming Lu* says that the way to keep good health is nothing but to avoid internal injuries from overstrain. Sun Simiao argued that it is not advisable to overwork and overrest, for either of them is harmful to health. A same statement can be also found in the book *Lao Zi Yang Sheng Yao Jue*.

Imbalance between work and rest is harmful to health in several ways. Internal injuries caused by overstrain may involve not only the physical and mental types but also that due to sexual intercourse. Injuries caused by too much leisure involve either of the mind and body. What traditional Chinese medicine has reiterated about work and rest is reflected in the respects mentioned above.

1.4.1 Avoiding Overwork

Traditional Chinese medicine believes that overwork may injure the body, causing tiredness and listlessness in light cases and resulting in relevant pathological changes in the severe cases. The book *Nei Jing* points out, "There are five kinds of overstrain that are responsible for internal injuries: Looking too long does harm to the blood; lying too long, the Qi; sitting too long, the muscles; standing too long, the bones and walking too long, the tendons." This shows that if one keeps any one of the above postures for a long time he can not stand and may hurt his body. How can working injure the body? This question was explained very well in the book *Peng Zu She Sheng Yang Xing Lun*. It says, "Doing physical labour beyond one's ability will hurt the body."

The book *Nei Jing* points out, "Overwork consumes the Qi.", which indicates that excessive physical or mental exertion is chiefly responsible for that of Qi. The shortage of Qi will cause tiredness, spiritlessness, asthenia and weakness. This is quite true in actual life. Fast walking for a long time may put the body and mind in an intense state, greatly consuming the primordial energy. As a result, with the vital energy hiding in the interior instead of spreading out, it is hard for the walking to be continued. Sitting quietly for too long may slow down the function of the spleen and the stomach. As the spleen relates to the movements of muscles, the stagnation of the spleen—Qi will weaken the muscles. Standing long keeps the waist stretched and bones burdened. The lumbus is the residence of the kidney, and the kidney is responsible for the bones. So standing for too long is liable to injure the lumbus, the kidney and the bones as well. Over-long lying makes it difficult for the lung to carry out its normal function. The lung is in charge of the Qi. Stagnation of the lung—Qi can slow down the circulation of the general Qi, and therefore, over-long lying harms the lung. The book *Yang Sheng Shu* states, "Over-long walking is harmful to the tendons and the liver, while over-long standing to the bones and the kidney. "This reveals the fact that overstrain is really a hazard to *Zang-Fu* organs. "Internal injury due to fatigue" has been always considered as an important cause of diseases by traditional Chinese medicine. Modern medical science also believes that when people are exhausted, the resistance to diseases may be remarkably reduced, and a variety of diseases will result.

According to the theory of traditional Chinese medicine, the internal injuries caused by overstrain not only refer to what has been mentioned above but also include those due to excessive diet, imbalance of metabolism and spiritlessness. The book *Nei Jing* states, "Sweat comes from the stomach when one eats his fill, from the heart when one is in great terror, from the kidney when one walks long distance with heavy load, from the liver when one is frightened or takes a fast walk, and from the spleen when one works with rocking movements." It is common knowledge that diseases are often caused by overfatigue regardless the season and no matter how Yin and Yang alternate.

Our ancients held the view that one must keep a proper balance between work and rest, and avoid overwork. After work, he should refresh himself with a short rest. The book *Yang Xing Yan Ming Lu* offers people very scientific and reasonable principles for body activities by saying this: those who want to keep good health should not spin with great force, nor walk too fast, nor use their ears and eyes too hard, nor sit too long, nor stand still tired and nor lie till muddled, etc.

The book *Bao Sheng Yao Lu* has it that those who are good at health care should work without becoming over-fatigued.

Flowing water stands fresh while stagnant water tends to turn stale. So proper work is beneficial to health. Those who want to keep healthy must, by doing work, keep the blood circulating freely just as the flowing water. But they should take a rest before getting tired when walking for too long a time, and should slow down for a rest when taking a long fast walk. This attaches the importance of moderate work to health-preservation and also points out that taking a rest at intervals during work is a way to prevent overstrain and thus worth following. Ge Hong, a famous medical scientist of the Jin Dynasty, suggested in his book *Bao Pu Zi* a set of ways of health care, some of which deal with work and rest. His points of view are similar to those mentioned above. Furthermore, he pointed out that people should not eat or drink unless they feel hungry and thirsty. Otherwise, they will injure their spleen and stomach. Moreover, they should work and eat regularly and get up between cocks crow and sunrise. Both the books *Nei Jing* and *Shou Qin Yang Lao Xin Shu* claim, "When weather and temperature are suitable, old people should take a walk of about 2—3 *Li* or 200—300 paces, they must be sure not to get out of breath. When relatives or friends visit each other they may, if convenient, have a walk, sitting, talking and chatting but must remember not to get too excited or too tired." This indicates that the old and weak people should walk or take other activities according to their capability and prevent exhaustion lest their health be damaged.

1.4.2 Avoiding Irritability

Traditional Chinese medicine considers that any of the seven emotions, if too intense, will harm the mind, affect health and reduce longevity. The book *Ling Shu* says, "Apprehensions and anxieties may injure the mind, thus making people weak and emaciated, with dried hair and pallid countenance."; "Continuous worry and anxiety may injure intention.", which leads to "debility of the limbs"; "Sorrow injures the soul, thus causing the decline of *Yin* and convulsion."; "Excessive joy may injure the spirit, leading to the withering of the hair."; "Excessive anger may injure the will, making it difficult for the spinal column to bend and stretch."; "Being in terror for long may injure the primordial energy, leading to debility of the bones.". All these indicate clearly that an excess of any of the seven emotions may injure not only the mind but also the physique. Spirit is the embodiment of the living activities of human beings, as Peng Zu once said, "Those who have vigorous spirit will live longer", while "those whose minds are injured will die young." The ancients also realized that injury of the mind would be the precursor of some diseases. Sun Simiao said, "Anger injures the *Qi* and the weakened *Qi* will be followed by disease." The book *Yang Sheng Lun* also points out, "Unrefrained excitement and anger may injure the vital energy." This shows that once the mind is injured, the vital energy will decline, and then exopathogen is likely to invade the body, resulting in various diseases.

    The injury of the mind will seriously affect the health, so the ancients took great care of the mind by preventing extremes of any of the seven emotions. The book *Suo Sui Lu* says, "Excessive sorrow or joy must be avoided." The book *She Sheng Si Yao* believes, "Less thinking can help nourish the mind." Traditional Chinese medicine has proposed the methods of spirit recuperation, including optimism, less anxiety and lust, refrainment from joy and anger, abstention from too much thinking and worrying and avoidance of terror. All the above methods are useful to prevent the mind from being injured.

1.4.3 Regulating Sexual Life

Sexual activity is an important part of human life. It is considered as essential as material and mental lives. Several thousands of years ago, the Chinese people began to study the subject of sexual life. In the book *Nei Jing* the relationship between sexual life and health was discussed in detail. Since then, medical scientists through the ages have put forward a lot of scientific views about the influence of sexual life on physiological function and pathological changes of the body.

Excess of sexual intercourse is harmful to health, which was well known to the ancients. The book *Nei Jing* points out, "Some people regard alcohol as tonic, the abnormal way of life as conventional. They enjoy their sexual life after being drunk, which will exhaust their genuine *Qi*. So those who indulge themselves in sexual life will become senile in their fifties." Sun Simiao said, "Those who indulge in sexual activities will have a short life span like morning dew." He also added vividly, "In palaces there are thousands of beautiful women, and in high officials' homes, hundreds of concubines. During the day they are drenched with good wine, watching and listening to what is obscene and pornographic ... At night they consume their *Qi* and blood by sexual activities, or have intercourse when diseased, thus reducing their primordial energy and blood ... This is why only few such people have achieved longevity." The face that emperors of successive dynasties in our country who indulged in sex and strong wine usually died very young is the evidence that the above statements are quite true.

Excess intercourse mainly consumes the primordial energy, which is the base of health. "Less primordial energy results in diseases and exhaustion of it leads to death." Zhang Jingyue said, "Sexual activities must be restricted, otherwise the primordial energy is bound to be exhausted; if so, the vital energy will be distracted. Primordial energy can transform into Qi which can in turn transform into spirit, thus nourishing the body." This indicates the importance of primordial energy to life. Excessive sexual activities consume the primordial energy and injure the spirit, thus destroying the basis of life. In such case, it is difficult to have a long life. Peng Zu said, "To have a single bed is better than a hundred doses of medicine. Improper intercourse for one night may shorten one's life by one year. Do be careful." This statement seems radical, however, it is necessary to restrict sexual life.

It is more important for the aged and invalid to control sexual life, otherwise troubles will arise. The book *Shou Shi Bao Yuan* says, "Old people are weak in blood and Qi, but occasionally, sexual desire comes strongly. In this case, it is better to drive such desire away by turning their attention to some other things." Being weak in the kidney–Qi, old people should not indulge themselves in sexual activities.

As stated above, since early times traditional Chinese medicine has realized that excess of sexual intercourse is harmful to health, and put forward a series of propositions and specific measures to check it.

1. Marrying at a Mature Age

Traditional Chinese medicine has been favouring and advocating marriage at a mature age, considering it harmful to the health to marry too young. The book *Yang Sheng Yi Yao Qian Shuo* says, "Marrying under mature age may hurt the primordial *Yang* and the vital energy so as to weaken the *Qi* and distract the spirit. Spermatorrhea, impotence and other consumptive diseases will follow. Most of the people who suffer from the diseases mentioned above will have no descendants." The book *Ge Zhi Yu Lun* also says, "Males develop semen at sixteen, and females have menstruation at fourteen. The ancients' age of marrige must have been next to thirty or at least over twenty." Different marriageable ages were then suggested according to different physiological development of both sexes. This has remained perfectly reasonable up to now. The book *Leng Lu Yi Hua* also maintains, "It is suitable for males to get married at thirty and females at twenty." The book *Shou Shi Bao Yuan* also has this that "Weak females are supposed to nourish the blood first before getting married while weak males are supposed to control sexual passion and not to get married until strong enough." These statements show the benefit of late marriage and the importance of restricting sex.

2. Regulating Sexual Life

Sex must be limited within right range. The book *Chun Qiu Fan Lu* points out the frequenoy of sexual act: "Once in ten days in people strong and young; once in 20 days in people of middle age; once in 40 days in people who are slightly weak; once in 80 days in people who are moderately weak and once in 10 months in very weak people." Sun Simiao maintained: "Those who are in their twenties may have sex once every 4 days, in their thirties once every 8 days, in their forties once every 16 days, in their fifties once every 20 days and in their sixties once a month if they are very strong. Those who are very healthy may not necessarily act according to the above principles so as not to suffer from carbuncle due to overrestraint". It is obvious that the frequency of sexual life varies greatly with age. The general trend is that the older, the less. It also varies with the individual's constitution and other concrete conditions of the same age. Modern medicine holds that whether or not a sexual act is normal depends on whether the person is still in high spirits and full of vigour next day. Most people believe that in general once or twice a week is normal and adequate, which can bring about satisfaction of sex rather than harmfulness to the health.

3. Taboos for Sexual Life

Sexual intercourse should be tabooed under some conditions. As Sun Simiao said, " Sexual intercourse must be avoided under the following conditions: just after a bath or a long journey, or in the state of fill or tipsiness or great joy or much sorrow, or in the course of febrile diseases, or in the menstruation or postpartum period." The book *Shou Shi Bao Yuan* points out, "Sexual intercourse after being full up or in tipsiness will cause men to have less and less sperm as well as impotence, and women to have less and less menstruation with blood extravasated and maligant boils developed for, after being full up, the blood—*Qi* is impaired; in tipsiness, the vital energy consumed and the *Qi* of the liver and intestines injured. Sexual intercourse in anger will make the essence of life deficient, resulting in boils; in terror, both *Yin* and *Yang* insufficient, resulting in spontaneous perspiration, night sweating, and even more serious disorders; after a long journey, the five kinds of impairments caused and disability of reproduction occur; during menstruation, cold invade the body, leading to pale skin and infertility; in the course of a wound, the blood–Qi damaged, making the wound worse; with the bladder full of urine, such disorders produced as stranguria, pain in the penis, pale complexion and winding of the womb towards the navel which causes great pain and even death; in case of infectious disease, the disease worse even up to death with the tongue stretched out." All the above statements show that sexual intercourse may be contraindicated in many cases. The following three points must be kept in mind.

(1) Sexual Intercourse with No Tipsiness

Sun Simiao said, "Sexual life in tipsiness is not advisable, it will cause dusky complexion, mild cough, and even death in severe cases by injuring the channels and organs." This statement shows the danger of sexual intercourse in tipsiness. Being drunk, people often lose self-control, which is liable to cause excessive sexual intercourse. injuring the kidney, consuming the primordial energy, damaging spirit and shortening life span. Meanwhile sexual intercourse in tipsiness makes sexual life inharmonious, hurting the feelings between husbands and wives, resulting in, if pregnancy occurs in such a moment, poor constitution and low intelligence of the coming baby, and even fetal malformation, mental retardation or dementia. Moreover, it is responsible for the disorders such as impotence and prospermia.

(2) Sexual Intercourse with No Anger, Terror and Tiredness

Traditional Chinese medicine pays special attention to the influence of seven emotions and tiredness on sexual life. Su Simiao, said "When people are angry their Qi and blood are unstable. If they have sex on this occasion, they tend to suffer from boils.", pointing out the harmfulness. If sexual intercourse in terror brings about pregnancy, the coming baby will suffer from epilepsy, as the book *Nei Jing* says.

(3) Sexual Intercourse in Usual Weather

Sexual intercourse must be avoided in such unusual weathers as those of thunderstorm and lightning or extreme coldness or hotness. Because sexual intercourse in such weathers is harmful not only to the mother but also, if pregnancy should occur, to the fetus. Su Simiao said, "The baby died at birth along with his mother, why? The mother had become pregnant on a stormy occasion."

Moreover, women shouldn't have sex during periods of menstruation, the first trimester and the third trimester of pregnancy. Nor should mothers within one hundred days after giving birth. Sexual life should be avoided when one is suffering from an illness, and should be controlled after one has recovered from a long illness.

1.4.4 Avoiding Excessive Leisure

One can be hurt either by overwork or by overleisure. Traditional Chinese medicine holds that people who want to keep fit should avoid not only overwork but also too easy and comfortable a life. When they are tired, it is positive to have a temporary rest to readjust themselves. However, excessive leisure will become the negative factor which is not beneficial to health. Experts in health care have warned people against overleisure. Confucius pointed out, "Addicting oneself to comfort is harmful to health." Ge Hong said, "Those who are good at keeping health adjust their muscles and tendons and bones by lying after getting tired, and get rid of diseases and pathogenic factors through doing breathing exercise." Viscera are constently in motion in order to play their physiological roles. Suitable activities can improve the body functions. Rest after work is needed. But too much leisure and comfort can slow down the circulation of *Qi* and blood, hold up the channels, reduce the functions of *Zang* and *Fu* organs, fatigue the limbs, thus leading to general deficiency of the body. Furtern once pointed out, "Life lies in movement." He considered movement as good medicine for keeping calm and strong.

    The first way to refrain from excessive leisure is to take physical exercise. The book *Lü Shi Chun Qiu* says, "Running water is never stale and a door—hinge never gets worm—eaten. The same is true of the body." Exercises in the exterior lead to those of *Qi* and blood in the interior. Both of them improve each other. The human body is powerful with the aid of nutrition from *Qi* and blood, while *Qi* and blood can travel freely by means of the body movements. Frequently moving the fingers and arms can make the joints move smoothly and frequently moving the feet, legs, thighs and knees can make the bones stronger and steps more vigorous. In daily life one should take proper exercise to keep fit. The second way is to avoid sitting or lying too long. Traditional Chinese medicine believes long sitting will hurt muscles, while long lying, the vital energy. In terms of sleep, the ancients thought, "It is very beneficial for people to have enough sleep, but excess of sleep will make people weak and muddleheaded." Sitting long will lead to the stagnation of *Qi* and blood, or even diseases. So long lying or sitting should be avoided, and regular exercise should be taken to adjust the flowing of *Qi* and blood. The third way is to use the brain frequently. The brain must be used frequently so as to prevent the declining of intelligence. This is imperative for old people. They need sufficient information to stimulate the cerebral cortex frequently so that their brains can be supplied with enough blood. Old people should often read books and newspapers, and keep active in thinking. In recent years, scientists have measured the brains of people living in different ways with ultrasonic waves and found that those who have made good use of their brains can keep the blood vessels of their brains in dilated state and their brain nerve cells well nourished, which prevents their brains from declining too early.

1.5 Health Care by Sports

Sport, an effective health care method, has caught great attention since the ancient time. The book *Yi Zhuan . Xiang Ci . Qian Xiang* has it that nature is in constant movement. Only in so doing, can man keep fit and achieve longevity. The book *Yan Xing Lu* says, "If one takes exercise, he will become stronger; so will a family; a nation; and the whole world." Hua Tuo, a famous physician in the Han Dynasty created a sport *Wu Qin Xi* (five-animal-minic boxing), which made great contribution to the development of ancient sports. Among the historical relics discovered from Mawangdui No.3 Han Tomb in Chang sha, Hunan Province, in 1975, there is a piece of silk on which such poses are painted as sitting, stretching arms, bending knees, holding legs in arms and squating. It shows that health care through physical exercise has a long history in our country.

Traditional Chinese medicine considers that sports can keep the primordial energy running within the body. The book *Shou Shi Bao Yuan* holds, "To keep healthy, one can neither lie down soon after a meal nor sit quietly all day long. Otherwise, *Qi* and blood will be stagnated and the life span will be shortened." Sports can also improve the digestive function of the spleen and stomach. Hua Tuo once said, "Sports help digestion, promote blood circulation and prevent disease." Sun Simiao stressed repeatedly, "One should have a walk of several *Li* after a meal and then massage his stomach for a while. In this way, he will have a good appetite and be in good health." The researches of modern medicine indicate that sports can increase the functions of the heart and blood vessels, improve the function of the respiratory system, exert a good effect on the nervous system, strengthen the muscles and bones, and prevent and control some diseases. Therefore, sports are essential to health and longevity.

Exercises can be divided into the active types such as labour and various sports, and the passive types such as massage. There are so many different forms of exercises, including labour, physical training, dance, *Dao Yin* (physical and breathing exercises) and seesawing, which can be chosen according to individual needs. Regular physical exercise can keep one fit and let him live long.

1.5.1 Participating in Physical Labour

Labour creates the world, It is an essential factor for people to survive. Regular and adequate physical labour is also one of the important forms of exercises. Traditional Chinese medicine maintains that physical labour can build up the body, adjust the spirit, regulate *Qi* and blood, relax the muscles and tendons and strengthen the bones. Hua Tuo once pointed out, "Human beings should take part in proper physical labour." Physical labour is especially important for mental workers and old people. It can not only train the body and improve health, but also mould one's temperament and cultivate one's sentiment. At the same time, physical labour offers a good rest to the brain, gives one spiritual pleasure and makes his mood steady. Sun Simiao stated that without physical labour and sports the functional activities of *Qi* may be out of order or even stagnated. People should make an arrangement to take part in certain amount of manual labour. For mental workers, labour, as a kind of rest and relaxation, is especially important.

1.5.2 Taking Part in Physical Training

Physical training is the most important form of sports. The ancients paid special attention to it, and created many items unique to our Chinese nation, such as *Tai Ji Quan, Wu Qin Xi, Ba Duan Jin*, etc., some of which are still popular all over the world. At present, physical training items are even richer and more colourful, such as jumping, running, walking, lifting, shooting, swimming, throwing and bouncing, etc. Most of them are practical and easy to learn. People can make a choice among them according to their own conditions.

1.5.3 Brief Introduction to Common Exercises

1. Walking

Walking is the easiest and most frequently used exercise. The ancients strongly held the view that people should take a walk in the early morning or after a meal, before sleep or during free time in order to build up their bodies, regulate *Qi* and blood, improve the transport and conversion of food, invigorate the mind and promote health. There is a special discussion on walking in the book *Lao Lao Heng Yan*, which says, "A walker should walk at a leisurely pace, stopping to rest at intervals."It also points out that walking has the effect of relaxing muscles and tendons, strengthening the limbs, promoting digestion, and tranquilizing the mind. It has been proved by practice that walking is a method which is indeed beneficial to health and easy to practise.

2. Dancing

Dancing is also one of the effective methods for building up one's body. In the book *Lü Shi Chun Qiu* there is an account that "Dancing can promote blood circulation, thus preventing the stagnation of *Qi* and the contraction and spasms of the tendons and muscles." The book *Hong Lu Dian Xue* says, "Dancing can benefit the blood vessels."It also stresses, "It is suitable to dance a little after meals." Modern investigations also suggest that lively dancing can indeed enhance one's constitution and invigorate one's mind.

3. Dao Yin

Dao Yin, combining physical and breathing exercise, is a method of preserving health which is handed down from ancient times. Examples of this are five–animal–mimic boxing and the twelve ways of Brahman *Dao Yin*. The ancients thought that *Dao Yin* bad the main effect of mediating the functional activities of *Qi*, promoting the flow of *Ying*, *Wei Qi* and blood, relaxing muscles and tendons, strengthening bones and relieving tiredness and restlessness. The book *Lao Lao Heng Yan* says, "There are many kinds of *Dao Yin* ... Their beneficial effects are nothing but promoting the flow of *Qi* and blood, and relaxing muscles and tendons."

4. **Shadow Boxing** (*Tai Ji Quan*)

Shadow boxing, which is a combination of some poses of Chinese boxing developed in the late Ming Dynasty with ancient *Dao Yin*, is also one of the commonly used methods. Although shadow boxing is included in dynamic *Qi Gong*, it is the combination of both dynamic and static exercises, training the body internally and externally. Shadow boxing is named after the diagram of *Tai Ji* which shows the relationship between *Yin* and *Yang*. the human body, like the universe, includes *Yin* and *Yang*, two respects which are opposite and unitive. If one wants to be healthy, *Yin* and *Yang* in his body must be kept in the state of dynamic balance. Practising shadow boxing will reach this goal. After 1949, the National Sports Committee published the diagram and captions of the simplified shadow boxing which is easy to learn and practise and highly favoured by people.

Besides the exercise mentioned above, there are still others beneficial to health such as massage. *Tian Zhu Guo* massage, running, *Wu Shu* (now a form of physical culture), etc. They will benefit the mind and body if one can master their essentials and persist in practising them.

1.6 Health Care by Conforming to Nature

Human beings live in nature. The changes of climate and surroundings are closely related to human health. Guided by the theory of *Tian Ren Xiang Ying* (correspondence between man and the universe), ancient medical scientists believed that human beings and the natural environments are in unity. Consistent changes of climate of the four seasons and environments affect not only the body's physiological function but also, under certain conditions, the occurence and development of the pathological process. The book *Ling Shu* says, "In hot weather heavy clothes open the striae between the skin and muscles and lead to sweating, while in cold weather, with the striae closed, *Qi* tends to be stagnated and water in the body will go down to the bladder to form urine to be expelled from the body." That is to say that the way of water excretion in the human body varies with the climate. If the six factors (wind, cold, heat, dampness, dryness and fire) change according to their laws, they will not harm the human body. If the climate changes abnormally, the six factors will become six exogenous pathogenic factors. If people do not adapt to the geographical changes, such as moving from the high land to the wet plain, or from the hot south to the cold north, they will develop diseases due to these changes. To gain and maintain health, people must adapt themselves to environmental changes and keep away from evil factors.

1.6.1 Conforming to the Four Seasons

The four seasons are spring, summer, autumn and winter, people should act in accordance with the changes of the four seasons. The book *Nei Jing* says, "The *Yin* and *Yang* in the four seasons are the essentials for all things to exist. The reason that the wise nourish *Yang* in spring and summer and nourish *Yin* in autumn and winter is simply for meeting the basic requirements of *Yin* or *Yang*. Human beings, like all the other living things, lead a certain length of life—neither die young nor live forever. Going against the regular changes of seasons means damaging the essentials and primordial *Qi*. So the changes of *Yin* and *Yang* of the four seasons are essential for making things appear or disappear, human beings come into being or pass away. Going against them means disasters; going with them means no severe diseases. This is the way to keep health. The wise will follow it, but the dull-witted won't." The book *Ling Shu* also says, "The wise who want to preserve their health should adapt themselves to the changeable weather of the four seasons, mediate their joy and anger, live a quiet life, regulate *Yin* and *Yang* and adjust their firmness and gentleness. In doing so, they can keep away from pathogenic factors and live a long life", stressing that only conforming with the changes of the four seasons can human beings live a long life.

1. Health Care in Spring

Traditional Chinese medicine holds that spring is the season when everything has a tendency to grow and develop, and when all plants are in bud and are flourishing. Human beings should conform to the season in daily life. The book *Nei Jing* says, "Spring is the season with active force. In spring everything is thriving. In this season people should go to bed and get up early. After getting up in the morning they should have a stroll in the court with their hair dishevelled, thus relaxing their bodies and invigorating their mind." The book *Qian Jin Yao Fang* claims, "In spring people should go to bed early and get up not before the cock-crow." The book *Nei Jing* holds that one who doesn't do this may hurt his liver in spring, and the troubled liver will in turn suffer from a pathologic change of cold nature in the coming summer."

In terms of diet, the book *Sun Zhen Ren Wei Sheng Ge* points out that in spring people should "have more sweet food and less sour food". The book *Yun Ji Qi Jian* says, "It is warm in spring, so people should have food cool in nature, and should not have any other kind of food warm in nature." The book *She*

Sheng Xiao Xi Lun holds, "People shouldn't drink too much alcohol or eat too much dough from rice or flour, which is hard to digest and may hurt the spleen and stomach." All these tell us that in spring people should have soft and easily-digested food with sweet taste rather than dry food sour and pungent in taste and warm in nature, in favour of the digestive function.

In terms of clothing, the book *Sun Zhen Ren Wei Sheng Ge* advocates, "One shouldn't wear cotton-padded clothes that is too thin when it is still chilly in spring." The book *She Sheng Xiao Xi Lun* points out, "The temperature is changeable in spring, so people should reduce gradually cotton-padded clothes. Old people are subject to general deficiency of *Qi* and weakness of the bones and the body. They are apt to be hurt by wind and cold. And they should get double-layer-cloth clothes ready and substitute them for the cotton-padded one when it is warm. The clothing worn should be reduced gradually, not suddenly." Although it gets warmer in spring, the weather is changeable, people, therefore, should be careful of wind and cold.

Besides, the book *She Sheng Xiao Xi Lun* also has the view that in spring every living thing has a tendency to grow. And people should adjust emotions in order to avoid spiritual depression. The above discussions have proved to be quite practical.

2. Health Care in Summer

Summer is the hottest season in a year. Every living thing is flourishing and the *Yang-Qi* in the body is also apt to be expelled. The book *Nei Jing* points out that in summer one should not go to bed too early at night but should get up early in the morning, should enjoy the longer daytime, should be full of energy and avoid getting angry, thus activating the function of

Qi. This is the way for health care in summer. Without following it one will have his heart impaired and shall be attacked by malaria or other disease in the coming autumn or winter.

As regards diet, the book *Qian Jin Yao Fang* says that in summer people should have less food with bitter taste and more food with acid taste to nourish the lung—*Qi,* otherwise flaring heart—*Qi* may disturb the dispersal of the lung—*Qi.* The book *Yang Sheng Lun* also tells that in summer it is suitable for people to have coarse cereals cold in nature other than wheat and rice hot in nature, and not to have greasy food. It points out, "In late summer or early autumn, many diseases are caused by too much greasy or fried food, which has the same effect as alcohol and fruit." The book *Yang Lao Feng Qin Shu* also has a discussion on avoiding eating some cold, raw or greasy food in summer.

With regard to clothing, the book *Sun Zhen Ren Wei Sheng Ge* says, "Clothes should be thinner and often be changed and washed in summer, because hot weather makes people sweat too much."

The ancients had strict claim on enjoying the cool. The book *Yang Lao Feng Qin Shu* holds, "In summer, it is hot and so is the earth. People should avoid enjoying the cool under the eaves, in a passageway or before a broken window for fear that the evil wind should harm the bodies." The book *She Sheng Xiao Xi Lun* has the same discussion as described above. It adds, "In summer it is appropriate for people to enjoy the cool at places such as in an empty room, a pavilion by the water or under a tree. Natural coolness there is more comfortable to the body and the mind. And people will feel as if there were a piece of ice at the heart and heat in the interior will then be cleared up." It continues, "People should not sleep in the open air during the night, or with the body fanned by somebody else." The book *Li Xu Yuan Jian* also points out, "People should avoid being attacked by coolness in summer and prevent wet pathogens in the whole course of summer." All that described above is the summary of the experience of our Chinese people in the long history and all are still instructive now.

3. Health Care in Autumn

The book *Nei Jing* says that in autumn all the living things are ripe and stop growing. The sky looks higher and the wind is stronger. People should adapt themselves to the climatic features by going to bed and getting up early in order that the mind be tranquilized, the vitality astringed and the lung—*Qi* kept pure and descending. If one goes against this, he will have his lung hurt and suffer diarrhea in the coming winter.

As to diet, the book *Yin Shan Zheng Yao* points out, "It is dry in autumn and sesame should be taken to moisten the dryness." Some people hold that it was suitable to eat gruel containing dried rehmannia root(Radix Rehmanniae) to nourish *Yin* and dampen dryness, and to eat less and less food with pungent taste and more and more food with sour taste lest the excess of the lung—*Qi* suppress the liver—*Qi*.

With regard to clothing, the book *Sun Zhen Ren Wei Sheng Ge* says that it is getting cooler and cooler in autumn and one should add his clothes in time in order not to catch cold.

4. Health Care in Winter

It is cold in winter and everything in the world is now in the state of storage. Man should be careful to keep warm and prevent coldness, store up the *Yin* essence in the interior and allow less *Yang* energy to be lost. In this way, one can adapt himself to the natural climate of winter. Just as the book *Nei Jing* says, "The winter months are such a season that all things hide, water ices and the earth cracks. One should be in good spirits and maintain *Yang*, go to bed early and get up after sunrise, think as if he had had what he wanted, avoid being exposed to cold and keep himself warm but not sweaty lest the *Qi* be affected. That is the way to take care of health in winter." The above words set forth the characteristics of winter climate and the principle of daily life and mental preservation. One going against it will have his kidney—*Qi* injured and suffer from flaccidity syndrome in the coming spring and his adaptability to the spring may be weakened.

In respect of diet, Qiu Chuji said that in winter man should nourish the heart—*Qi* by taking food which tastes less sour and more bitter. About clothing, he said that one shouldn't put on cotton—padded clothes until it is extremely cold, and add clothes gradually. As for getting oneself warm in winter, our forefathers had clear requirements, just as Qiu Chuji claimed, "It is all right if the house is not cold. One must not use stoves of various sizes too frequently, otherwise, he will be greatly hurt. One can't heat his hands over fire, which can affect the heart through the hands and cause irritability. It is said that hands and feet are associated with the heart." These ideas accord with the fact.

In brief, the ancient medical practioners have made great contributions to human health. Their statements on the conservation of health in the four seasons still have practical and guiding significance today.

1.6.2 Adjusting the Environment

Man has realized since ancient time that the geographic environment is closely related to human health. Different conditions of natural environment and climate have different influences on man's health. The book *Nei Jing* says, "People living at the same place under the same climate have different life spans. why?" Qi Bo said, "It is because terrain can be classified as high and low. The *Yin-Qi* is dominant in higher places where living things die later. The *Yang-Qi* is dominant in lower places where living things die early. And people living in a higher place live a longer life than people living in a lower place. The life span differs with terrain." This explains why different elevations affect man's health and life expectancy. Our forefathers also had clear realization about the effect of climate on geographical conditions. the book *Nei Jing* says, "The changes of climate are closely related to those of geographic environment. Too much dryness of climate makes the earth dry; too much heat, the earth hot; too much wind, the earth shake; too much dampness, the earth muddy; too much cold, the earth crack; too much fire, the earth hard, etc."

A great deal of research material indicates that longevity is closely related to the geographical features. Those who live in the mountainous areas with fresh air and cold climate usually have long lives while those who live in the plains with foul air and hot climate usually have short lives. Of course, highness or lowness of terrains is relative. The investigation in the areas Duan and Bama of Guangxi province—the famous longevity area of China shows that all the fifty-one people who were above one-hundred years old had lived in the countryside, and most of them lived about half way up the mountains. Another investigation in Hubei province also shows that of 125 long-living people aged 90 years old, over 96% lived in the countryside. Certainly, this is not absolute, but the result of all the investigations show that our forefathers' exposition is in accord with the facts.

Since environment has a close relationship with the human health, people should properly adjust it and make it beneficial for our health and longevity. The adjustment mainly lies in the choice and improvement of the living environment.

1. Choice of Environment

Our forefathers have always attached great importance to the choice of environment, thinking that the houses built in the lower, wet and dirty places will cause various diseases, while those built in higher, clean and dry places will make man healthy and live long. The book *Shi Shu* records, "A house should be built on a carefully chosen site." The book *Bo Wu Zhi* points out that a house should not be built in a place near stagnant water or cemetery or in too lonely a place where wild animals such as foxes often haunt, but should be built in a place before a hill, by a river, with crisp air, sufficient sunshine, clean spring water, green trees, but without dense smoke and dirty fog, sandy or black dust, dirty mud and water, and loud noise. Generally speaking, mountain areas are preferable to the plains, country is better than city. Country people should build their houses according to the above stated principles. The retired workers or cadres who live in cities should move to the country, conditions permitting. The residential quarters should not be situated in the central or industrial district full of smoke and with loud noise from heavy traffic.

2. Adjustment of Environment

The choice of living environment is certainly important, but owing to actual circumtances, the chances of being able to choose ideal conditions are slim, sometimes even impossible, especially in densely populated cities. The choice, therefore, is quite limited. But where possible, it is praticable and very good to health to make necessary adjustments and improvements to the living environment.

(1) Improvement of a Room

A room is one used for people to prevent the attack of wind, storm, heat and cold from the outside, and to maintain people's normal physiological function. A nice micro-climate is formed in a room where people can rest, sleep and be refreshed. Half of man's life is spent in his room. Whether or not its structurs is reasonable and its sanitary conditions are good exerts direct effects on his health. Sun Simiao once said, "The room should be in a condition good enough not to have any cracks through which wind comes in." Chen Zhi, a famous physician, also said, "The room should be clean, graceful, open in summer and closed in winter." He also told us the necessary requirements for a micro-climate in our rooms, by saying, "The room should be warm in winter and cool in summer. The bed with screens on three sides should not be too high and too large and the bed-clothes should be soft and smooth." The ancients were fastidious about the facing of a room, the location of a bed, the height of a room and the brightness in it, whether a window is to be opened or closed, etc. For example, the book *Tian Yin Zi Yang Sheng Shu* says, "What is a good room to live in? It is not a hall with a large bed and thick bed clothes. A good room should face south with the bed put in the east of it. It is half bright and half dim, with moderate *Yin* (dimness) and *Yang* (brightness). It is not to be too high, otherwise it will be too bright. Neither is it to be too low, or else it will be too dim. Too much light in it is harmful to human body, too much dimness will hurt man's spirit. Man's spirit belongs to *Yang* while human body to *Yin*. If *Yin* and *Yang* are not balanced, one will be ill. The room I live in has windows on every wall, They are closed when there is wind and opened when the wind stops. The room has curtains in the front of it and screens at the back. I put down the curtains when too bright in order to make the light soft and pull them up when too dim in order to let light in. As a result, both my heart and eyes are eased and I feel comfortable. The above ideas and requirements are quite practicable and possess much referential value.

Modern research also shows that several factors of a room such as dimensions, volume, height and width are very important. A room should not be too small or too low. The volume of a room for one person to live in is at least $15m^3$ which is a breathing space big enough for him. The height should be 2.6—3.5 metres and the width should not be over 2.0—2.5 times of the height from the floor to the upper limit of the windows. The temperature in it should be kept within 17—22℃ in winter and 17—25℃ in summer. The relative humidity should be within 40—60%. Circumstances permitting, one should improve his room according to the requirements mentioned above in order to preserve man's health.

(2) Improvement of Surroundings

The surroundings of a room, including the surroundings of the court-yard, are closely related to man's health, therefore, they should be improved and beautified. The experts in health care in ancient times attached great importance to the living surroundings. Most of their houses were situated in the places where there were green hills, clean water and plenty of sunshine. In our country, the houses in most districts face south, with the doors and windows facing the sun, thus causing the rooms to be bright, to have fresh air in, and to be kept warm in winter and cool in summer. People plant trees, flowers and grass around the houses. This not only makes the surroundings beautiful but also prevents wind and dust and conditions the air. This kind of environment is undoubtedly good to man's health and longevity. The famous expert in health care in the Qing Dynasty, Cao Cishan paid great attention to the living surroundings. He lived in a city but he could create good micro-environment. He built a garden in which his house faced a clear pool, and planted many pine trees around it. He could hear the soughing of the wind between the trees as if being in a valley ... He survived until he was over 90. In his book *Lao Lao Heng Yan*, he advocated that old people should plant dozens of flowers and trees of various kinds by themselves. They needn't be the exotic or rare types, if only they could be with us in every season. Before the steps of his house a water vat was placed with some goldfish in. This not only beautified the surroundings but also moulded his temperament. It was really beneficial to his health and longevity.

The way of beautifying surroundings is mainly through planting trees, flowers and grass extensively. Modern research has indicated that afforestation can adjust the temperature, humidity and the content of carbon dioxide in the air, purify the air, prevent wind and dust, kill bacteria, eliminate noise and have good effects on the organs of our bodies.

Improving surroundings also includes eliminating the noise and harmful industrial toxic gases so as to create a fine living environment and to promote man's health and longevity.

(3) Improvement of Cleanliness and Sanitation

Keeping the living surroundings clean is one of the important measures to prevent illness and keep one's health. In China's earliest inscriptions on bones or tortoise shells of the Shang Dynasty, there are records of general cleaning. The book *Li Ji* says, "When the cock crows for the first time, one should clean the house and sweep the yard." This shows that 2000 years ago our forefathers paid great attention to the environmental sanitation. The book *Meng Liang Lu* says, "In December, every family, rich or poor, sprays and sweeps the room and yard, removes dust in order to make all things clean." Here it refers to the general cleaning before the Spring Festival. Besides, people sprayed red orpiment liquor to the courtyard and bed-clothes at the Dragon Boat Festival. All of those are very necessary folk measures for sanitation. Our forefathers also knew the way of preventing pestilence by clearing away dirty water through ditches. The book *Zhou Shu Mi Ao Zao Ce Jing* says, "If the irrigation canals and ditches are not blocked, the house is clean and there is no dirty gas, there will be no pestilence." Our forefathers also had discussed how to sterilize the air. The book *Ju Jia Yi Ji* says, "One should burn incense in front of the bed in order to ward off the dirty gases and other ominous things." This method of fumigating the air to prevent diseases is still practicable now.

2 Practical Chinese Materia Medica for Health Care

2.1 Commonly Used Chinese Material Medicines for Health Care

Chinese material medicines for health care are those which can supplement the body with nutrients, enhance the body's functions, strengthen resistance, build up health or promote recovery and increase longevity. They are also called tonics for their tonifying properties. According to their effects and indications, they are classified as the following five kinds: *Qi* tonics, blood tonics, *Yang* tonics, *Yin* tonics, and other tonics.

2.1.1 *Qi* Tonics

Drugs that have the action of replenishing *Qi* and eliminating or relieving syndromes due to *Qi* deficiency are defined as *Qi* tonics.

All life activities, such as growth, development and metabolism, are dependent on *Qi*. The spleen, being the material basis of the acquired constitution, is the source of *Qi* and blood, while the lung is the dominator of the *Qi* of the whole body. As a result, whether the spleen and lung function normally or not is closely related to the formation and circulation of *Qi* in the body. Dysfunction of the spleen and lung due to one cause or another will result in the syndrome of *Qi* deficiency, the body becoming weak, manifested as such symptoms of asthenic type as fatigue, lassitude, listlessness, poor appetite, languor and spontaneous sweating. *Qi* tonics can remove or relieve the syndrome of *Qi* deficiency and promote recovery. Some *Qi* tonics, such as *Ren Shen* (Radix Ginseng), *Da Zao*(Fructus Jujubae), *Feng Huang Jiang*(royal jelly), *Ci Wu Jia* (Radix Acanthopanacis Senticosi) *Yi Tang* (Saccharum Granorum), *Mi* (Mel), etc., may play a role in maintaining good health and prolonging life when any of them is taken in small dose by the old or middle aged with delicate constitution in autumn and winter.

Appropriate tonics are chosen according to different symptoms of *Qi* deficiency, and the syndrome of *Qi* deficiency should be treated on the basis of overall analysis of its main symptoms and accompanying symptoms. Excessive intake of *Qi* tonics must be avoided, or *Qi* will be stagnated.

1. *Ren Shen* (Radix Ginseng)

Ren Shen is named according to its original growing area. That from Jilin province of China is called *Jilin Shen*; from Korea, *Gaoli Shen*, etc. The best is that produced at Fusong county in Jilin province of China. *Ren Shen* is also named according to the process. That dried in the sun is known as *Gan Shen;* that immersed in syrup before being dried, Tang Shen; that steamed and then dried, *Hong Shen. Ren Shen,* sweet and a little bitter in taste and slightly warm in nature, is a good tonic in winter. It has the potency to invigorate primordial *Qi,* reinforce the spleen, benefit the lung, promote the production of body fluid, quench thirst, tranquilize the mind and develop intelligence. People who are infirm with age or people who are overstrained may take small doses of *Ren Shen* when they have no appetite, feel tired and sleepy but have difficulty falling asleep. In so doing, their *Qi* will be invigorated; their minds, tranquilized; their appetite, improved; their bodily strength, restored. In clinical practice, *Ren Shen* is often administered to patients whose *Qi* is deficient due to prolonged disease, those in various kinds of shock or those whose *Qi* and *Yin* are both deficient. Pharmacological studies have proved that *Ren Shen*, with ginsenoside as its main active component, can improve the functions of various organs, especially those of the nervous, circulatory and endocrine systems, enhance the immune system and the adaptability of the body to the natural environment, thus strengthening the body and contributing to longevity.

Ren Shen is applicable to the syndrome due to *Qi* deficiency. Overintake of it in those with strong constitution is contraindicated. It is incompatible with *Li Lu* (Rhizoma et Radix Veratri), *Wu Ling Zhi* (Faeces Trogopterori), and *Zao Jia* (Spina Gleditsiae). It is decocted in water for oral use. The usual dosage is 5—10 g. While it is being taken, radish and tea are to be avoided.

2. *Xi Yang Shen* (**Radix Panacis Quinquefolii**)

Xi Yang Shen, bitter and slightly sweet in taste and cold in nature, has the potency to invigorate *Qi*, nourish *Yin*, clear away heat and promote the production of body fluid. With slower drug action, it is most suitable for children's high fever, excessive thirst, dehydration due to diarrhea, and fever of deficiency-type and irritating dry cough due to pulmonary tuberculosis. In addition, it may be used to treat disorders due to the damage of both *Qi* and *Yin*, regardless of the cause. If one infirm with age takes a suitable dose, he will have his body function and his resistance improved. Studies have shown that *Xi Yang Shen* contains such main active components as panasenoside and ginsenoside, which work together to exert the following pharmacological actions: reducing fever, promoting the formation of antibodies, improving the immune function and strengthening the body.

Xi Yang Shen is decocted in water for oral use. Its usual dosage is 3—6 g. Be sure not to administer it together with *Li Lu* (Rhizoma et Radix Veratri), nor to parch it on ironwork.

3. *Tai Zi Shen* (**Radix Pseudostellariae**)

Tai Zi Shen, sweet in taste and neutral in nature, has the potency, similar to that of *Ren Shen*, to invigorate *Qi*, promote the production of body fluid, reinforce the spleen and tonify the lung. Bing a mild and not-too-greasy tonic, it is often administered to those who have just recovered from illness but remain delibitated and those who are old or weak or feel listless or have no appetite. In addition, it is often used as a substitute for *Xi Yang Shen* to treat those who have less saliva and feel thirsty when their febrile diseases are in the late stage, their *Qi* and *Yin* have been both consumed, and the pathogenic factors of their diseases have not been cleared away completely.

Tai Zi Shen is known to contain the following main active elements: saponin, fructose and starch. It is decocted in water for oral use, with the usual dosage boing 10—30 g.

4. *Ci Wu Jia* (**Radix Acanthopanacis Senticosi**)

Ci Wu Jia, acrid and slightly bitter in taste and warm in nature, has the potency to replenish *Qi*, invigorate the spleen, tonify the kidney, tranquilize the mind, expel wind and remove dampness. Being an important tonic for strengthening the body resistance and / or restoring normal functioning of the body to consolidate the constitution, when it is used for inexplicable debility, senile disorders, menopausal syndrome, primary hypertension, hypotension, paralytic or excitatory impotence and toxicant poisoning, good curative effects will be achieved. Furthermore, it is suitable for athletes, divers and people working at high altitudes. *Ci Wu Jia* is known to contain a variety of eleutherosides and organic acids, and some tens of trace elements as its main active components, and to have the following pharmacological actions: double regulation of the central nervous system and blood pressure, relieving fatigue, increasing the efficiency of mental and manual labour, enhancing longevity, improving the immune function, building up the body's resistance to harmful factors, stimulating the sexual and adrenal glands, lowering blood sugar level, restraining the growth of tumors, resisting diuresis and inflammation, and playing an adaptagen−like part through adjusting the function of the whole body, all of which are almost the same as, or even more potent than, those of *Ren Shen*.

Ci Wu Jia is decocted in water for oral use or put in other dosage forms and then taken. The usual dosage is 9−30 g.

5. *Dang Shen* (**Radix Codonopsis**)

Shangdang district of Shanxi province of China is the habitat of *Dang Shen*. The wild type is named *Ye Tai Dang*; the cultivated, *Lu Dang Shen*. *Dang Shen*, sweet in taste and neutral in nature, has the potency to promote the production of body fluid, nourish the blood, invigorate the spleen and replenish *Qi*. With saponin, protein, vitamins, etc. as its main active components, it is a longevity−promise tonic without any toxicity and suitable for such disorders due to *Qi* deficiency as asthenia of any type and various kinds of anemia. The syndrome due to the general deficiency of *Qi* and exopathic effects or due to interior excess and the weakened body resistance may be treated with *Dang Shen* administered together with diaphoretic or purgative, for the coadministration will ensure the curative effect of strengthening the body resistance to eliminate the pathogenic factors.

Dang Shen has been known to act in stimulating the central nervous system, relieving fatigue, lowering blood pressure, raising blood sugar level, promoting the production of red blood cells and hemoglobin, improving the immune function and enhancing the resistance to disease.

Dang Shen is incompatible with Li Lu (Rhizoma et Radix Veratri) and while it being taken, radish and tea are avoided. It is decocted in water for oral use, the usual dosage being 10—30 g.

6. *Huang Qi* **(Radix Astragali)**

Huang Qi, sweet in taste and slightly warm in nature, has the potency to replenish *Qi*, keep *Yang—Qi* ascending, supplement the defensive—*Qi*, consolidate superficial resistance, promote pus discharge and tissue regeneration, cause diuresis and relieve edema. It is a commonly used *Qi* tonic suitable for such syndromes as *Qi* deficiency of the spleen and lung or sinking of the *Qi* in middle—*Jiao* and spontaneous sweating due to exterior deficiency, and such disorders as carbuncles difficult to degenerate or boils slow in healing and edema due to oliguria. Pharmacological researches have proved that *Huang Qi* mainly contains such active components as coumarin, flavone and saponin, and plays a role in lowering blood pressure, tonifying the heart, inhibiting bacteria, protecting the liver, relieving the pathogenic change of the kidney, stimulating the central nervous system, functioning as sexual hormone, and strengthening the body. So, it is advisable to prescribe *Huang Qi* in the treatment of gastroptosis, hysteroptosis, proctoptosis, long-standing diarrhea and dysentery, incontinence of urine and chronic nephritis.

Huang Qi is decocted in water for oral use. The usual dosage is 10–30 g.

7. Bai Zhu (Rhizoma Atractylodis Macrocephalae)

Bai Zhu, bitter and sweet in taste and warm in nature, is a choice tonic, which has the potency to replenish *Qi,* invigorate the spleen, eliminate dampness, promote diuresis, arrest profuse or spontaneous sweating and prevent miscarriage. It is often used to treat chronic dyspepsia, chronic nonspecific colitis, edema due to hypofunction of the spleen, nephrogenic edema, alimentary, edema, edema of pregnancy, miscarriage, spontaneous sweating due to general deficiency of *Qi,* and chronic rheumatic arthritis. *Bai Zhu* is known to contain atractylol, atractylone and vitamin A, and to exert such pharmacological actions as reducing blood sugar level, improving blood coagulation, stimulating peristalsis harmonizing the internal environment with the external, inhibiting cell mutation, and building up health.

Bai Zhu is decocted in water for oral use. The usual dosage is 5–15 g.

8. Gan Cao (Radix Glycyrrhizae)

Gan Cao, sweet in taste and neutral in nature, has the potency to invigorate the spleen, replenish *Qi,* moisturize the lung, arrest cough, relieve spasm and pain and moderate the properties of other drugs. Clinically, it finds wide usage in harmonizing the properties of the drugs in various kinds of prescriptions and in treating gastro-duodenal ulcer, infective hepatitis, Addison's disease, bronchial asthma, pulmonary tuberculosis, thrombocytopenic purpura, thrombotic phlebitis, etc. Research has proved that *Gan Cao* mainly contains glycyrrhizin, glycyrrhetinic acid, liquiritigenin, liquiritin, etc., being highly efficacious for peptic ulcer. Its effect is like that of adrenocortical hormone, acting in improving the function of the digestive system, detoxifying, lowering fever, relieving cough and asthma, resisting inflammation and allergy, reducing cholesterol, bettering the condition of atherosclerosis, and combatting bacteria in vitro.

Gan Cao is incompatible with *Hai Zao* (Sargassum), *Da Ji* (Radix Knoxiae), *Gan Sui* (Radix Kansui) and *Yuan Hua* (Flos Genkwa). It is decocted in water for oral use. The usual dosage is 3—15 g. Larger doses tend to cause edema and the elevation of blood pressure.

9. *Shan Yao* (Rhizoma Dioscoreae)

Shan Yao is sweet and mild-natured and has the potency to supplement *Qi*, nourish *Yin* and tonify the spleen, the lung and the kidney. That produced at Xinxiang county in Henan province of China is the finest in quality and called *Huai Shan Yao*. Its main active elements are known to be saponin, phlegm, choline, glucoprotein, amino acids, vitamin C and dopamine; and its pharmacological actions are inducing the formation of interferon, enhancing the immunologic function, promoting the flow of blood in the coronary arteries and micrangium, relieving cough and asthma, removing sputum, and strengthening the body. The disorders that *Shan Yao*, a mild tonic for nourishing the spleen and stomach, should be prescribed to treat are as follows: diarrhea due to the hypofunction of the spleen, cough due to the hypofunction of the lung, diabetes, spermatorrhea, frequent urination, chronic nephritis and emaciation due to consumption.

Shan Yao is decocted in water for oral use, The usual dosage is 10—30 g.

10. *Huang Jing* **(Rhizoma Polygonati)**

Huang Jing, sweet in taste and neutral in nature, is a longevity-enhancing tonic with the potency of invigorating the spleen, replenishing *Qi*, moisturizing the lung and nourishing *Yin*. It is often used to treat copos, chronic malnutrition, pulmonary tuberculosis, the syndrome of insufficiency of primordial energy due to the kidney deficiency and the syndrome of weakness of the spleen and stomach. Furthermore, it can be treated as a tonic for building up the health of those who are infirm with age. *Huang Jing* mainly contains nicotinic acid, quinone, phlegm, sugar, and alkaloid, and has many pharmacological actions, such as decreasing blood sugar level, lowering blood pressure, inhibiting bacteria, resisting tuberculosis, preventing atherosclerosis, increasing the number of T cells and enhancing their function, prolonging the life of somatic cells, strengthening the body to retard ageing and boosting longevity.

Huang Jing is decocted in water for oral use. The usual dosage of the dried is 10—20 g, the dosage of the fresh being 30—60 g.

11. *Da Zao* **(Fructus Jujubae)**

Da Zao, sweet in taste and warm in nature, is a longevity enhancing tonic with the potency to invigorate the spleen, replenish *Qi*, nourish the blood, calm the mind, and moderate the properties and tastes of other drugs. It is suited to the case with weakened spleen and stomach. Taking the decoction of *Da Zao*, a healthy person will have his acquired constitution strengthened.

Studies have proved that *Da Zao* mainly contains protein, sugar, organic acids and vitamins, and has such pharmacological actions as increasing the strength of the muscles, protecting the liver, improving the symptoms of allergic or primary thrombocytopenic purpura, tranquilizing the mind and promoting urination.

Da Zao is decocted in water for oral use. The usual dosage is 3—12 dates or 10—30 g.

12. Yi Tang (Saccharum Granorum)

Yi Tang, sweet in taste and warm in nature, is a fine tonic with the potency to invigorate the spleen, replenish Qi, relieve spasm and pain, moisturize the lung and arrest cough. Its indications are gastric ulcer, duodenal bulbar ulcer, chronic gastritis, cough due to the lung deficiency, chronic bronchitis and pulmonary tuberculosis. *Yi Tang* can detoxify and benefit a healthy person. Modern pharmacological research has also proved that *Yi Tang*, with maltobiose and a small proportion of protein as its main active composition, has the power to strengthen the stomach, moisten the lung and arrest cough.

Yi Tang is dissolved in a decoction and taken 2—3 times. The usual dosage is 30—60 g.

13. Feng Mi (Mel)

Feng Mi, sweet in taste and neutral in nature, has the potency to reinforce the function of the spleen and stomach, alleviate spasm, moisten the lung, arrest cough and relax the bowels. It is a tonic rich in medical and health-protection value, and suitable for ulcerous disorders, chronic hepatitis and for the syndromes such as infirmity with age, lack of body fluid during convalescence, constipation due to dry feces and prolonged cough due to consumption. Applied externally, it may be used to treat skin and external diseases and scalds, while taken orally, to detoxify the decoction which has been taken and contains the elements of *Chuan Wu* (Radix Aconiti), *Fu Zi* (Radix Aconiti) and the like with toxicity. It is often used to help process other Chinese drugs or as an ingredient of other preparations. Pharmacological studies have proved that *Feng Mi,* with sugar, inorganic salt, enzyme, protein, pigment and pollen grain as its main active principles, has the power to inhibit bacteria and strengthen the body. Those infirm with age will be considerably benefited by taking *Feng Mi* frequently.

Feng Mi is taken after being infused in boiled water, the usual dosage being 15—30 g.

2.1.2 Blood Tonics

Drugs that have the action of enriching the blood and improving or eliminating the syndrome due to blood deficiency are all named blood tonics.

Why one becomes senile is a very complicated question but blood deficiency is, undoubtedly, a major factor. The main symptoms and signs of blood deficiency are sallow complexion, pale lips and tongue, giddiness, numbness of the extremities and palpitation. Blood tonics play an active part in promoting the general circulation of blood and harmonizing the functions of internal organs, thus slowing down senility.

Most blood tonics are viscid and greasy. Overintake of any of them will affect appetite.

1. *E Jiao* (Colla Corii Asini)

E Jiao is named after Donge county and Donge town of Pingyin county, both of which are in Shandong province of

China. *E Jiao* originated in Shandong province. But more and more have appeared in many other provinces such as Zhejiang and Jiangsu. In terms of quality, *E Jiao* produced by the Refineries at Pingyin and Donge counties of Shandong province is the best and is also world-famous. Of late years, the *E Jiao* Refinery at Dingtao County of Shandong Province has also been awarded a prize for its fine product.

E Jiao, sweet in taste and neutral in nature, has the potency to tonify the blood, arrest bleeding, nourish *Yin* and moisten the lung. As an essential tonic used to treat the syndrome of blood deficiency, it has wide indications such as various kinds of anemia and hemorrhage and gynecopathy as well. For example, when it is administered to treat the disorder of postpartum blood deficiency, remarkable curative effects will be attained. Taken in suitable dosage it will greatly benefit those infirm with age, nourishing and strengthening them. Pharmacological experiments have proved that *E Jiao*, with amino acids, calcium and sulfur as its main active components, can raise the number of red blood cells and the amount of hemoglobin, prevent and treat progressive dystrophy, promote calcium equilibrium in the body, improve the immunological function, and elevate blood pressure.

E Jiao is dissolved in boiled water or yellow rice wine, or melted in a decoction before taking. The usual dosage is 5—10 g.

2. *Dang Gui* (**Radix Angelicae Sinensis**)

Dang Gui is mainly produced at Min county (Qinzhou) in the southeast of Gansu province of China. It is an effective tonic with sweet and pungent tastes and warm nature, which can nourish the blood, promote blood circulation, alleviate pain and moisten the intestines, the chief active components being sugar, amino acids, some tens of inorganic elements and vitamins, with the pharmacological effects of tonifying the heart, dilating coronary arteries, lowering blood pressure and cholesterol level, relieving atherosclerosis, ·resisting pernicious anemia, tranquilizing the mind, easing pain, combating bacteria, protecting the liver and dually—regulating the uterus, and with wide indications of hypertension, coronary heart disease, cerebral arteriosclerosis, various kinds of anemia, thromboangiitis obliterans, constipation, gynecopathy such as irregular menstruation and all the syndromes due to blood deficiency.

The middle part of *Dang Gui* is used to nourish the blood; the tips, to remove blood stasis; and the total, to enrich the blood and promote blood circulation. Processed with liquor, *Dang Gui* will have stronger effects in promoting flowing of the blood. It is decocted in water for oral use, the usual dosage being 5—15 g.

3. *Shu Di Huang* (Radix Rehmanniae Praeparata)

Shu Di Huang is a vegetable tonic for prolonging life, being sweet in taste, slightly warm in nature, and able to nourish blood, replenish *Yin* and invigorate marrow. It's main active components are β—sitosterol, mannitol, rehmannin, alkaloid, fatty acid, glucose, amino acid and vitamin A. The pharmacological actions are resisting inflammation, combating bacteria, protecting the liver, inducing diuresis, functioning as sexual hormone, improving the circulatory system, lowering blood sugar concentration, and preventing leukopenia due to chemotherapy. The usual indications are the syndrome due to blood deficiency marked by pale complexion, dizziness, palpitation, insomnia, irregular menstruation, metrorrhagia, metrostaxis, the syndrome due to *Yin* deficiency of the liver and kidney, diabetes, infective hepatitis, rheumatic arthritis and rheumatoid arthritis.

Shu Di Huang is decocted for oral dose, the usual dosage being 10—30 g.

4. *He Shou Wu* (**Radix Polygoni Multiflori**)

He Shou Wu bitter, sweet and astringent in taste, and slightly warm in nature, is a good tonic with the potency to nourish the blood, replenish the vital essence, prevent the attack of malaria, relax the bowels, strengthen the bones and tendons, keep hair black and promote longevity. It acts on the syndrome due to *Yin* and blood deficiency, early—greying of hair, prolonged malaria, pyogenic infections, skin and external diseases, constipation, hypertension, coronary heart disease and hypercholesterolemia. With chrysophanol, emodin, rhein, phscion and lecithin as its main active components, *He Shou Wu* exerts the following pharmacological actions: reducing blood—fat, alleviating atherosclerosis, functioning as adrenocortical hormone, strengthening the heart, relieving constipation and inhibiting bacteria.

He Shou Wu is decocted in water for oral use. The usual dosage is 10—30 g. *Zhi* (prepared) *He Shou Wu* is prescribed to tonify blood and vital essence.

5. *Bai Shao* (**Radix Paeoniae Alba**)

Bai Shao, bitter and sour in taste and slightly cold in nature, is a commonly used blood tonic with the power to nourish the blood, astringe *Yin,* calm the liver, arrest pain and suppress hyperactivity of the liver—*Yang,* and is often administered to treat spasm of the limbs and irregular menstruation due to blood deficiency, abdominal pain due to the stagnation of the liver—*Qi,* spontaneous perspiration and night sweating due to blood deficiency and hyperactivity of the liver, ulcerative diseases and gastroenteritis. Modern parmacological studies have proved that *Bai Shao* mainly contains paeoniflorin, paeonol, β–sitosterol, volatile oil, resin, fatty oil, sugar, starch, phlegm, protein and triterpenes, and plays a role in anti–inflammation, ulcer–prevention, anti–spasm, anti–bacteria, sedation, analgesia, dilation of coronary arteries, enhancement of body resistance, anti–perspiration and diuresis.

Bai Shao is decocted in water for oral use. The usual dosage is 10–30 g.

6. *Long Yan Rou* (Arillus Longan)

Long Yan (longan) is an appetizing fruit, the aril of which (*Long Yan Rou*) is a choice tonic for those infirm with age to build up their health and prolong their lives. *Long Yan Rou,* sweet in taste and warm in nature, has the power to tonify the heart and spleen and replenish *Qi* and blood. It is often prescribed to treat neurosism due to the deficiency of both the heart and spleen, the syndrome due to *Qi* and blood deficiency, chronic bleeding due to general deficiency, profuse menstruation due to blood deficiency, postpartum edema, pulmonary tuberculosis, hypertension and coronary heart disease. Studies have shown that the main active components of *Long Yan Rou* are saponin, fatty oil, fatty acid, sugar, vitamins and choline, and the pharmacological actions are anti–bacteria, anti–cancer, sedation, lowering of blood–fat, enrichment of coronary blood flow and enhancement of constitution.

Long Yan Rou is made into a decoction or liquid extract, soaked in liquor, or made into pills, all for oral use. The usual dosage is 10–15 g.

7. *Sang Shen* (Fructus Mori)

Sang Shen is an effective tonic for nourishing the blood and

Yin. It is able to replenish *Yin* and blood, promote the production of body fluid and moisturize the intestines. And it is suitable for the treatment of the syndrome due to blood and *Yin* deficiency, marked by dizziness, tinnitus, imsomnia, premature-greying of hair and constipation, as well as diabetes, hypertension, artheriosclerosis, various kinds of anemia and neurosism. Studies have proved that *Sang Shen* mainly contains rutin, anthocyanin, carotin, vitamin, nicotinic acid, sugar and fatty oil, and contributes to the increase of the number and the function of T cells, the improvement of the immunologic function, good health and long life.

Sang Shen is eaten raw, or decocted in water into a decoction or a liquid extract, or soaked in liquor, all for oral dosage. The usual dose is 10—15 g.

2.1.3 *Yang* Tonics

Yang Tonics refer to all the Chinese drugs which have the potency to support *Yang—Qi* of the body and relieve or eliminate the syndromes due to *Yang* deficiency.

Yang deficiency includes the deficiency of the heart—*Yang*, the spleen—*Yang* and the kidney—*Yang*. Of all the three kinds of *Yang—Qi*, the most important is the kidney—*Yang* which *Zang* and *Fu* organs depend on to be warmed and to give full play of their physiological functions. For this reason deficiency of kidney—*Yang* is closely related to various syndromes due to *Yang* deficiency. The syndrome of the kidney—*Yang* deficiency is mainly manifested as aversion to cold, cold limbs, weakness and soreness of the loins and knees, weak constitution, listlessness, asexuality, nocturia and watery leukorrhea. *Yang* tonics have the potency to alleviate or remove the syndrome due to *Yang* deficiency and retard senility because they have the power to tonify the kidney—*Yang*, nourish the marrow and strengthen the bones and tendons. Modern pharmacological researches have proved that *Yang* tonics can regulate adrenocortical function, adjust energy metabolism, improve gonadal function, promote growth and development and enhance the resistance of the body.

Healthy persons should be discreet in taking *Yang* tonics, for most of them are warm and dry in nature.

1. Lu Rong (Cornu Cervi Pantotrichum)

As one of the rare Chinese drugs, *Lu Rong* sweet and salty in taste and warm in nature, is an important and powerful tonic which has the potency to invigorate the kidney—*Yang*, replenish the vital essence and blood, and strengthen the bones and tendons. It is often administered to treat impotence, spermatorrhea, infertility, children's maldevelopment, severe anemia, rheumatic heart disease, neurosism and unhealing ulcer. *Lu Rong* is known to contain such main active components as pantocrine, calcium phosphate, calcium carbonate, colloids, protein, phosphorus, magnesium, cholesterol and vitamin A, and to have such pharmacological effects as functioning like a powerful androgenic hormone, promoting protein synthesis, raising the number of white blood cells, enhancing body functions, benefiting hematopoiesis, promoting growth and development, stimulating rapid healing of fractures and ulcers, strengthening the heart, inducing diuresis, increasing the womb's expansion and contraction strength and improving the energy metabolism of the patients with the syndrome of *Yang* deficiency.

Lu Rong is ground into powder and taken with boiled water. The usual dosage is 1–3g, divided into thirds and taken at intervals.

2. Ge Jie (Gecko)

Ge Jie is an animal *Yang* tonic produced mainly in Guangxi province of China. Salty in taste and neutral in nature and with the potency of invigorating the lung−*Qi*, tonifying the kidney−*Yang*, relieving asthma and cough and replenishing the vital essence and blood, it is often administered to treat prolonged cough with blood due to pulmonary tuberculosis, bronchial asthma, pulmonary emphysema, impotence, frequent urination and neurosism. Studies have shown that *Ge Jie*, with protein, fat and starch as its main active composition, can stimulate, directly or indirectly, the sex glands, enhance the body functions and promote growth and development.

Ge Jie is decocted in water, or ground into powder or soaked in liquor, all for oral use. If decocted in water, the usual dosage is 3−7g; if ground into powder, the powder is taken with boiled water three times a day, 1−2g each time; if soaked in liquor, 1−2 pairs of *Ge Jie* (geckoes) are soaked each time and the medicated liquor is drunk according to the doctor's orders.

3. *Ba Ji Tian* **(Radix Morindae Officinalis)**

Ba Ji Tian, acrid and sweet in taste and slightly warm in nature, is an essential drug for tonifying the kidney. Its medicinal power is reinforcing the kidney, supporting *Yang*, expelling wind, removing dampness and prolonging life; its indications are impotence, incontinence of urine, frequent urination, infertility, and irregular menstruation; its main active elements are morindin, vitamin C, sugar and resin; and its pharmacological effects are functioning like adrenocortical hormone, strengthening the heart, dilating the coronary arteries, lowering blood pressure, combating bacteria, removing phlegm, relieving cough and asthma, enhancing the immunologic function and preventing leukopenia due to chemotherapy.

   Ba Ji Tian is decocted in water for oral use. The usual dosage is 10—15g.

   4.   *Du Zhong* **(Cortex Eucommiae)**

   Du Zhong is not only a traditional *Yang* tonic but also a safe natural hypotensor. With sweet taste and warm nature and the action of tonifying the liver and kidney, strengthening the bones and tendons and preventing abortion, it is a highly effective drug for strengthening the body and prolonging life, and suitable for the treatment of the syndrome due to the deficiency of the liver and kidney, weakness and soreness of the loins and knees, hypertension, sequel of poliomyelitis, threatened abortion and habitual abortion. *Du Zhong* contains mainly gutta-percha, resin, glucoprotein, organic acids and vitamin C, and plays a part in lowering blood pressure, inducing diuresis, reducing the amount of cholesterol absorbed, relaxing the womb and tranquilizing the mind through restraining the central nervous system.

   Du Zhong is decocted in water for oral use. Stir-fried *Du Zhong* is more efficacious.

   5.   *Dong Chong Xia Cao* **(Cordyceps)**

   Dong Chong Xia Cao is a famous and precious tonic. With sweet taste and warm nature, and the potency to nourish the kidney, tonify the lung, arrest bleeding, resolve phlegm, restore *Qi*, consolidate constitution and enhance longevity, it is suited to those who are weak and susceptible to cold and those who are infirm with age and need to consolidate their constitutions through strengthening their body resistance and/or restoring normal functioning of their bodies, as well as to the treatment of copos, anemia, impotence, spermatorrhea, weakness and soreness of the loins and knees, asthma and cough with blood due to pulmonary tuberculosis. It is known that *Dong Chong Xia Cao* contains mainly the following active elements: cordycepic acid, cordycepin, protein, fat, vitamin B_{12}, amino acids, cordypolysaccharide, uracil and adenosine, and has the following pharmacological effects: tranquilizing the mind, relieving spasm, resisting inflammation, combating bacteria, removing phlegm, preventing cough, alleviating asthma, resisting the development of neoplasm, lowering blood pressure, dilating the coronary arteries, reducing blood-fat and enhancing hypoxia tolerance under ordinary pressure.

The usual dose of *Dong Chong Xia Cao* is 5−10g. It is boiled in water and taken orally as a decoction or made into pill or powder form to be taken with boiled water, or stewed and eaten with chicken or duck or fish.

6. · *Zi He Che* (Placenta Hominis)

A *Zi He Che* refers to a woman's placenta, which is an excellent tonic for warming the kidney and strengthening *Yang*. Sweet and salty in taste and warm in property, it acts in replenishing vital essence, nourishing blood and invigorating *Qi*. And it is used to build up the constitutions of those infirm with age, prevent hepatitis and influenza, and treat infertility, impotence and spermatorrhea due to the deficiency of kidney−*Qi*, vital essence and blood, as well as emaciation, lassitude, sallow complexion and inability to lactate after giving birth due to deficiency of both *Qi* and blood, asthma due to deficiency of both the lung and kidney. *Zi He Che* has been found to contain amino acids, immune factors and hormones, and to play a part in promoting the development of the sex glands and reproductive organs, preventing leukopenia due to chemotherapy, activating the immune system, stimulating the body to function fully and bringing about an advance in the growth and development of the body.

* *Zi He Che* is ground into powder and put into capsules to be taken with boiled water. The usual dose is 1.5–3g, taken 2–3 times daily. Alternatively, a whole or half *Zi He Che* may be boiled in water and eaten together with the broth.

7. *Tu Si Zi*(**Semen Cuscutae**)

Tu Si Zi,acrid and sweet in taste and neutral in nature, can invigorate *Yang*, replenish *Yin*, control spontaneous emission, arrest diuresis, relieve diarrhea and improve acuity of sight. And it is a tonic commonly used for tonifying the kidney–*Yang* and enhancing longevity, and is suitable for the treatment of weakness and soreness of the loins and knees due to kidney deficiency, enuresis, frequent urination, spermatorrhea, habitual abortion, hypertension, hypoposia and diabetes. Pharmacological research has proved that *Tu Si Zi*, of which the main active elements are resinous glucoside, β–sitosterol, sugar, amylase and vitamin A, has the power to lower blood pressure, strengthen the heart, inhibit bacteria, stimulate the uterus, regulate the immune function, enhance the function of the whole body and adjust and raise the metabolic function of the body.

Tu Si Zi is decocted in water for oral dosage. The usual dosage is 10–15 g.

8. *Hu Tao Ren* (**Semen Juglandis**)

Hu Tao Ren is not only a popular food with higher nutritive value but also a tonic suitable for the aged and the debilitated. Sweet in taste and warm in property, it can tonify the kidney, warm the lung, moisturize the intestines and consolidate the constitution. It is used to treat chronic asthmatic bronchitis, lumbago due to kidney deficiency, weak legs, habitual constipation and urinary calculus. *Hu Tao Ren* is known to contain fatty oil, protein, carbohydrate, calcium, phosphorus, iron, carotin and ovoflavin, and to act strongly in lowering blood pressure and controlling inflammation.

Hu Tao Ren is decocted in water for oral use or eaten raw. The usual dosage is 10—30 g.

9. *Yang Qi Shi* (Actinolitum)

With magnesium silicate and calcium silicate as its main active principles and with salty taste and slightly—warm nature, *Yang Qi Shi* can warm the kidney and invigorate *Yang*. It is a mineral tonic applicable to the treatment of such disorders as cold penis and impotence due to the deficiency of the kidney—*Yang*, cold uterus, women's pruritus genitalium of dampness—type and cold loins and knees as well.

Yang Qi Shi is processed into pills or powder and taken orally with boiled water. The usual dosage is 3—6 g. Prolonged administration of it is avoided.

10. *Bu Gu Zhi* (Fructus Psoraleae)

Bu Gu Zhi, bitter and acrid in taste and greatly warm in nature, can invigorate the kidney—*Yang*, control spontaneous emission, arrest enuresis, warm the spleen and treat diarrhea. It is a commonly used kidney—*Yang* tonic suitable for the treatment of impotence, spermatorrhea, enuresis, frequent urination, cold—pain of the loins and knees, diarrhea due to *Yang* deficiency, endometrorrhagia, psoriasis and vitiligo. *Bu Gu Zhi* is known to contain saponin, resin, organic acids, psoralen, psoralidine and ispsoralene, and to have such pharmacological actions as functioning like female sex hormone, dilating the coronary arteries, strengthening the heart, tranquilizing the mind, relieving spasms, stimulating the smooth muscles, combating bacteria, promoting the formation of pigment cells of the skin and enhancing the immunologic function of the body.

Bu Gu Zhi is decocted in water for oral dosage, but contraindicated in pregnant women. The usual dosage is 5—10 g.

11. *Yin Yang Huo* (Herba Epimedii)

Yin Yang Huo, acrid and sweet in taste and warm in nature, can invigorate the kidney—*Yang*, expel wind and remove dampness. It is a highly potent tonic for health care and suited to the treatment of impotence, spermatorrhea, frequent urination, weakness and soreness of the loins and knees, rheumalalgia, numbness of the limbs, poliomyelitis, women's climacteric hypertension, coronary heart disease and chronic bronchitis. Pharmacological studies have shown that *Yin Yang Huo*, with icariine, glucoside of flavone, sterol volatile oil and vitamin E as its main active principles, has male sex hormone—like action, and plays a part in lowering blood pressure, strengthening the heart, dilating the coronary arteries, inhibiting bacteria, combating viruses, reducing blood sugar level, regulating the immunologic function and enhancing the adrenocortical function.

Yin Yang Huo is decocted in water, taken as a liquid extract, soaked in liquor or put into a pill or powder form, taken orally. The usual dosage is 10—15 g.

2.1.4 *Yin* Tonics

Yin tonics refer to all the Chinese drugs which have the action of nourishing *Yin*, promoting the production of body fluid, moisturizing dryness, and improving or eliminating the syndromes due to *Yin* deficiency. *Yin* deficiency includes the deficiency of the lung—*Yin*, the stomach—*Yin* the liver—*Yin* and the kidney—*Yin*. The syndrome of *Yin* deficiency is often seen in those infirm with age, in the advanced stage of febrile disease and in the course of a number of chronic diseases. In general, it is manifested as thirst with dry mouth, dry cough with little sputum, afternoon fever, night sweating, irritability, insomnia, spermatorrhea, dizziness and dry sensation of the eyes. *Yin* tonics have the role of promoting the production of body fluid, moisturizing dryness and strengthening the body by way of improving sucroclastic metabolism to return hyperfunctional energy metabolism to normal, enhancing immunologic function and regulating the body fluid metabolism.

Yin tonics are contraindicated in the cases with syndromes of weakness of the spleen and stomach or internal stagnation of phlegm—dampness or abdominal distension and loose stools, because most of them are sweet in taste and cold, viscid and greasy in nature.

1. *Sha Shen* (**Radix Adenophorae or Radix Glehnia**)

Sha Shen refers to *Nan Sha Shen* (Radix Adenophorae) and *Bei Sha Shen* (Radix Glehnia), the latter being more efficacious than the former. Both of them are sweet in taste and slightly cold in nature, and can clear away the lung—heat, nourish *Yin*, replenish the stomach and promote the production of body fluid. They are more nutritious tonics used to treat dry cough with little sputum caused by the lung—*Yin* deficiency due to the lung—heat, cough with blood due to pulmonary tuberculosis, dry mouth and tongue, and poor appetite due to the overconsumption of body fluid caused by febrile diseases. Pharmacological studies have shown that *Sha Shen* contains mainly saponin, volatile oils, triterpenoid acid, stigmasterol, β-sitosterol and alkaloids, and has the potency to reduce fever, remove phlegm and ease pain.

Sha Shen is decocted in water for oral use. The usual dosage, if dried, is 10—15 g; and if fresh, 15—30 g. It is incompatible with *Li Lu* (Rhizoma et Radix Veratri)

2. *Tian Dong* (**Radix Asparagi**)

Tian Dong is a tonic for strengthening the bones, building up health, delaying senility and prolonging life. Sweet and bitter in taste and greatly cold in nature, it can remove heat from the lung, replenish *Yin* and moisten dryness. It is administered to treat the following disorders: consumption of *Yin* due to febrile diseases, dry cough due to lung deficiency, senile chronic bronchitis, pulmonary tuberculosis, whooping cough, mammary tumor, constipation and spermatorrhea. *Tian Dong* contains mainly 19 kinds of amino acids such as glutamic acid and asparagine, glucose and steroid saponin, and has many pharmacological actions, such as relieving cough, removing phlegm, combating bacteria, restraining the growth to tumors, improving the function of the heart and lung, enhancing the ability of the body to adapt to the environment and decreasing the mutation of body cells.

Tian Dong is decocted in water for oral use, but contraindicated in the cases with loose stools. The usual dosage is 10—15 g.

3. *Shi Hu* (**Herba Dendrobii**)

Shi Hu, sweet in taste and slightly cold in property, can nourish the stomach, promote the production of body fluid, replenish

Yin and remove heat. Being a commonly used tonic for nourishing the stomach—*Yin*, it is administered to treat such disorders as the damage of body fluid due to febrile disease, deficiency of the stomach—*Yin*, consumption of body fluid due to the deficiency of *Yin*, persistent fever of *Yin* deficiency—type, chronic gastritis and diabetes. *Shi Hu* mainly contains dendrobine, phlegm and nobilonine, and acts in reducing fever, easing pain, promoting digestion, strengthening the heart, lowering blood pressure, preventing leukopenia due to chemotherapy, enhancing the immunologic function of the body, improving the metabolism within the body and regulating the balance of body fluid.

Shi Hu is decocted in water for oral use. If administered as an ingredient of a prescription, it must be the first to be decocted. The usual dose of the dried is 6—15 g, and of the fresh, 15—30 g.

4. *Mai Dong* (**Radix Ophiopogonis**)

Mai Dong, sweet and slightly bitter in taste and a little cold in nature, can remove dryness from the lung, nourish *Yin*, reinforce the stomach, promote the production of body fluid, clear away heat from the heart and ease mental anxiety. Being a tonic for preventing senility and promising longevity, it is suitable for such disorders as dry cough due to lung—dryness, deficiency of stomach—*Yin*, irritability, insomnia, constipation due to intestinal dryness, expectoration of blood, apostaxis, chronic pharyngitis and coronary heart disease. *Mai Dong* has been found to contain steroid saponins, β—sitosterol, amino acid, glucose and vitamin A—like substance, and to act in improving the function of islet cells and cardiovascular system, enhancing the ability of the body to adapt to the environment, restraining the mutation of body cells, increasing remarkably the capacity of the hypoxiatolerance under ordinary or decompressed pressure and combating bacteria.

Mai Dong is decocted in water for oral use. The usual dosage is 10—15 g.

5. Yu Zhu (Rhizoma Polygonati Odorati)

Yu Zhu, sweet in taste and neutral in nature, can replenish *Yin,* remove heat from the lung, promote the production of body fluid and nourish the stomach. It is weak in potency and non−greasy in nature, and used as a general tonic for those infirm with age. It is suitable for the treatment of *Yin* damage of the spleen and stomach, heart failure, coronary heart disease, pulmonary tuberculosis and diabetes. *Yu Zhu* contains mainly convallamarin, convallarin, kaempferitrin, quercitrin, vitamin A and nicotinic acid, all of which act as the active elements. Its tonic action is based on its broad pharmacological effects, such as strengthening the heart, dilating the coronary arteries, reducing blood sugar concentration, combating bacteria, working like adrenocortical hormone, enhancing the immunologic function of the body, bettering the function of the heart and lung and the ability of the body to adapt to the environment, improving the function of islet cells and vasomotor centers.

Yu Zhu is decocted in water for oral use. The usual dosage is 10−15 g.

6. Bai He (Bulbus Lilii)

Bai He, sweet in taste and slightly cold in nature, can moisten the lung to arrest cough, and clear away heart−fire to tranquilize the mind. As a commonly used *Yin* tonic having the action of preventing senility and prolonging life, it is applicable to the treatment of cough due to lung−heat, fidgeting of deficiency—type, insomnia or heavy dreaming, chronic nephritis, pulmonary tuberculosis, hypertension, bronchial asthma and chronic bronchitis. Pharmacological studies have proved that *Bai He* mainly contains colchicine, starch, protein, fat, sugar, calcium, phosphorus and iron, and plays a part in removing phlegm, arresting cough, relieving asthma, enhancing or improving the immunologic function and the function of the heart and lung, and preventing leukopenia due to chemotherapy.

Bai He is decocted in water for oral use, or taken in gruel or as a vegetable dish. The usual dosage of the dried is 10—30 g, and that of the fresh, 30—50 g.

7. *Gou Qi Zi* (Fructus Lycii)

Gou Qi Zi, sweet in taste and neutral in nature, can nourish the liver and kidney, improve acuity of sight and moisten the lung. As a good tonic for replenishing *Yin* and the kidney, preventing diseases and prolonging life, it is suitable for the treatment of *Yin* deficiency of the liver and kidney, cough due to *Yin* deficiency, chronic nephritis, chronic hepatitis, cirrhosis, diabetes and tumors. The main active principles of *Gou Qi Zi* are betaine, carotene, zeaxanthin, nicotinic acid and vitamins, and the pharmacological actions are as follows: lowering blood sugar level and blood—fat level and blood pressure, enhancing the immunologic function, protecting the liver and improving remarkably leukopenia due to chemotherapy.

Gou Qi Zi is decocted in water for oral use. The usual dosage is 5—10 g.

8. *Nü Zhen Zi* (Fructus Ligustri Lucidi)

Nü Zhen Zi, sweet and bitter in taste and cool in nature, can tonify and nourish the liver and kidney, remove heat and improve acuity of sight. It is a commonly used tonic having the action of preventing senility, retarding ageing and enhancing longevity. This tonic mainly contains triterpenoid oleanolic acid, mannitol, glucose, oleic acid, linoleic acid, ligustrin and fatty acids, all of which work together to play an active part in strengthening the heart, inducing diuresis, protecting the liver, inhibiting bacteria, increasing the number of white blood cells, reducing blood-fat and enhancing the immunologic function of the body. Thus, it is used to treat the following disorders: *Yin* deficiency of the liver and kidney, dizziness, weakness and soreness of the loins and knees, early-greying of hair, blurred vision, chronic nephritis, chronic hepatitis, coronary heart disease, central choroido-retinitis and leukopenia.

Nü Zhen Zi is decocted in water for oral use. The usual dosage is 10-15 g.

9. *Hei Zhi Ma* (Semen Sesami Nigrum)

Hei Zhi Ma, sweet in taste and neutral in nature, can replenish vital essence and blood, moisten dryness and relieve constipation. To both the old and the young, it is not only a good health care tonic for eliminating diseases and building up health but also a tasty food. Pharmacological studies have shown that *Hei Zhi Ma* contains mainly protein, fatty oil, sugar, fibrin, calcium, phosphorus, iron, vitamin B_{12} and vitamin E, sesamin and sesamol, all of which work together in preventing senility, lowering blood pressure and blood sugar concentration and blood-fat level, and relaxing the bowels. Naturally, it is suitable for the treatment of hypertension, coronary heart disease, arteriosclerosis, neurosis, constipation due to intestinal dryness, *Yin* deficiency of the liver and kidney, dizziness, early-greying of hair, anemia and agalactosia.

Hei Zhi Ma is decocted in water for oral dose, or stir-baked and taken as a cooked food. The usual dosage is 10-30 g.

10. *Bie* (Trionycis)

Bie refers to fresh-water turtle. the flesh of it is sweet in taste and neutral in nature; the shell, salty and cold. *Bie,* of which both the blood and flesh are potent, is an effective tonic for replenishing vital essence and nourishing the blood. For nourishing action, however, the flesh is best. Modern research has shown that *Bie* contains mainly protein, fat carbohydrate, calcium, phosphorus, iron, vitamin, animal gum, keratin and iodine, and can play an important role in nourishing the body and building up health. Thus it can nourish *Yin,* suppress hyperactive *Yang,* remove heat from the blood and resolve mass, and can be used to treat the following disorders: *Yin* deficiency of the liver and kidney, copos, hectic fever, night sweating, wind stirring due to *Yin* deficiency and hypertension. Those infirm with age, and even healthy persons, will benefit from eating *Bie.*

One *Bie* is stewed and eaten each time. Alternatively, 10-13g of its shell is decocted in water for oral use.

11. *Yin Er* (Tremella)

Yin Er, sweet, tasteless and mild-natured, can nourish *Yin,* moisten the lung and replenish *Qi* and blood. As a rare tonic, it may be used to treat hemoptysis due to pulmonary tuberculosis, hypertension, arteriosclerosis, leukopenia, cancer and general debility due to chronic diseases. This tonic is suitable for those infirm with age and also benefits the healthy. Studies have shown that the main active elements of *Yin Er* are protein, gummy substance, enzyme, polysaccharide, inorganic salts and vitamin B, and the tonic pharmacological effects of it are as follows: enhancing the immunologic function, activating the hematopoietic function, promoting the synthesis of protein and nucleic acid, resisting tumors and improving pathogenic changes of the respiratory system.

Yin Er is stewed, or cooked into a thick soup with other food and eaten. The usual dosage is 3—10 g.

2.1.5 Other Chinese Medicines for Health Care

These Chinese medicines which are not classified as tonics in the works —*Zhong Yao Xue* (The Chinese Materia Medica) but may be used, according to their tonifying action, to treat debility, prevent diseases and prolong life are included in the medicines of this type.

With the development of modern pharmacological research, the health care functions of many Chinese medicines have been progressively discovered. These medicines, with strong and newly—discovered health care functions, are perfectly edible and have few side or toxic effects.

1. *Suan Zao Ren* **(Semen Ziziphi Spinosae)**

Suan Zao Ren, sweet and mild—natured, can nourish the heart, ease the mind and arrest sweating.

Traditionally, it has been only regarded as a sedative. But modern pharmacological studies have shown that *Suan Zao Ren* can act not only in tranquilizing the mind, lulling one to sleep, easing pain, relieving spasm, preventing convulsion, but also in reducing fever, lowering blood pressure, improving the function of the cardiovascular and immune systems, stimulating the uterus, arresting shock, alleviating local edema and invigorating the body.

As a result, it is often used as a tonic for those infirm with age. The main active elements of *Suan Zao Ren* are jujubogenin, sterol, triterpenoid, high proportion of vegetable oil, vitamin C and protein.

Suan Zao Ren is decocted in water for oral dose, or eaten raw, or taken in other dosage forms or nutriments such as wine or non-alcoholic beverage for health care. The usual dosage is 6—15 g.

2. *Shan Zha* (Fructus Crataegi)

Shan Zha, sour and sweet in taste and slightly warm in nature, can remove food stagnation to promote digestion and eliminate blood stasis to activate blood flow. It is not only a nutritious and tasty fruit but also a good tonic for the patients with hypertension or coronary heart disease and for those infirm with age.

Shan Zha contains mainly triterpenes, flavonoid, β-sitosterol, stearic acid, vitamin C and carotene. It has the potency to lower blood-fat level, increase blood flow in the coronary arteries and prevent arrhythmia, in addition to its long-term effects of lowering blood pressure, its long-term and potent action of strengthening the heart and its more powerful action of inhibiting bacteria and promoting digestion.

Shan Zha is decocted in water for oral use, or eaten raw, or taken in the form of flake, cake, jam, juice, extract or wine. The usual dosage of the dried is 6—15 g, and the fresh, 30—50 g.

3. *Lian Zi* (Semen Nelumbinis)

Lian Zi, sweet and puckery in taste and neutral in nature, can invigorate the spleen to treat diarrhea, tonify the kidney to arrest spontaneous emission and nourish the heart to calm the mind. It is traditionally used as an astringent to treat the following disorders: dreamfulness, spontaneous emission, spermatorrhea, frequent urination due to kidney deficiency, prolonged diarrhea due to spleen deficiency, palpitation, restlessness of deficiency-type and insomnia. Either people old and infirm or people in good condition will have their health enhanced and their life prolonged if they often take *Lian Zi*. It is known that the main active elements *Lian Zi* contains are starch, melitose, protein, fat, carbohydrate, calcium, phosphorus and iron, and the pharmacological actions it exerts are treating tumor, lowering blood pressure, etc.

Lian Zi is decocted in water for oral use, or eaten in a gruel or thick soup, or taken in other dosage forms. The usual dosage is 6—15 g.

4. *Ling Zhi* **(Ganoderma Lucidum seu Japonicum)**

Tasteless and slightly bitter and warm-natured, *Ling Zhi* can tranquilize the mind and invigorate the spleen and stomach. As a rare drug having the power to consolidate the constitution through strengthening the body resistance and/or restoring normal functioning of the body and as a good tonic for people old and infirm, it is suitable for such disorders as angina pectoris due to coronary heart disease, infectious hepatitis, leukopenia, neurosism and anemia. It is known that *Ling Zhi* contains mainly alkaloids, peptides, sugar, sterol, triterpenes, volatile oil, resin, 13 kinds of inorganic elements, and 15 kinds of amino acids such as lysine and leucine, all of which work together to exert the following pharmacological actions: strengthening the heart, dilating coronary arteries, preventing atherogenesis, relieving cough, removing phlegm, alleviating asthma, inhibiting bacteria, enhancing the immunologic function, protecting the liver, tranquilizing, easing pain, resisting cancer and activating hematopoietic system.

1.5–3 g of *Ling Zhi* is decocted in water for oral use, or 0.9–1.5 g of it is ground into powder and swallowed with boiled water. It may also be soaked in, and taken with, liquor. It may also be taken in others dosage forms.

5. *Fu Ling* (Poria)

Fu Ling, sweet and tasteless and mild–natured, can promote water metabolism, remove dampness, strengthen the spleen and stomach and ease mental stress. In the case of the main active elements, *Fu Ling* contains pachymic acid, β–pachman, choline, protein, fat, ergosterin, kalium, natrium and lecithin. As one of the commonly used Chinese medicinal herbs and a good, nutritious tonic for health care and boosting longevity, it is suitable for the treatment of edema, difficult urination, deficiency of the spleen and stomach, chronic diarrhea, palpitation, insomnia, and Meniere's disease. Studies have indicated that *Fu Ling* has the following pharmacological actions: inducing diuresis, tranquilizing, inhibiting bacteria, resisting tumor, strengthening the heart, reducing blood sugar level, improving the function of the digestive system and enhancing the immunological function.

Fu Ling is decocted in water for oral use, or prepared into pills or powder, or taken in gruel or cake. The usual dosage is 10–15 g.

6. *Yi Yi Ren* (Semen Coicis)

Sweet, tasteless and slightly cold–natured, *Yi Yi Ren* can promote water metabolism, remove dampness, strengthen the spleen, relieve the stagnation–syndrome of *Qi* and blood, clear away heat and discharge pus. It is administered in the treatment of urinary difficulty, edema, diarrhea due to spleen deficiency, rheumatic arthritis, pulmonary abscess, pulmonary tuberculosis and cancer. Furthermore, *Yi Yi Ren* may be used as a tonic for health care, suitable for people old and infirm especially with stiff limbs. Often taking this medicine will promote body vigour. Modern research has shown that the main active components *Yi Yi Ren* contains are protein, fat, carbohydrate, vitamin B_1, coixol and coixenolide, all of which work together to act in reducing fever, easing pain, strengthening the heart, resisting tumor and improving the function of the respiratory system.

Yi Yi Ren is decocted in water for oral dose, or eaten in a gruel. The usual dosage is 10—30 g.

7. *Qian Shi* **(Semen Euryales)**

sweet and puckery and mild—natured, *Qian Shi* can replenish the kidney, check spontaneous emission, invigorate the spleen, remove dampness and treat diarrhea. Its main active elements are protein, starch, sugar, fat, vitamin B_1, B_{12} and C, nicotinic acid, carotene, calcium, phosphorus and iron, thus containing the five main types of nutrients beneficial to health. Being an excellent tonic for curing diseases and prolonging life, *Qian Shi* is easy to digest and suitable for the treatment of prolonged diarrhea due to spleen deficiency, spontaneous emission due to kidney deficiency, incontinence of urine and leukorrhagia.

Qian Shi is decocted in water for oral dose, or eaten in a gruel. The usual dosage is 10—15 g.

8. *Xiang Gu* **(Lentinus Edodes)**

By *Xiang Gu* here is meant the edible variety used as a herbal medicine. Sweet and mild—natured, it has the potency to restore *Qi*, strengthen the stomach and promote the eruption of rash, and is used to treat poor appetite, vomitting, diarrhea, lassitude, dribbling urination, turbid urine, pox or measles, cancer, hyperlipemia, rickets and anemia. Pharmacological studies have shown that the main active elements *Xiang Gu* contains are protein, fat, carbohydrate, vitamin, calcium, phosphorus, iron and nicotinic acid, all of which work together to play a role in resisting tumor, reducing blood-fat, enhancing the immunologic function and preventing rickets. Recently, people have become more aware of the nutritive and health care value of *Xiang Gu* and have used it as an effective tonic for curing disease and prolonging life.

Xiang Gu is decocted in water for oral use, or stewed with pork, chicken or fish. The usual dosage is 6—9 g.

9. *Mu Er* (Auricularia)

Mu Er, sweet in taste and neutral in nature, has the potency to invigorate *Qi,* remove the pathogenic heat from the blood and arrest bleeding, and it is used to treat hypertension, coronary heart disease and various kinds of hemorrhage. Studies have shown that *Mu Er,* with protein, sugar, lipid, sterol, inorganic salt and vitamin as its main active composition, exerts such pharmacological functions as hemostasis, prevention and treatment of atherosclerosis, activation of the body and mind, and can retard the onset of senility. It is not only a suitable food for the dinner-table but is also a good tonic for preventing diseases, protecting health and enhancing longevity.

Mu Er is cooked and eaten as a dish or in a thick soup. The usual dosage is 15—30 g.

10. *Ju Hua* (Flos Chrysanthemi)

Sweet, better and cool-natured, *Ju Hua* has the potency to

expel wind, clear away heat, calm the liver, improve acuity of sight, subdue inflammation and expel toxic substances, and it has been used as an exterior−syndrome−relieving drug, pungent in flavor and cool in property, to treat wind−heat syndrome due to exopathogen, furuncle, carbuncle and swelling. Recently, it has been used to treat coronary heart disease and hypertension. Research has shown that the main active principles *Ju Hua* contains are volatile oil, chrysanthmin, choline, amino acid, vitamins, adenine and trace elements, all of which ensure the following pharmacological actions: improving the function of the cardiovascular system, preventing thrombosis, preventing and treating cardiovascular diseases, reducing fever, tranquilizing the mind, inhibiting bacteria, combating virus, retarding the onset of senility and enhancing longevity.

Ju Hua is decocted in water or soaked in liquor and taken orally. Alternatively, it may be infused in boiling water and taken as tea. The usual dosage is 6−9 g.

11. *Dan Shen* **(Radix Salviae Miltiorrhizae)**

Bitter and slightly cold, *Dan Shen* has the potency to cool and nourish the blood, remove blood stasis, promote the circulation of blood, heal skin and external disorders and tranquilize the mind, and is used as a blood−flow−promoting drug to treat abdominal pain due to blood stasis, abdominal mass, irregular menstruation, amenorrhea due to blood stagnation, skin and external disorders and the syndrome due to the invasion of the blood system by pathogenic heat. Recently, it has been used effectively in the treatment of coronary heart disease, thromboangiitis obliterans, chronic hepatitis, hepatosplenomegaly, infantile pneumonia of persistent type.

Pharmacological studies have shown that the main active components *Dan Shen* contains are tanshinone, cryptotanshinone, miltirone, β-sitosterol, vitamin E, etc., all of which act together in delaying senility, enhancing the immunologic function, dilating coronary arteries, strengthening the heart, lowering blood pressure, regulating the function of blood platelets, resisting tumor, combating bacteria and tranquilizing the mind. Thus it is prescribed as a tonic for building up health, retarding senility and prolonging life.

Dan Shen is decocted in water for oral dose, or taken in other dosage forms. The usual dosage is 5—15 g.

12. San Qi (**Radix Notoginseng**)

Sweet and slightly bitter in taste and warm in nature, *San Qi* has the power to arrest bleeding, promote blood flow, remove blood, stasis, relieve pain and strengthen the body. It is used as a traditional blood—arresting drug to treat various kinds of hemorrhage, traumatic injury, pain due to blood stasis and swelling. Recently, it has been used effectively in the treatment of anemia, debility, coronary heart disease, hyperlipemia and hyperkinetic syndrome. Modern research has found that *San Qi* contains the following main active elements similar to those of *Ren Shen* (Radix Ginseng): saponin, styptic active mass, flavenoids, alkaloids, protein, sugar, fatty oil, volatile oil, resin, nucleoside and carotene, and it has almost the same pharmacological actions as *Ren Shen,* such as, nourishing the blood, improving the function of the cardiovascular system, regulating the immunologic function, bidirectional adjustment of blood sugar, arresting bleeding, resisting imflammation, tranquilizing the mind and relieving pain. In short, *San Qi* is a good tonic for nourishment and health care.

Dried or prepared *San Qi* is ground into powder to be taken with boiled water, 1—1.5 g of the powder made of the dried or 3—5 g of the prepared each time. Alternatively, it may be soaked in liquor or infused in boiling water and taken as tea. The usual dosage is 3—10 g.

13.　*Tian Ma* (**Rhizoma Gastrodiae**)

Sweet and mild—natured, *Tian Ma* has the potency to calm internal wind, relieve convulsions, subdue the exuberant *Yang* of the liver and tranquilize the mind. It has been traditionally used as a liver—wind—calming drug to treat dizziness, numbness of the limbs and hemiplegia. The main active elements *Tian Ma* contains are as follows: gastrodine, vanillyl alcohol, succinic acid, β—sitosterol, vitamin A—like substance, glucose, alkaloids, etc. Pharmacological studies have indicated that *Tian Ma* has the power to enhance longevity because in addition to its actions of tranquilizing the mind, alleviating pain and relieving convulsions, it can act in enhancing the immunologic function of the body, improving the nutritive blood flow in the cardiac muscles and increasing the hypoxia tolerance of experimental animals.

Tian Ma is decocted in water for oral use or ground into powder and swallowed in amounts of 1—1.5 g with boiled water. Alternatively, it may be soaked in liquor or put into other dosage forms. The usual dosage of *Tian Ma* is 3—10 g.

14.　*Hua Fen* (**Pollen**)

The reproductive cells in the stamens of flowers are collected and pollinated to the pistils by bees. The reproductive cells of the pistils are inseminated and a kind of pollen of nectar source is developed. By *Hua Fen* (pollen) here is meant the pollen of nectar source. Pollen of nectar source is an ideal tonic for people old and infirm or even people in good condition, and used to prevent diseases, build up health, postpone senility and promise longevity. It is especially fit for athletes, for improving a woman's looks and for the treatment of neurosism, anemia, prostatic hyperplasia, diabetes, angiocardiopathy, ulcerous disorders and menopausal syndrome. Research has proved that pollen of nectar source contains such main active components as 20 kinds of amino acids, 14 kinds of vitamins, 24 kinds of inorganic elements, 18 kinds of natural organized enzymes, fat, hormone and aromatic substances, all of which work together to exert the following pharmacological actions: activizing the hematopoietic function, regulating the cardiovascular function, combating bacteria, resisting tumor and delaying senility.

Hua Fen(pollen of nectar source) on sale is often in the form of a prepared product to be taken according to the accompanying instructions.

2.2 Commonly Used Chinese Patent Medicines for Health Care

2.2.1 Patent Medicines for Tonifying *Qi*

1. *Bu Zhong Yi Qi Wan*
Main Ingredients
Huang Qi (Radix Astragali)
Dang Shen (Radix Codonopsis)
Gan Cao (Radix Glycyrrhizae)
Dang Gui (Radix Angelicae Sinensis)

Chen Pi (Pericarpium Citri Reticulatae)
Sheng Ma (Rhizoma Cimicifugae)
Chai Hu (Radix Bupleuri)
Bai Zhu (Rhizoma Atractylodis Macrocephalae)

Dosage Form

Honeyed bolus or water—paste pill, 1 bolus weighing 9 g; 1 bag of the pills, 19 g.

Dosage and Administration

Taken orally, 1 bolus or 9 g of the pills each time, twice daily.

Effect

Reinforcing the middle—*Jiao*, replenishing *Qi*, elevating the clear *Qi* and sending down the turbid Indications

Headache and languor due to the hypofunction of both the spleen and the lung, spontaneous sweating due to *Yin* deficiency, aversion to wind, anorexia, chills or fever in malaria with general debility, protracted diarrhea or dysentery, gastroptosis, metroptosis, syndromes of asthenia, various kinds of anemia, chronic gastritis, etc.

Source

The book *Pi Wei Lun*

2. Shen Ling Bai Zhu Wan

Main Ingredients

Ren Shen (Radix Ginseng)
Fu Ling (Poria)
Bai Zhu (Rhizoma Atractylodis Macrocephalae)
Bai Bian Dou (Semen Dolichoris Album)
Shan Yao (Rhizoma Dioscoreae)
Gan Cao (Radix Glycyrrhizae)

Lian Zi (Semen Nelumbinis)
Jie Geng (Radix Platycodi)
Sha Ren (Fructus Amomi)
Yi Yi Ren (Semen Coicis)

Dosage Form

Water-paste pill, 1 bag of the pills weighing 18 g.

Dosage and Administration

Taken orally, once or twice daily, 6—9 g each time.

Effect

Nourishing the spleen and stomach and adjusting their functions.

Indications

Dyspepsia due to weakness of the spleen and stomach and manifested as vomiting or diarrhea, sallowness and emaciation, lassitude and hypodynamia, chronic nephritis, Pulmonary tuberculosis, etc.

Source

The book *Tai Ping Hui Min He Ji Ju Fang*

3. *Si Jun Zi Wan*

Ingredients

Dang Shen (Radix Codonopsis)
Bai Zhu (Rhizoma Atractylodis Macrocephalae)
Fu Ling (Poria)
Gan Cao (Radix Glycyrrhizae)

Dosage Form

Water-paste pill, 1 bag of the pills weighing 18 g.

Dosage and Administration

Taken 3 times daily, 6 g each time.

Effect

Invigorating the spleen and replenishing *Qi*.

Indications

Weakness of the spleen and stomach, manifested as poor appetite, loose stools, sallow complexion, dizziness and debility, including chronic gastroenteritis, gastric and duodenal ulcers, protracted or chronic hepatitis, anemia and leukocytopenia, etc.

Source

The book *Tai Ping Hui Min He Ji Ju Fang*

4. Shi Quan Da Bu Wan

Ingredients

Dang Shen (Radix Codonopsis)
Huang Qi (Radix Astragali)
Rou Gui (Cortex Cinnamomi)
Shu Di (Rhizoma Rehmanniae Praeparata)
Bai Zhu (Rhizoma Atractylodis Macrocephalae)
Dang Gui (Radix Angelicae Sinensis)
Bai Shao (Radix Paeoniae Alba)
Chuan Xiong (Rhizoma Chuanxiong)
Fu Ling (Poria)
Gan Cao (Radix Glycyrrhizae)

Dosage Form

Honeyed bolus, 1 bolus weighing 9 g.

Dosage and Administration

Taken orally, twice daily, 1 bolus each time.

Effect

Invigorating the spleen and replenishing *Qi*, enriching the blood and regulating the nutrient system.

Indications

Syndrome due to deficiency of both *Qi* and blood, marked

by general debility, sallow complexion, asthma and cough due to consumption, lassitude, spermatorrhea, impairment of blood, weakness of the loins and knees, etc.

Source

The book *Tai Ping Hui Min He Ji Ju Fang*

5. *Liang Shen Jing*

Main Ingredients

Ren Shen (Radix Ginseng)

Wu Jia Shen (Radix Acanthopanacis Senticosi)

Dosage Form

Oral liquid, 1 ampoule containing 10 ml.

Dosage and Administration

Taken orally before breakfast, 1 ampoule each day.

Effect

Replenishing *Qi*, enriching the blood, strengthening constitution.

Indications

Neurosism, infirmity with age, general debility after illness, anorexia, heart failure, hepatitis, anemia, etc.

Manufacturer

Yanji No. 2 Pharmaceutical Factory

Notes

Regular intake can promote the function of the body and enhance the resistance to disease.

6. *Ren Shen Feng Wang Jiang (Shuang Bao Su Kou Fu Ye)*

Main Ingredients

Ren Shen (Radix Ginseng)

Feng Wang Jiang (royal jelly)

Feng Mi (Mel)

Dosage Form

Heoneyed jelly, 1 ampoule containing 10 ml.

Dosage and Administration

Taken orally, twice daily, 1 ampoule each time.

Effect

Building up the body, replenishing *Qi,* strengthening the spleen.

Indications

Weak constitution, debility after illness, malnutrition, neurosism, lassitude, poor appetite, decline of neurometabolism, etc.

Manufacturer

Beijing Dong Feng Pharmaceutical Factory, Hangzhou No. 2 Pharmaceutical Factory of Traditional Chinese Medicines, etc.

Notes

Regular intake will have the effect of promoting growth and development, improve physical and mental ability, prevent disease and prolong life.

Shuang Bao Su Kou Fu Ye is manufactured by Hangzhou No. 2 factory of Traditional Chinese Medicines. Its ingredients and effects are basically the same as those of *Ren Shen Feng Wang Jiang.*

7. Bei Jing *Feng Wang Jing*

Ingredients

Feng Wang Jiang (royal jelly)

Ren Shen (Radix Ginseng)

Dang Shen (Radix Codonopsis)

Gou Qi Zi (Fructus Lycii)

Wu Wei Zi (Fructus Schisandrae)

Dosage Form

Oral liquid, each ampoule containing 10 ml.

Dosage and Administration

Taken orally after getting up in the morning or before going to bed in the evening, 1 ampoule daily.

Effect

Invigorating the spleen, replenishing *Qi*, promoting the production of body fluid.

Indications

Anorexia, neurosism, anemia, gastric ulcer, senilism, hepatitis, arthritis, angiitis, etc.

Manufacturer

Beijing Nutrient Medicine Factory

Notes

This medicine has proved to be a tonic of high quality.

8. *Yan Nian Yi Shou Jing*

Ingredients

The same as those in the prescription of *Yan Nian Yi Shou Dan*, a secret recipe of the Institute of Imperial Physicians in the Qing Dynasty.

Dosage Form

Oral liquid, 1 ampoule containing 10 ml.

Dosage and Administration

Taken orally, after getting up in the morning or before going to bed in the evening, 1–2 times daily, 1 amoule each time.

Effect

Regulating metabolism of the body, slowing down histiocytic decay and senility of the old.

Indications

Senility, general debility.

Manufacturer

Wuhan Zhonglian Pharmaceutical Factory

Notes

Produced according to traditional extractive process.

9. Wu Jia Shen Chong Ji

Main Ingredients

Wu Jia Shen (Radix Acanthopanacis Senticosi)

Dosage Form

Granules in lumps for infusing, each lump weighing 12.25 g.

Dosage and Administration

Taken orally after being infused with boiling water, twice daily, 1 lump each time.

Effect

Strengthening the body resistance and / or restoring normal functioning of the body to consolidate the constitution, tranquilizing the mind, improving mental power.

Indications

Neurosism, debility after illness, lassitude, insomnia or dreamfulness, anorexia, coronary heart disease, leukopenia, etc.

Manufacturer

Haerbin No. 1 Pharmaceutical Factory of Traditional Chinese Medicines

10. Da Li Shi Bu Ye

Main Ingredients

Wu Jia Shen (Radix Acanthopanacis Senticosi)

Huang Qi (Radix Astragali)

Dan Shen (Radix Salviae Miltiorrhizae)

Dosage Form

Syrup, each bottle containing 500 ml.

Dosage and Administration

Taken orally, 3 times daily, 20 ml each time.

Effect

Strengthening the body, improving mental power, tranquilizing the mind.

Indications

Weak constitution, debility after illness, lassitude, soreness and weakness of the loins and knees, dizziness, severe palpitation, insomnia, etc.

Manufacturer

Experimental Pharmaceutical Factory of Heilongjiang Institute of Traditional Chinese Medicine

11. *Ren Shen* Vitamin C *Zi Bu Pian*

Main Ingredients

Ren Shen (Radix Ginseng)

Vitamin C

Dosage Form

Tablet

Dosage and Administration

Taken orally, 3 times daily, 3—5 tablets each time.

Effect

Invigorating *Qi* to build up health

Indications

Infirmity with age, disorders in the convalescence, dyspnea due to deficiency of the lung, diarrhea due to deficiency of the spleen, neurosism, amnesia, anorexia, chronic hepatitis, diabetes, anemia, hypertension, syndrome due to deficiency of Vitamin C, etc.

Manufacturer

Beijing Pharmaceutical Factory

12. Qing Chun Bao

Main Ingredients

Ren Shen (Radix Ginseng)

Tian Dong (Radix Asparagi)

Shu Di Huang (Rhizoma Rehmanniae Praeparata)

Effect

Invigorating *Qi,* nourishing *Yin,* replenishing vital essence and blood.

Indications

Deficiency of vital essence, *Qi* and blood in the middle—age and the aged, general debility, weakness in the convalescence.

Manufacturer

Hangzhou No. 2 Pharmaceutical Factory of Traditional Chinese Medicine

13. Wan Nian Chun Zi Bu Jiang

Main Ingredients

Ren Shen (Radix Ginseng)

Tai Zi Shen (Radix Pseudostellariae)

Dang Shen (Radix Codonopsis)

Feng Wang Jiang (royal jelly)

Mai Dong (Radix Ophiopogonis)

Zhi Shou Wu (Radix Polygoni Multiflori Preparata)

Dang Gui (Radix Angelicae Sinensis)

Dosage Form

Oral liquid, 1 ampoule containing 10 ml.

Dosage and Administration

Taken orally, once daily, 1 ampoule each time.

Effect

Invigorating the spleen, replenishing *Qi,* nourishing *Yin,* enriching blood.

Indications

Deficiency of both *Qi* and blood, *Yin*-deficiency of the liver and kidney, insufficiency of body fluid, weakness in the convalescence, infirmity with age, etc.

Manufacturer

Wuxi Pharmaceutical Factory of Traditional Chinese Medicine.

2.2.2 Patent Medicines for Nourishing Blood

1. *Ba Zhen Wan*

Source

The book *Rui Zhu Tang Jing Yan Fang*

Ingredients

Ren Shen (Radix Ginseng)

Shu Di Huang (Rhizoma Rehmanniae Praeparata)

Dang Gui (Radix Angelicae Sinensis)

Bai Shao (Radix Paeoiae Alba)

Chuan Xiong (Rhizoma Chuanxiong)

Fu Ling (Poria)

Bai Zhu (Rhizoma Atractylodis Macrocephalae)

Gan Cao (Radix Glycyrrhizae)

Dosage Form

Bolus, each bolus weighing 9 g.

Dosage and Administration

Taken orally, twice daily, 2 boluses each time. Effect

Regulating and invigorating *Qi* and blood

Indications

Pallid countenance and thin shape, anorexia, weakness of the limbs, dizziness, blurring of vision, all due to deficiency of Qi and blood; irregular menstruation, various kinds of anemia, primary thrombocytopenic purpura, rheumatic heart disease, etc.

2. *Fu Fang E Jiao Jiang*

Main Ingredients

E Jiao (Colla Corii Asini)

Ren Shen (Radix Ginseng)

Shan Zha (Fructus Crataegi)

Dosage Form

Honeyed jelly

Dosage and Administration

Taken orally, 3 times daily, 20 ml each time.

Effect

Replenishing Qi, nourishing blood.

Indications

Syndrome due to deficiency of both Qi and blood, various kinds of anemia, leukopenia.

Intake of it in the old, the weak and athletes may have the effect of building up health, resisting disease and prolonging life.

Manufacturer

Shandong Donge Ejiao Factory

3. *Kang Bao*

Main Ingredients

Ci Wu Jia (Radix Acanthopanacis Senticosi)

Feng Wang Jiang (royal jelly)

Yin Yang Huo (Herba Epimedii)

Gou Qi (Fructus Lycii)

Huang Jing (Radix Polygonati)
Shu Di (Rhizoma Rehmanniae Praeparata)
Huang Qi (Radix Astragali)
Shan Zha (Fructus Crataegi)

Dosage Form

Honeyed jelly, each bottle containing 100 ml.

Dosage and Administration

Taken orally, 5–10 ml each time.

Effect

Invigorating *Qi*, enriching the blood, warming the kidney, replenishing vital essence, resisting senility.

Indications

Syndrome due to deficiency of both *Qi* and blood, various kinds of anemia, infirmity with age, debility in the convalescence, etc.

It may be used by the healthy to prevent disease and preserve health.

Manufacturer

Shandong Yantai Pharmaceutical Factory of Traditional Chinese Medicines

4. *Shen Qi Wang Jiang Yang Xue Jing*

Main Ingredients

Feng Wang Jiang (royal jelly)
Ren Shen Jing (extracts of the ingredient Radix Ginseng)
Huang Qi Jing (extracts of the ingredient Radix Astragali)

Dosage Form

Oral liquid, each ampoule containing 10 ml.

Dosage and Administration

Taken orally before breakfast, once daily, 1 ampoule each

time.

Effect

Enriching the blood, replenishing *Qi,* strengthening the heart, invigorating the spleen.

Indications

Anemia, general debility, infirmity with age, neurosism, hepatitis, baldness, etc.

Manufacturer

Yanji No. 2 Pharmaceutical Factory in Jilin Province

5. Ren Shen Shou Wu Jing

Main Ingredients

Hong Shen (Radix Ginseng Rubra)

He Shou Wu (Radix Polygoni Multiflori)

Dosage Form

Oral liquid, each ampoule containing 50 ml.

Dosage and Administration

Taken orally, 3 times daily, 10 ml each time.

Effect

Enriching the blood, replenishing *Qi,* tranquilizing the mind, improving mental power.

Indications

Deficiency of both *Qi* and blood, amnesia, insomnia, anorexia, lassitude, impotence, prospermia, etc.

6. E Jiao Zi Bu Jing

Main Ingredients

E Jiao (Colla Corii Asini)

Dang Shen (Radix Codonopsis)

Shu Di (Rhizoma Rehmanniae Praeparata)

Dosage Form

Granules for infusing

Dosage and Administration

Taken orally after being infused with boiling water, twice daily, 20 g each time.

Effect

Nourishing the liver and kidney, invigorating greatly *Qi* and blood.

Indications

Deficiency of both *Qi* and blood, weakness of the body, infirmity with age, etc.

7. *Liang Yi Chong Ji*

Main Ingredients

Dang Shen (Radix Codonopsis)

Shu Di (Rhizoma Rehmanniae Praeparata)

Dosage Form

Granule for infusing, each tube containing 250 g.

Dosage and Administration

Taken orally after being infused with boiling water, twice daily, 20 g each time.

Effect

Replenishing *Qi*, nourishing blood.

Indications

Deficiency of both *Qi* and blood, general debility, weakness in the convalescence.

8. *Yi Shou Zi Bu Jiang*

Main Ingredients

Ren Shen (Radix Ginseng)

He Shou Wu (Radix Polygoni Multiflori)

Quan Dang Gui (Radix Angelicae Sinensis)

Bai Fu Ling (Poria)

Jin Ying Zi (Fructus Rosae Laevigatae)

Dosage Form

Syrup, each bottle containing 300 ml.

Dosage and Administration

Taken orally, twice daily, 20 ml each time.

Effect

Replenishing *Qi*, nourishing blood, strengthening the spleen, tonifying the kidney.

Indications

Deficiency of *Qi* and blood, general debility, early-greying of hair.

Regular intake of it will have the effect of enriching blood, nourishing the heart, strenthening the tendons and bones, darkening hair and regulating menstruation.

9. Bu Xue Ning Shen Pian

Main Ingredients

Shou Wu Teng (Caulis Polygoni Multiflori)

Ji Xue Teng (Caulis Spatholobi)

Shu Di (Rhizoma Rehmanniae Praeparata)

Dosage Form

Tablet

Dosage and Administration

Taken orally, 3 times daily, 5 tablets each time.

Effect

Enriching the blood, tranquilizing the mind, nourishing *Yin*, tonifying the kidney.

Indications

Insomnia, amnesia, nocturnal emission, frequent urination,

soreness and weakness of the loins and knees, irregular menstruation, etc.

Manufacturer

Guangzhou Hongwei Pharmaceutical Factory

10. Shen Gui Zao Zhi

Main Ingredients

Hong Zao (Fructus Jujubae)

Tai Zi Shen (Radix Pseudostellariae)

Dang Gui (Radix Angelicae Sinensis)

Dosage Form

Honeyed syrup

Dosage and Administration

Taken orally with warm boiled water, 2—3 times daily, 10—20 ml each time.

Effect

Nourishing the blood, promoting the production of body fluid, replenishing *Qi,* strengthening the spleen.

Indications

Deficiency of both *Qi* and blood, listlessness, general debility, poor appetite, various consumptive disorders.

Manufacturer

Bengbu Pharmaceutical Factory of Traditional Chinese Medicines in Anhui Province

2. 2. 3   Patent Medicines for Supporting *Yang*

1. *Jin Kui Shen Qi Wan*

Source

The book *Jin Kui Yao Lile*

Ingredients

Shu Di (Rhizoma Rehmanniae Praeparata)
Shan Yao (Radix Dioscoreae)
Rou Gui (Cortex Cinnamomi)
Dan Pi (Cortex Moutan)
Fu Ling (Poria)
Fu Zi (Radix Aconiti Lateralis Preparata)
Shan Yu Rou (Fructus Corni)
Ze Xie (Rhizoma Alismatis)
Dosage Form
Honeyed bolus, each bolus weighing 9 g.
Dosage and Administration
Taken orally, twice daily, 1 bolus each time.
Effect
Warming the kidney—*Yang*
Indications
Syndrome due to deficiency of the kidney—*Yang* and cold of deficiency type in the spleen and stomach, marked by soreness and weakness of the loins and legs, spasmodic sensation of the lower abdomen, seminal emission, loose stools, frequent urination, edema of the lower limbs, etc.

2. Hai Long Ge Jie Jing
Main Ingredients
Hai Long (Syngnathus)
Ge Jie (Gecko)
Bei Qi (Radix Astragali)
Ren Shen (Radix Ginseng)
Shou Wu (Radix Polygoni Multiflori)
Dang Gui (Radix Angelicae Sinensis)
Qi Zi (Fructus Lycii)

Chen Xiang (Lignum Aquilariae Resinatum)
Dosage Form
Oral liquid, each ampoule containing 10 ml.
Dosage and Administration
Taken orally, 1-2 times daily, 1 ampoule each time.
Effect
Tonifying the body, replenishing *Qi,* enriching the blood, strengthening, the heart, brightening the face, improving eyesight.
Indications
Neurosism, overstrain, deficiency of *Qi* and blood, soreness of the loins, pain in the back, weakness of the limbs, dizziness, blurring of vision, etc.
Notes
This medicine is a tonic of high-quality especially suitable for those infirm with age.
Manufacturer
Jinan Pharmaceutical Factory of Traditional Chinese Medicines in Shandong Province, China

3. *Nan Bao*
Main Ingredients
Lü Shen (Peniet Testes Asini)
Gou Shen (Peniet Testes Canini)
Hai Ma (Hippocampus)
Ren Shen (Radix Ginseng)
Lu Rong (Cornu Cervi Pantotrichum)
E Jiao (Colla Corii Asini)
Huang Qi (Radix Astragali)
Shan Yu Rou (Fructus Corni)
Dosage Form

Capsule, each weighing 0.3 g.

Dosage and Administration

Taken orally, twice daily, 2—3 capsules each time.

Effect

Warming the kidney—*Yang*, replenishing *Qi*, building up the body.

Indications

Syndrome due to deficiency of the kidney—*Yang*, marked by impotence, spermatorrhea, weakness and soreness of the loins and knees, cold and damp feeling of scrotum, listlessness, anorexia, etc.

Manufacturer

Houma Pharmaceutical Factory of Traditional Chinese Medicines in Shanxi Province

4. *Shen Rong Bian Wan*

Main Ingredients

Ren Shen (Radix Ginseng)

Lu Rong (Cornu Cervi Pantotrichum)

Diao Bian (Peniet Testes Martes)

Hai Ma (Hippocampus)

Du Zhong (Cortex Eucommiae)

Gou Qi (Fructus Lycii)

Rou Gui (Cortex Cinnamomi)

Dosage Form

Water—paste pill

Dosage and Administration

Taken according to the instructions

Effect

Tonifying the kidney, supporting *Yang*, strengthening vital essence, promoting the production of marrow.

Indications

Weakened *Qi* due to deficiency of the kidney, marked by neurosism, impotence, prospermia, emission, and all disorders due to deficiency of the kidney in men or women.

Manufacturer

Dalian Pharmaceutical Factory of Traditional Chinese Medicines

5. *Yang Chun Yao*

Main Ingredients

Shui Diao Bian (Peniet Testes Martes)
Mei Lu Bian (Peniet Testes Cervi)
Guang Gou Bian (Peniet Testes Canini)
Lu Rong (Cornu Cervi Pantotrichum)
Yin Yang Huo (Herba Epimedii)
Ba Ji Tian (Radix Morindae Officinalis)
Huang Qi (Radix Astragali)
Fei Yang Qi Shi (Actinolitum refined with water)
Tu Si Zi (Semen Cuscutae)
He Shou Wu (Radix Polygoni Multiflori)
Rou Cong Rong (Herba Cistanchis)
Shan Yao (Rhizoma Dioscoreae)

Dosage Form

Capsule

Dosage and Administration

Taken orally, twice daily, 2 capsules each time.

Effect

Strengthening the loins, supporting *Yang*, restoring *Qi*, building up health.

Indications

Weak constitution, emission due to physical debility, lassitude, dizziness, tinnitus, palpitation caused by fright, amnesia, soreness and weakness of the loins and knees, decline of memory, neurosism, insomnia, anorexia, etc.

6. *Yi Shen Tang Jiang*

Main Ingredients

Gou Qi Zi (Fructus Lycii)

Fu Pen Zi (Fructus Rubi)

Wu Wei Zi (Fructus Schisandrae)

Dosage Form

Syrup

Dosage and Administration

Taken orally, twice daily, 5–10 ml each time.

Effect

Reinforcing the kidney–*Yang*, replenishing vital essence, supplementing the marrow.

Indications

General debility, impotence due to deficiency of the kidney, nocturnal emission, turbid urine.

Manufacturer

Tianjin No. 1 Pharmaceutical Factory of Traditional Chinese Medicines

7. *Shen Rong Da Bu Wan*

Main Ingredients

Sheng Shai Shen (dried Radix Ginseng)

Lu Rong (Cornu Cervi Pantotrichum)

Rou Cong Rong (Herba Cistanchis)

Lu Jiao Jiao (Colla Cornus Cervi)

Suo Yang (Herba Cynomorii)
Chen Xiang (Lignum Aquilariae Resinatum)
Rou Gui (Cortex Cinnamomi)
Fu Zi (Radix Aconiti Lateralis Preparata)
Tu Si Zi (Semen Cuscutae)
Gou Qi Zi (Fructus Lycii)
Du Zhong (Cortex Eucommiae)
Shou Wu (Radix Polygoni Multiflori)
Shan Yao (Rhizoma Dioscoreae)
Fu Ling (Poria)
Yuan Zhi (Radix Polygalae)

Dosage Form

Honeyed bolus, each bolus weighing 3.2 g.

Dosage and Administration

Taken orally, 1−2 times daily, 1 bolus each time.

Effect

Tonifying the kidney−*Yang*, promoting the production of vital essence, replenishing marrow.

Indications

Cold syndrome of the stomach due to *Yang*−deficiency, soreness and weakness of the loins and knees, impotence, emission, prospermia, spermatorrhea, frequent urination, etc.

Notes

It is prepared according to the prescription from Zhejiang.

8. *Chu Feng Jing*

Main Ingredients

Ji Tai (chicken's embryo)
Yang Bian (Peniet Testes Caprae seu Ovis)
Ren Shen (Radix Ginseng)

Sha Ren (Fructus Amomi)
Huang Qi (Radix Astragali)
Gou Qi (Fructus Lycii)
Yin Yang Huo (Herba Epimedii)
Lu Rong (Cornu Cervi Pantotrichum)
Rou Gui (Cortex Cinnamomi)
Dang Gui (Radix Angelicae Sinensis)
Rou Cong Rong (Herba Cistanchis)

Dosage Form

Oral liquid, each ampoule containing 10 ml.

Dosage and Administration

Taken orally, twice daily, 1 ampoule each time.

Effect

Tonifying the kidney—*Yang*, strenghtening the loins, building up health, replenishing *Qi*, enriching the blood.

Indications

Syndrome due to deficiency of the kidney—*Yang*, marked by anemia, soreness of the loins, pain in the back, weakness of the limbs, dizziness, tinnitus, neurosism, insomnia, palpitation, overtaxation of the mind, decline of memory, poor appetite, reduced sexual function, or coldness in the womb, irregular menstruation; etc.

Manufacturer

Jinan Pharmaceutical Factory of Traditional Chinese Medicines in Shandong Province of China

Notes

This medicine is a strong tonic of high quality.

9. *Hai Ma Bu Shen Wan*

Main Ingredients

Hai Ma (Hippocampus)
Ren Shen (Radix Ginseng)
Hua Long Gu (Os Draconis)
Gou Qi Zi (Fructus Lycii)
Hei Lü Shen (Peniet Testes Asini)
Lu Jin (Ligamentum Cervi)
Bu Gu Zhi (Fructus Psoraleae)
Fu Ling (Poria)
Huang Qi (Radix Astragali)
He Tao Ren (Semen Juglandis)
Lu Rong (Cornu Cervi Pantotrichum)
Ge Jie Wei (tails of gecko)
Hai Gou Shen (Peniet Testes Callorhini)
Xian Dui Xia (fresh prawns)
Hu Gu (Os Tigris)
Hua Lu Shen (Peniet Testes Cervi)
Shan Yu Rou (Fructus Corni)
Dang Gui (Radix Angelicae Sinensis)

Dosage Form

Pills, every 10 pills weighing 2.7 g.

Dosage and Administration

Taken orally on an empty stomach, twice daily, 10 pills each time.

Effect

Supplementing the kidney—*Yang*, reinforcing the brain, strengthening the body.

Indications

Syndrome due to deficiency of both *Qi* and blood as well as insufficiency of the kidney—*Qi*, marked by general debility, sallow complexion, emaciation, palpitation, short breath, weakness of the loins and legs, impotence, emission, etc.

Manufacturer

Tianjin No. 3 Pharmaceutical Factory of Traditional Chinese Medicines

Notes

It is prepared according to a prescription established by a famous physician.

10. Mei Hua Lu Rong Xue

Main Ingredients

Lu Rong Xue (Sanguis Cervi)

Mei Hua Lu Rong (Cornu Cervi Pantotrichum)

Wu Jia Shen (Radix Acanthopanacis Senticosi)

Dosage Form

Oral liquid, each ampoule containing 10 ml.

Dosage and Administration

Taken orally before breakfast, once daily, 1 ampoule each time.

Effect

Warming the kidney—*Yang*, promoting the production of vital essence, enriching the blood.

Indications

Male hypogonadism, irregular menstruation, coldness in the womb, leucorrhagia with reddish and whitish discharge, copos, postpartum debility, infirmity with age, weakness of the heart, malnutrition, anemia, overtaxation of the mind, hypomnesis, soreness and weakness of the loins and knees, dizziness, insomnia, etc.

11. Hai Shen Wan

Main Ingredients

Hai Shen (Holothuriae)

Hu Tao Rou (Semen Juglandis)

Yang Yao Zi (peniet Testes Caprae seu Ovis)

Zhu Ji Sui (spinal cord of pig)

Lu Jiao Jiao (Colla Cornus Cervi)

Gui Ban (Carapax et Plastrum Testudinis)

Du Zhong (Cortex Eucommiae)

Niu Xi (Radix Achyranthis Bidentatae)

Ba Ji Tian (Radix Morindae Officinalis)

Tu Si Zi (Semen Cuscutae)

Bu Gu Zhi (Fructus Psoraleae)

Gou Qi Zi (Fructus Lycii)

Dang Gui (Radix Angelicae Sinensis)

Dosage Form

Honeyed bolus, each bolus weighing 9 g.

Dosage and Administration

Taken orally, twice daily, 1 bolus each time.

Effect

Reinforcing the kidney–*Yang*, nourishing the blood, replenishing vital essence.

Indications

Syndrome due to deficiency of the kidney–*Yang* manifested as impotence, emission, soreness and weakness of the loins and knees, dizziness, tinnitus, weakness of the limbs, etc.

2.2.4 Patent Medicines for Nourishing *Yin*

1. *Liu Wei Di Huang Wan*

Source

The book *Xiao Er Yao Zheng Zhi Jue*
Ingredients
Shu Di Huang (Rhizoma Rehmanniae Praeparata)
Shan Yao (Rhizoma Dioscoreae)
Shan Yu Rou (Fructus Corni)
Fu Ling (poria)
Ze Xie (Rhizoma Alismatis)
Dan Pi (Cortex Moutan)
Dosage Form
Honeyed boluses, 1 bolus weighing 9 g.
Dosage and Administration
Taken orally, twice daily, 1 bolus each time.
Effect
Tonifying the liver and kidney
Indications
Syndrome due to *Yin*—deficiency of the liver and kidney, marked by soreness and weakness of the loins and legs, dizziness, tinnitus, insomnia, nocturnal emission, dry mouth in diabetes, hectic fever, night sweating, dysphoria with feverish sensation in the chest, palms and soles, etc.

2. *Ren Shen Gu Ben Wan*
Ingredients
Ren Shen (Radix Ginseng)
Shan Yao (Rhizoma Dioscoreae)
Shu Di Huang (Rhizoma Rehmanniae Praeparata)
Tian Dong (Radix Asparagi)
Mai Dong (Radix Ophiopogonis)
Shan Zhu Yu (Fructus Corni)
Feng Mi (Mel)

Fu Ling (Poria)

Dosage Form

Honeyed bolus, 1 bolus weighing 9 g.

Dosage and Administration

Taken orally, twice daily, 1 bolus each time.

Effect

Nourishing *Yin,* supplementing the blood, replenishing *Qi,* promoting the production of body fluid.

Indications

Syndrome due to *Yin*-deficiency and weakened *Qi,* marked by general debility, palpitation, shortness of breath, pain in the loins, tinnitus, soreness and weakness of the limbs, hectic fever due to consumption, etc.

3. Jian Nao Chong Ji

Main Ingredients

Gou Qi Zi (Fructus Lycii)

Suan Zao Ren (Semen Ziziphi Spinosae)

Dosage Form

Granule for infusing, each bag containing 14 g.

Dosage and Administration

Taken orally before going to bed in the evening, once daily, 1 bag each time.

Effect

Replenishing the kidney—*Yin,* strengthening the brain, nourishing the heart, calming the mind.

Indications

Yin—deficiency of the liver and kidney, neurosism, insomnia, amnesia, dizziness, tinnitus, soreness and weakness of the loins and knees, etc.

4. Shen Qi Feng Huang Jiang

Feng Ru (Lac Regis Apis)
Feng Mi (Mel)
Dang Shen (Radix Codonopsis)
Gou Qi Zi (Fructus Lycii)

Dosage Form

Honeyed jelly, each ampoule containing 10 ml.

Dosage and Administration

Taken orally, 1—2 times daily, 1 ampoule each time.

Effect

Tonifying the liver and kidney, replenishing *Qi*, improving acuity of vision.

Indications

Yin—deficiency of the liver and kidney, dizziness, blurring of vision, soreness and weakness of the loins and knees, poor appetite, lassitude, infirmity with age, debility in the convalescence, etc.

5. Zi Yin Bai Bu Wan

Main Ingredients

Dang Gui (Radix Angelicae Sinensis)
Fu Ling (Poria)
Yuan Zhi (Radix Polygalae)
Niu Xi (Radix Achyranthis Bidentatae)
Mai Dong (Radix Ophiopogonis)
Zhi Mu (Rhizoma Anemarrhenae)
Rou Cong Rong (Herba Cistanchis)
Gou Qi Zi (Fructus Lycii)
Nü Zhen Zi (Fructus Ligustri Lucidi)
Tu Si Zi (Semen Cuscutae)

Suo Yang (Herba Cynomorii)
Ba Ji Tian (Radix Morindea Officinalis)
Bai Zi Ren (Semen Biotae)
Shan Yu Rou (Fructus Corni)

Dosage Form

Honeyed bolus, each weighing 3 g.

Dosage and Administration

Taken orally, twice daily, 6—9 g each time.

Effect

Tonifying the kidney, replenishing Yin, controlling nocturnal emission, calming the mind.

Indications

Interior heat due to *Yin*—deficiency, dizziness, lassitude, soreness in the loins, weakness of the limbs, night sweating, emission, infirmity with age, etc.

6. Kang Fu Wan

Main Ingredients

Tai Zi Shen (Radix Beudostellariae)
Dang Gui (Radix Angelicae Sinensis)
Wu Wei Zi (Fructus Schisandrae)
Zhen Zhu Mu (Concha Margaritifera Usta)
Shan Yao (Rhizoma Dioscoreae)
Shu Di (Rhizma Rehmanniae Praeparata)
Chuan Duan (Radix Disaci)

Dosage Form

Water—pills

Dosage and Administration

Taken orally, 3 times daily, 10 pills each time.

Effect

Tonifying the kidney, restoring *Qi*, nourishing the blood to control nocturnal emission, building up health.

Indications

General debility, in the convalescence, *Yin*-deficiency of the liver and kidney, dizziness, tinnitus, lassitude in the loins, insomnia, amnesia, emission, night sweating, etc.

Manufacturer

Xian pharmaceutical Factory of Traditional Chinese Medicines

7. Qing Gong Shou Tao Wan

Main Ingredients

Yi Zhi Ren (Fructus Alpiniae Oxyphyllae)

Da Sheng Di (Radix Rehmanniae)

Gou Qi Zi (Fructus Lycii)

Tian Dong (Radix Asparagi)

Ren Shen (Radix Ginseng)

Dang Gui (Radix Angelicae Sinensis)

He Tao Rou (Semen Juglandis)

Dosage Form

Honeyed boluses, each weighing 6 g.

Dosage and Administration

Taken orally, twice daily, 1 bolus each time.

Effect

Reinforcing the kidney, invigorating primordial *Qi*, nourishing *Yin*, supporting *Yang*, enriching blood, prolonging life.

Indications

Infirmity with age, debility in the convalescence, various disorders of deficiency type.

Manufacturer

Darentang Pharmaceutical Factory in Tianjin City

Notes

This medicine is a roborant patent one produced according to a secret prescription for health care from the Palace of the Qing Dynasty. It is a good tonic for resisting senility and enhancing longevity.

2.2.5 Other Patent Medicines for Health Care

1. Ling Zhi Pian

Main Ingredients

Ling Zhi (Ganoderma Lucidum seu Japonicum)

Dosage Form

Tablets or granule for infusing; 1 tablet weighing 1 g; granule being in lumps, each lump weighing 13 g, whose effect is equal to that of 3 g of herbal medicine.

Dosage and Administration

The tablet is taken twice daily, 1—2 tablets each time. Or the granule is taken after being infused with boiling water, once daily, 1 lump each time.

Effect

Tonifying the heart, calming the mind, strengthening the spleen, regulating the stomach, building up health, prolonging life.

Indications

Neurosism, dizziness, insomnia, anorexia, coronary heart disease, hyperlipemia, etc.

Manufacturer

The Pharmaceutical Factory of Guangxi College of Traditional Chinese Medicine

Notes

It is a good tonic for those infirm with age.

2. Yi Nao Fu Jian Wan

Main Ingredients

San Qi (Radix Notoginseng)

Xi Hong Hua (Stigma Croci)

Chuan Xiong (Rhizoma Chuanxiong)

Dosage Form

Capsule, each capsule weighing 0.3 g.

Dosage and Administration

Taken orally, 3 times daily, 6—8 capsules each time.

Effect

Supplementing the brain to benefit the mind, smoothing the channels and collaterals, activationg blood circulation to remove stasis, eliminating phlegm to induce resuscitation.

Indications

Distortion of the face, hemiparalysis and dysphasia due to acute ischemic apoplexy

3. Nao Ling Su

Main Ingredients

Ren Shen (Radix Ginseng)

Lu Rong (Cornu Cervi Pantotrichum)

Gui Ban (Carapax et Plastrum Testudinis)

Lu Jiao Jiao (Colla Cornus Cervi)

Suan Zao Ren (Semen Ziziphi Spinosae)

Gou Qi Zi (Fructus Lycii)

Wu Wei Zi (Fructus Schisandrae)

Fu Ling (Poria)

Yuan Zhi (Radix Polygalae)

Dosage Form

Sugar-coated tablets, each weighing 0.5 g.

Dosage and Administration

Taken orally, twice daily, 2—3 tablets each time.

Effect

Supplementing both *Qi* and blood, nourishing the heart and kidney, strengthening the brain, calming the mind.

Indications

Neurosism, amnesia, insomnia, dizziness, blurring of vision, palpitation, shortness of breath, lassitude, general debility, spontaneous sweating, impotence, seminal emission, etc.

Manufacturer

Jiamusi Pharmaceutical Factory of Traditional Chinese Medicines, Linyi Health Pharmaceutical Factory in Shandong Province, to name but a few.

4. *You Kang Ping*

Main Ingredients

Yin Er (Tremella)

Wu Jia Shen (Radix Acanthopanacis Senticosi)

Wu Wei Zi (Fructus Schisandrae)

Dan Shen (Radix Salviae Miltiorrhizae)

Ban Lan Gen (Radix Isatidis)

Gan Cao (Radix Glycyrrhizae)

Dosage Form

Malt extract in lumps, eachlump weighing 5.2 g.

Dosage and Administration

Taken orally, 2—3 times daily, 1—2 lumps each time.

Effect

Restoring normal function of the body to consolidate constitution, enriching the blood, tranquilizing the mind, clearing away heat and toxic material, enhancing body resistance, combating and preventing influenza and hepatitis, promoting growth and development, invigorating primordial *Qi* and building up constitution in adults and the aged who take it regularly, etc.

Manufacturer

Weihai Pharmaceutical Factory of Traditional Chinese Medicines in Shandong Province

Notes

It is prepared according to an ancient prescription.

5. An Shen Bu Xin Wan

Main Ingredients

Dan Shen (Radix Salviae Miltiorrhizae)

Wu Wei Zi (Fructus Schisandrae)

Shi Chang Pu (Rhizoma Acori Graminei)

He Huan Pi (Cortex Albiziae)

Mo Han Lian (Herba Ecliptae)

Nü Zhen Zi (Fructus Ligustri Lucidi)

Shou Wu Teng (Caulis Polygoni Multiflori)

Sheng Di (Radix Rehmanniae)

Zhen Zhu Mu (Concha Margaritifera Usta)

Dosage Form

Pills

Dosage and Administration

Taken orally, 3 times daily, 15 pills each time.

Effect

Replenishing *Yin,* nourishing the blood, tonifying the heart, calming the mind.

Indications

Palpitation, insomnia, dizziness, tinnitus, etc.

Manufacturer

Shanghai No. 1 Pharmaceutical Factory of Traditional Chinese Medicines

6. Yi Chun Bao Kou Fu Ye

Main Ingredients

Lu Rong (Cornu Cervi Pantotrichum)

Feng Wang Jiang (royal jelly)

Ci Wu Jia (Radix Acanthopanacis Senticosi)

Dosage Form

Oral liquid, each ampoule containing 10 ml.

Dosage and Administration

Taken orally after getting up in the morning or before going to bed in the evening, once daily, 1 ampoule each time.

Effect

Reinforcing the heart, strengthening the spleen, tonifying the kidney, calming the mind, replenishing *Qi,* nourishing the blood.

Indications

Neurosism, deficiency of the enery, poor appetite, dysplasia, infirmity with age, postpartum debility, copos, etc.

Notes

This medicine may be used for health care of athletes and children.

7. Ling Zhi Qiang Ti Pian

Main Ingredients

Ren Shen (Radix Ginseng)

Ling Zhi (Ganoderma Lucidum seu Japonicum)

Dosage Form

Tablets

Dosage and Administration
Taken according to the instructions
Effect
Replenishing *Qi,* nourishing the blood, strengthening health.
Indications
Neurosism, dizziness, tinnitus, restlessness, insomnia, poor appetite, anemia, sallow complexion, general debility, etc.

8. *Dan Qi Pian*
Main Ingredients
San Qi (Radix Notoginseng)
Dan Shen (Radix Salviae Miltiorrhizae)
Dosage Form
Tablets
Dosage and Administration
Taken orally, 3 times daily, 3 tablets each time.
Effect
Reinforcing the heart, dilating the coronary arteries activating blood circulation, removing stasis
Indications
Angina pectoris due to coronary heart disease, neurosism, etc.
Manufacturer
Tongrentang Pharmaceutical Factory in Beijing
Notes
It can also afford a tonic and roborant effect.

9. *Nü Bao*
Main Ingredients
Ren Shen (Radix Ginseng)
Lu Tai (Fetus Cervi)

Lu Rong (Cornu Cervi Pantotrichum)
Hong Hua (Flos Carthami)
Dan Shen (Radix Salviae Miltiorrhizae)
Dan Pi (Cortex Moutan)
Chuan Xiong (Rhizoma Chuanxiong)
E Jiao (Colla Corii Asini)

Dosage Form

Capsules, each weighing 0.3 g.

Dosage and Administration

Taken orally, 3 times daily, 4 capsules each time.

Effect

Replenishing *Qi*, activating blood circulation, nourishing *Yin*, supporting *Yang*, regulating menstruation, treating leukorrhagia.

Indications

Irregular menstruation, dysmenorrhea, amenorrhea, leukorrhagia, sterility due to cold uterus, postpartum disorders, deficiency of vital essence due to consumption in male, man's soreness and weakness of the loins and knees, etc.

Manufacturer

Pharmaceutical Factory of Changchun College of Traditional Chinese Medicine and Dongfeng Pharmaceutical Factory in Jilin Province

Notes

It is a newly-developed medicine for women's health care.

10. Geng Nian An

Main Ingredients

Shu Di (Rhizoma Rehmanniae Praeparata)
He Shou Wu (Radix Polygoni Multiflori)

Ze Xie (Rhizoma Alismatis)
Fu Ling (Poria)
Wu Wei Zi (Fructus Schisandrae)
Zhen Zhu Mu (Concha Margaritifera Usta)
Ye Jiao Teng (Caulis Polygoni Multiflori)
Xuan Shen (Radix Scrophulariae)
Fu Xiao Mai (Fructus Tritici Levis)

Dosage Form

Tablets, each weighing 0.3 g.

Dosage and Administration

Taken orally, 2-3 times daily, 6 tablets each time.

Effect

Nourishing *Yin*, removing heat, relieving restlessness, calming the mind, building up health, prolonging life.

Indications

Male and female climacteric syndromes, various gerontal diseases due to deficient *Yin* and hyperactive *Yang*.

Manufacturer

Tianjin No. 3 Pharmaceutical Factory of Traditional Chinese Medicines

2.3 Chinese Medicated Liquor for Health Care

Chinese medicated liquor (medicated liquor for short), a combination of liquor and traditional Chinese medicinal herbs, is a liquid form of medicine. It may be prepared in two ways: A, by steeping or bo ling the herbs in Chinese white liquor, millet wine or rice wine and then removing the residues to get the medicated liquor; B, by putting a distiller's yeast into the mixture of herbs and a cereal such as rice, polished glutinous rice or husked sorghum and fermenting the mixture and then romoving the residues to get the medicated liquor. There are two types of medicated liquor: one for oral intake, the other for external application. Medicated liquor is used for the treatment and prevention of diseases as well as for health care. Among various types of medicated liquor, those used for nourishment, longevity, prophylaxis and convalescence constitute the majority. The application of medicated liquor to health care is one of the characteristics of TCM.

In ancient times, Chinese medicated liquor was called *Lao Li* (sweet wine with drugs). In the book *Nei Jing*, there is a chapter entitled "On Lao Li", giving a description of how it was made and used clinically. It was recorded in the book *Jin Gui Yao Lüe* by Zhang Zhongjing in the late Easten Han Dynasty (25 B. C. — 220 A. D.)that *Hong Lan Hua Jiu* was used for relieving women's abdominal stabbing pain. Since the Tang Dynasty, medicated liquor has been extensively used in medical practice. A great number of prescriptions for medicated liquor were recorded in the book *Bei Ji Qian Jin Yao Fang* and the book *Wai Tai Mi Yao*. Great numbers of formulae for medicated liquor were found in medical works in the years that followed. For instance, Li Shizhen presented 69 kinds of prescriptions for medicated liquor in his works *Ben Cao Gang Mu*. Since 1949, mass-produced medicated liquors such as *San Bian Jiu* and *Gui Ling Ji Jiu* have won great popularity both at home and abroad. With the development of both moral and material civilization, medicated liquors, especially those for health care, will be further improved and better utilized, contributing more to people's health.

2.3.1 Health-care Effects of Chinese Medicated Liquor

Liquor is a beverage widely accepted by people. As a form of beverage, Chinese medicated liquor is convenient to be taken over a long term, To take medicated liquor has become an acceptable way for health care. And if chosen and taken properly, medicated liquor will exert the following benefits:

1. Regulating *Yin* and *Yang*

Good health and longevity is based on the harmony of *Yin* and *Yang*. One tends to contract illness or quicken the process of ageing if there exists incoordination between *Yin* and *Yang* in his body. Chinese medicated liquor is good either for tonifying *Yang* or nourishing *Yin*, or for both. Regular intake of an appropriate medicated liquor according to one's specific case of imbalance of *Yin* and *Yang* will help harmonize *Yin* and *Yang* and keep them in well dynamic equilibrium, thus maintaining health and longevity.

2. Invigorating *Qi* and blood

Qi and blood are the vital material basis of life. *Qi* is reflected by the functional activities of internal organs. The maintenance of vital activities relies on *Qi*'s functions of warming, dynamic, vitalization, prevention, nutrition and consolidation, and on the functions of blood in nourishing *Zang* and *Fu* internally and moistening the skin, hair, muscles and joints externally. Deficiency of *Qi* and blood will result in illness and quicken senility. It is suitable for those with deficient *Qi* and blood to take medicated liquor which is good for invigorating their *Qi* and nourishing their blood. This will strengthen their body resistance to diseases and slow down the process of senility.

3. Tonifying the Five *Zang*

The liver, heart, spleen, lung and kidney have the physiological functions of transforming and storing such refined nutritious substances as vital essence, *Qi*, blood and body fluid. Man's growing, developing and becoming strong or senile depend to a great extent on whether the physical function of the five *Zang* organs is normal and whether their *Qi*, especially the kidney–*Qi* is sufficient. Deficiency of the five *Zang* organs is the cause of internal diseases and senility. Each organ performs its own functions. The deficient organ can be detected from the symptoms and signs manifested when it is diseased. If proper medicated liquor is taken, the function of a dysfunctioning organ will be restored to normal. Thus, one can keep strong. TCM holds that the kidney is the origin of the congenital constitution while the spleen and stomach provide the material basis of the acquired constitution. Those two are most closely related to health and longevity. Among all the tonifying medicated liquors for health care, those for tonifying the kidney, aiding the essential *Qi* and strengthening the spleen and stomach are most commonly seen and used. The medicated liquor for tonifying the heart and soothing the mind is often used, too, for the heart, the vital important internal organ, controls mental activities and blood circulation.

4. Eliminating illness and expelling evils

In addition to various sorts of medicated liquor for tonification, there has been since ancient times some medicated liquors for expelling wind, cold and dampness or for invigorating blood circulation by warming the channels and collaterals. This kind of liquor is utilized for the treatment of illnesses and for health care as well. It is beneficial for those who are prone to be attacked by wind, cold and dampness or to have their channels obstructed due to blood stasis to take relevant medicated liquor for expelling the evils and resisting diseases. It is advisable for those suffering from *Bi* syndrome due to wind, cold or dampness, from hemiplegia caused by stroke or from cardialgia caused by obstruction in the chest to take certain medicated liquor in proper amount in the convalescence after having been treated with herbal decoction, pills and powder. This can help the takers restore normal health and prevent the relapse of their diseases; assist them to combat disease, keep fit or prolong their lives even when they have been suffering from incurable diseases.

5. Prolonging life

Becoming senile is caused by the incoordination between *Yin* and *Yang*, the deficiency of the five *Zang* organs, the insufficiency of *Qi* and blood, and the over-consumption of the essence of life. The tonic medicated liquor has the action of delaying the process of becoming senile. In the thousands of years' research for resistance to senility and for longevity, it was found out that certain traditional Chinese medicines and medicated liquors do have the action of slowing down the process of senility. Taking them frequently makes one's bones strong, hair black, skin smooth, face bright, eyes and ears in good condition so that one may enjoy health and longevity.

2.3.2 Mechanism of Chinese Medicated Liquor

The active elements of many traditional Chinese medicines are soluble in alcohol, which is the material basis for medicated liquor to take effect. Thousands of years' clinical experience and modern research have proved that the commonly used medicines and their active principles do play a part in medicated liquor in preserving health and prolonging life. For example, *Ren Shen* (Radix Ginseng) has quite a good effect on resisting senility, reinforcing immunity, regulating internal secretion, promoting the synthesis of protein, strengthening resistance to fatigue, resisting myocardial ischemia, reducing the blood sugar level and enhancing the hematopoietic function. *Huang Qi* (Radix Astragali) prolongs the life of cells in vivo, reinforces immunity, strengthens the muscle contractility and the capacity of stress reaction, promotes the synthesis of protein, dilates blood vessels and decreases high blood pressure. *Ling Zhi* (Ganoderma Lucidum seu Japonicum) has the action of strengthening immunity and tolerance of oxygen deficiency, resisting myocardial ischemia, regulating the metabolism of nucleic acid and protein and removing the free radicals of hydroxyls to lead to resistance to senility. *Dang Gui* (Radix Angelicae Sinensis) has the action of increasing the blood production, strengthening immunity, reinforcing the muscle contractility and body resistance to cold, protecting the liver, increasing the volume of blood flow in the heart muscles, resisting myocardial ischemia and arrhythmia, hindering the accumulation of blood platelets to prevent thrombosis, and leading to the delay of senility by means of anti-oxidation. *He Shou Wu* (Radix Polygoni Multiflori) has the action of resisting atherosclerosis and myocardial ischemia, strengthening cellular immunity, checking lipid peroxide and promoting the activity of diverged peroxidase to resist senility. *Gou Qi Zi* (Fructus Lycii) decreases the blood sugar and cholesterol levels, relieves atherosclerosis and protects the liver. *Shan Zha* (Fructus Crataegi) lowers high blood pressure and blood lipid, resists myocardial ischemia and promotes digestion. *Ju Hua* (Flos Chrysanthemi) increases the volume of blood flow in the coronary arteries, resists myocardial ischemia and thrombosis, contains a microelement, selenium, which is good for delaying the process of becoming senile. The medicated liquors made of these traditional Chinese medicines, such as *Ren Shen Jiu, Ling Zhi Jiu, Shou Wu Jiu, Gou Qi Jiu, Ju Hua Jiu* and *Dang Gui Jiu*, and many other medicated liquors play an important role due to their mechanism mentioned above in health protection and life prolongation.

In recent years, experiments and research have been made on some medicated liquors compound. The study on *Shi Quan Da Bu Jiu* made by Shanghai Medical Industry Institute reveals that this medicated liquor strengthens the non-specific immunity, enhances the gastrointestinal movement, increases the volume of blood flow in the coronary arteries, reinforces the tolerance of oxygen deficiency. Those advantages help explain in part why this medicated liquor is effective in invigorating *Qi* and activating the functional activities of the spleen. Shanxi Traditional Medicine Factory has made investigations on *Gui Ling Ji Jiu*. The findings suggest that it promotes the specific and non-specific immunity by the action of strengthening the activating of macrophages, the function of the reticuloendothelial system to remove foreign bodies, and increasing the production of antibody. Furthermore, it betters the central nervous system, enhances the memory, and serves as a cardiac tonic and tranquilizer, which suggests that it regulates both the excitation and inhibition of the cerebral cortex. The results of the research made by the First Military Medical University shows that *Ren Shen Feng Wang Jiang Jiu*, containing nutrients such as various free amino acids and water-soluble vitamines, strengthens sexual functions and resistance to fatigue. It also has the action of strengthening the cellular immunity, the body fluid immunity, the specific and non-specific immunity of the body whose immunity is normal or subnormal. Work of this sort needs further effort on a broader and deeper scale. Modern scientific investigation will not only affirm the actions of the medicated liquor but help to reveal its mechanism, leading to the correct utilization of the liquor.

2.3.3 Characteristics of Health Care with Chinese Medicated Liquor

1. Liquor Helps Potentiate Medicines

Liquor has the potency to promote blood circulation, resist cold and potentiate medicines. A saying in the works *Ben Cao Gang Mu* states: "By regulating *Qi* and blood, proper drinking makes people vigorous and warm." The book *Ming Yi Bie Lu* says, "Liquor helps spread the medicinal effect over the whole body. With its nature of warming up and regulating *Qi* and blood, liquor potentiates medicine in tonifying, dispelling cold, warming up and invigorating blood circulation. The main component of liquor is alcohol, an effective solvent which is apt to penetrate the tissues of crude drugs to dissolve certain elements of them. In crude medicinal materials, a lot of active elements such as alkaloids and their salts, volatile oils, glucoside, tannin, organic acids, resins, sugars, and some pigments can be easily dissolved in liquor. An experiment done with mice to compare the different immune effects of *Gui Ling Ji Jiu* and the crude or refined powder of *Gui Ling Ji* proved that the effect of *Gui Ling Ji Jiu* is much better.

2. Wide Indications and Easy Preparation

Medicated liquor is accepted widely. For healthy people, it makes them stronger and free from illness. For the middle-aged and the aged, it helps them delay the process of ageing. It serves as a supplementary treatment for patients with chronic diseases due to the imbalance of *Yin* and *Yang*, *Qi* and blood, *Zang* and *Fu*, promoting the restoration of their health. According to the individuals conditions, seasons and sources of medicinal substances, the prescription of a medicated liquor may be easily readjusted and its preparation may be readily made.

3. Stable Effect and Convenient Administration

Liquor can serve as a preservative. It can delay the hydrolysis of certain effective elements of medicines when its alcohol content is more than 40%. So medicated liquor keeps long and is convenient for patients to take. The herbal medicines often used to prepare medicated liquor are: *Long Yan* (Arillus Longan), *Shan Zha* (Fructus Crataegi), *Sang Shen* (Fructus Mori), *Gou Qi* (Fructus Lycii), *Yi Mi* (Semen Coicis), *Ju Hua* (Flos Chrysanthemi), etc., which can be taken as food or medicines. Most medicines chosen in medicated liquor are mild in nature. And they are quite safe when taken properly.

2.3.4 Indications of Chinese Medicated Liquor for Health Care

1. Indications of Medicated Liquor for Replenishing *Qi*

Symptoms due to *Qi* deficiency, such as lassitude, low voice, languor, weakness in the limbs, poor appetite, spontaneous sweating, pale and corpulent tongue sometimes with teeth prints, and feeble pulse.

2. Indications of Medicated Liquor for Nourishing Blood

Symptoms due to blood deficiency, such as pale or sallow complexion, dizziness, blurring of vision, darkness before the eye when rising suddenly, pale lips and nails, numbness of the hands and feet, whitish tongue and thready pulse.

3. Indications of Medicated Liquor for Nourishing *Yin*

Syndrome due to *Yin* deficiency, manifested as heat in the five centres (palms, soles and chest), afternoon fever, dryness in the mouth and throat, insomnia, dizziness, blurring of vision, night sweating, constipation, brown urine, reddish tongue or tongue with little coating, thready and rapid pulse.

4. Indications of Medicated Liquor for Reinforcing *Yang*

Syndrome due to *Yang* deficiency, manifested as general or local intolerance of cold, or cold limbs, edema of the face and feet, impotence, cold semen, frequent night urination, loose stools, watery urine, whitish and plump tongue with moist fur, faint and retarded pulse.

5. Indications of Medicated Liquor for Tonifying the Five *Zang* Organs

Symptoms due to heart deficiency such as palpitation, insomnia or dreaminess, amnesia, slow and weak pulse with regular intervals or slow pulse with irregular intervals or thready and faint pulse;

Symptoms due to spleen deficiency such as poor appetite, abdominal distension after meals and a feeling of comfort from pressure on the abdomen, sallow complexion, feeble muscles and loose stools;

Symptoms due to lung deficiency such as asthma and shortness of breath, prolonged cough, whitish sputum, frequent catching of cold;

Symptoms due to kidney deficiency such as soreness of the back, weakness of the legs and knees or pain in the heels, tinnitus, deafness, falling of teeth and hair, dripping after urination or incontinence of urine, retrogression of sexual function and sterility.

6. Indications of Medicated Liquor for Prolonging Life

Early senility. This type of liquor is good for the middle-aged and the aged. It has the action of tonifying the kidney, reinforcing the spleen and nourishing Qi and blood.

7. Indications of Medicated Liquor for Preventing Diseases and Building up Health

Prevention and supplementary treatment of certain special diseases and rehabilitation of them.

In addition, there is a medicated liquor for tonifying both Qi and blood, which is suitable for the symptoms and signs due to deficiency of both Qi and blood; and a medicated liquor for reinforcing both Yin and $Yang$, suitable for the syndrome due to deficiency of both Yin and $Yang$.

2.3.5 Preparation of Medicated Liquor

There is a variety of methods for preparing medicated liquor, such as cold-steeping, hot-steeping; brewing, percolating, circular-heating, etc. The first two are mainly for home-making medicated liquor; the last two, for industrial manufacture, which will not be introduced here. Drug materials, process and implements play a key role in the preparation of high-quality medicated liquor.

1. Raw Materials

(1) Liquor

It is important to make a choice of liquor, which is a solvent with its own medical effect. The commonly used solvent is Chinese white liquor or millet wine or yellow rice wine.

White liquor includes various hard liquor and spirit on sale. It is prepared through distillation and contains 40%−60% of alcohol. Medicated liquor made up of such liquor maintains medicinal effects, it is suitable for those fond of strong drinking, but unsuitable for those who don't like strong drinking very much. They should not take too much, as this will impair their health. Ideally, they should take a medicated liquor prepared from a liquor whose alcohol content is 40% or so or from yellow rice wine.

Yellow rice wine is prepared through fermentation. *Shao Xing Jiu* is such an example. It contains less than 20% alcohol, glucose, malt sugar and amino acids, being nutritious. Medicated liquor prepared from millet wine or yellow rice wine is suitable for those who don't like drinking very much, those who are infirm with age or those who are in poor health. For the unsteady medicinal effects due to its low alcohol content, it is not fit to be kept too long, so it is advisable to take this kind of medicated liquor regularly soon after it is prepared.

Grape wine is also prepared through fermentation. Its alcohol content is 7−8 per cent.

(2) Crude Medicines

The crude medicines in their proper amount selected in the light of the prescription should be processed in conventional ways so as to ensure their medicinal action and reduce their side effects. It should be noted to remove the impurities from them or have them. washed when necessary. It is preferable to have them sliced or ground to widen their contacting surface with the liquor. But, it is inadvisable to crush them too small lest the medicated liquor be turbid. Sometimes, crystal sugar or honey is added into the liquor to improve the palatability.

2. Process

(1) Cold-steeping

Put the cut or broken crude medicines and then the liquor (or wine) into a suitable container according to the prescribed amount. Seal the container. Stir or agitate it once a day for seven days, then with less frequency. After 15—20 days (in winter more time is needed), obtain the clear liquid and combine it with that from the pressed medicinal residue, have the combination kept still and then filtered, thus the medicated liquor is obtained.

(2) Hot-steeping

This is nearly the same as the cold-steeping. Heat the water in which a container stands until the liquid surface in the container becomes foamy. Take out the container, seal it and keep it for over half a month. Obtain the clear liquid and combine it with that from the pressed medicinal residue, have it kept still and filtered. Thus the medicinal liquor is obtained.

Whether cold-steeping or hot-steeping process is used, the crude medicines can be wrapped in a cloth bag, which suspends in the liquor.

Another method is to decoct the crude medicines and get the decoction by filtering. Heat the decoction until it becomes a concentrated extract. Put the extract into the liquor after it is cooled. Seal the container. Some days later, filter the mixed liquid to obtain the liquor. This method is not advisable for crude medicines containing aromatic and volatile elements.

(3) Brewing

Soak glutinous rice (or round-grained non-glutinous rice or husked sorghum) in water and then steam it until cooked. Cool it to 30℃, add distiller's yeast and the prepared crude medicines (or concentrated extr act from decoction), mix them evenly, put the mixture into a suitable container, seal it, keep it at a suitable temperature for 1-2 weeks, this being the brewing process. Press the brewed mixture and filter the liquid. Pour the liquid into a container which is to be heated in the water until the liquid's temperature reaches 75℃ -80℃ to kill saccharomycete and ot her harmful bacteria for storage and good quality. The medicated liquor obtained by this method has a mild nature suitable to be taken permanently by the aged and the weak.

3. Implements

The principle in selecting implements is to ensure that no chemical reactions should occur between the container and the medicinal substances. Commonly used are pottery, porcelain or glass jars, bottles or earthware pots, each container with a lid on. No metal containers should be used but those made of stainless steel.

2.3.6 Cautions for Taking Medicated Liquor

1. Correct Administration

TCM lays stress on "diagnosis and treatment based on the differentiation of symptoms and signs", so does the administration of medicated liquor. Good healing power results from the correct choice of medicated liquor that suits one's specific constitution and the symptoms and signs observed through differentiation of deficiency and excessiveness, cold and heat, *Zang* and *Fu*, *Qi* and blood, and *Yin* and *Yang*. Any medicated liquor should be administrated according to its therapeutic effect and indications. And not everyone is fit for taking tonic liquor or longevity-enhancing liquor.

2. Contraindications and Dosage

Medicated liquor contains a certain amount of alcohol. Small amounts of alcohol intake will do one more good than harm. The findings of some researches show that small amount of liquor intake (less than 30 g a day) helps lessen the danger of death caused by coronary heart disease. It is suggested that for safety the amount of alcohol intake be controlled under 45 g per day. Prolonged heavy drinking will do harm to the liver, the heart and the nerve system, and even make the drinkers deformative. The hazards of overdrinking are dwelt on in our ancient medical works. For instance, the book *Ben Cao Gang Mu* points out, "Light drinking leads to invigorating *Qi* and blood, making one warm and in high spirits, dispelling sorrow and bringing about cheerfulness; while heavy drinking results in the impairment of essence, blood and the stomach, and the promotion of phlegm and fire. Indulgence in heavy drinking may cause one to be ill or degenerative, even to ruin his own family and nation, or to die of it. Aren't these hazards terrible?" So, it is important to bear in mind the dosage and contraindications of medicated liquor. Generally, medicated liquor is not advisable for those who suffer from liver diseases, severe heart diseases, cardiac insufficiency, peptic ulcer, active TB, chronic nephritis, chronic enteritis and severe hypertension; for children; for women in pregnancy and lactation; and for those who are allergic to alcohol. In addition, it is contraindicated, because of certain medicinal ingredients, for women to take medicated liquor during menstruation and for patients with excessive fire due to *Yin* deficiency. The dosage is determined in the light of the nature of medicated liquor, the constitutions of patients and the condition of the disease. The amount prescribed should not be exceeded. Special care should be taken in taking medicated liquor made up of drastic or toxic drugs, beginning with small amounts and gradually increasing the dosage when no side effects occur. Medicated liquor with mild nature can be taken in larger dosage. A larger dosage is also suitable for patients young and strong or in severe condition; while, small dosage for the aged, the weak, women or mild cases. Light drinkers take it in small amounts or take medicated liquor made of yellow rice liquor or liquor with small ratio of alcohol. Those who take it regularly for longevity take the tonic liquor also in small amounts.

3. Othe Precautions

The administration of medicated liquor is associated with the seasons. It is proper to take medicated liquor warm in nature, especially the tonic type, in winter, and the dosage should be reduced if taken in summer. The time of administration varies with the location of the disease. It is taken after meals if the disease is located above the diaphragm, while before meals if below it. It is advisable to take at night the medicated liquor for nourishing the heart and soothing the mind or for regulating men struation.

Medicated liquor should be stored hermetically in a cool and dry place.

2.3.7 Commonly Used Medicated Liquor

There has been a large variety of medicated liquor since ancient times. Here only some will be recommended with their advantages such as convenience of being made at home, reliable therapeutic effect, mild medicinal nature, readily available drug materials and simpler prescriptions. Most of the prescriptions are based on historical medical books or modern clinical reports. But some of them are readjusted in the light of the author's experience. Some of the prescriptions are made by the writers themselves.

1. Medicated Liquor for Tonifying *Qi*

(1) *Ren Shen Jiu*

Ingredients

Ren Shen (Radix Ginseng in the form of coarse powder)	30 g
Bai Jiu (Chinese white liquor)	500 g

Process

Cold-steeping or hot-steeping

Dosage and Administration

Taken twice daily, 10–15 ml each time, in the morning and evening.

Effect

Tonifying *Qi*, the spleen and lung, promoting the production of body fluid, soothing the mind.

Indications

Shortness of breath, lassitude, poor appetite, dizziness, palpitation, impairment of body fluid, spontaneous sweating, impotence, diabetes, all caused by *Qi* deficiency after a prolonged disease.

Notes

When the liquor is all drunk, the residus may be steeped a second time in proper amount of white liquor. The residue may be eaten finally.

(2) Shen Qi Yi Qi Jiu

Ingredients

Huang Qi (Radix Astragali)	45 g
Dang Shen(Radix Codonopsis)	45 g
Chen Pi (Pericarpium Citri Reticulatae)	9 g
Da Zao(Fructus Jujubae)	10 dates
Bai Jiu(Chinese white liquor)	1000 g

Process

Cold-steeping or hot-steeping

Dosage and Administration

Taken warm, twice daily, 10—20 ml each time, in the morning and evening.

Effect

Replenishing *Qi*, invigorating the spleen, inducing appetite and digestion.

Indications

Syndrome due to *Qi* deficiency, marked by lassitude, lanquor, poor appetite, etc.

Notes

This medicated liquor is mild in nature, it is not as potent as *Ren Shen Jiu*.

(3) San Sheng Jiu

Ingredients

Ren Shen(Radix Ginseng)	21 g
Shan Yao(Rhizoma Dioscoreae)	21 g
Bai Zhu(Rhizoma Atractylodis Macrocephalae)	21 g
Bai Jiu(Chinese white liquor)	500 g

Process

Cold-steeping or hot-steeping

Dosage and Administration

Taken warm on an empty stomach, three times a day in the morning, at noon and in the evening, 10-20ml each time.

Effect

Tonifying primordial *Qi*, strengthening the spleen and stomach.

Indicatiors

General debility, *Qi* deficiency, lassitude, anorexia, sallow complexion, emaciation.

Source

The book *Sheng Ji Zong Lu*

(4) *Huang Qi Sheng Mai Jiu*

Ingredients

Ren Shen (Radix Ginseng)	30 g
Huang Qi (Radix Astragali)	60 g
Mai Dong (Radix Ophiopogonis)	18 g
Wu Wei Zi (Fructus Schisandrae)	12 g
Bai Jiu (Chinese white liquor)	1000 g

Process

Cold-steeping or hot-steeping

Dosage and Administration

Taken in the morning and evening, 10-20 ml each time.

Effect

Tonifying primordial *Qi* with the effect of nourishing *Yin* and promoting the production of body fluid, consolidating superficial resistance to astringe perspiration.

Indications

Qi deficiency accompanied by impairment of body fluid due to *Yin* deficiency, such as *Yin* deficiency of the heart and lung marked by asthma, cough, spontaneous sweating, thirst, reddened and dry tongue with little coating, feeble pulse, or promordial *Qi* impaired by heat marked by shortness of breath, spontaneous sweating, thirst, reddish tongue with little coating, feeble pulse.

Notes

This prescription is based on the famous prescription of *Sheng Mai San,* to which *Huang Qi* is added so as to enhance the effect of replenishing *Qi* to consolidate superficial resistance.

(5) *Chang Sheng Gu Ben Jiu*

Ingredients

Ren Shen (Radix Ginseng)	60 g
Gou Qi Zi (Fructus Lycii)	60 g
Shan Yao (Rhizoma Dioscoreae)	60 g
Wu Wei Zi (Fructus Schisandrae)	60 g
Tian Dong (Radix Asparagi)	60 g
Mai Dong (Radix Ophiopogonis)	60 g
Sheng Di (Radix Rehmanniae)	60 g
Shu Di (Rhizoma Rehmanniae Praeparata)	60 g
Bai Jiu (Chinese white liquor)	1500 g

Preparation

All the herbs are cut into slices and put into a silk bag and steeped in the liquor within a container. The container is sealed up with indocalamus leaves and heated in water for half an hour and buried in the earth and kept there for a few days to expel the evil fire. Finally the liquor is filtered.

Dosage and Administration

Taken twice daily in the morning and evening, 10—20 ml each time.

Effect

Replenishing *Qi,* reinforcing *Yin,* nourishing the liver and kidney.

Indications

Syndrome due to deficiency of both *Qi* and *Yin,* marked by lassitude, soreness and weakness of the loins and legs, upset, dry mouth, dizziness, blurred vision, palpitation, dreamfulness, early—greying of hair, etc.

Source

The book *Shou Shi Bao Yuan*

Notes

The home—made type of this liquor may have lower amounts of the herbs and liquor and is prepared in cold—steeping or hot—steeping way.

2. **Medicated Liquor for Nourishing Blood**

(1)　*E Jiao Jiu*

Ingredients

E Jiao (Colla Corii Asini)	75 g
Huang Jiu (millet wine)	500 g

Preparation

E Jiao is cut into small pieces and put into a container, into which an appropriate amount of *Huang Jiu* is poured until *E Jiao* is totally immersed. The container is heated over mild fire while the rest *Huang Jiu* is added little by little until all the *Huang Jiu* is poured into the container and all the *E Jiao* is melted. Finally the container is cooled and the wine in it is put into a bottle.

Dosage and Administration

Taken Warm, on an empty stomach, in the morning, at noon and in the evening, 20—30 ml each time.

Effect

Tonifying blood, nourishing *Yin*, arresting bleeding, clearing away lung—heat, moistening dryness.

Indications

Deficiency of *Yin*—blood manifested as sallow complexion, dizziness, blurring of vision, palpitation, fidgeting, insomnia, dry cough due to *Yin* deficiency.

This wine is also used in the convalescence of women who have suffered such bleeding disorders as uterine bleeding, menorrhagia, vaginal bleeding during pregnancy, bleeding after miscarriage.

(2) *Long Yan Sang Shen Jiu*

Ingredients

Long Yan Rou (Arillus Longan)	30 g
Sang Shen (Fructus Mori)	30 g
Bai Jiu (Chinese white liquor)	500 g

Process

Cold—steeping

Dosage and Administration

Taken twice daily in the morning and evening, 10—20 ml each time.

Effect

Nourishing *Yin* and blood, tonifying the heart and spleen, soothing the mind, promoting the production of body fluid.

Indications

Deficiency of the blood, *Yin*, the heart and kidney, marked by dizziness, blurred vision, palpitation, insomnia, poor appetite, lassitude, forgetfulness, early-greying of hair, etc.

Notes

Bai Jiu may be substituted for *Huang Jiu* (millet wine or yellow rice wine) when it is prepared by cold-steeping. It may be prepared by brewing In this case *Bai Jiu* is replaced with round-grained non-glutinous rice and distiller's yeast.

The ingredients *Long Yan Rou* and *Sang Shen* are both dried fruit with the action of tonifying the heart and spleen and soothing the mind. Therefore, this liquor may be taken by the healthy.

(3) *Gui Yuan Jiu*

Ingredients

Ju Hua (Flos Chrysanthemi)	250 g
Gou Qi Zi (Fructus Lycii)	500 g
Dang Gui (Radix Angelicae Sinensis)	250 g
Long Yan Rou (Arillus Longan)	1500 g
Bai Jiu (Chinese white liquor)	15 kg
Jiu Niang (fermented glutinous rice)	5 kg

Process.

Cold-steeping or hot-steeping

Dosage and Admnistration

Taken twice in the morning and evening, 10-20 ml each time.

Effect

Nourishing blood and vital essence, tonifying the heart, spleen, liver and kidney, calming the mind, improving eyesight.

Indications

Deficiency of blood and vital essence, weakness of the heart, spleen, liver and kidney, sallow complexion, dizziness, blurring of vision, dim eyesight, palpitation, insomnia, general debility, amnesia, etc.

Source

The book *Ji Yan Liang Fang* and the book *Hui Zhi Tang Jing Yan Fang*, etc.

Notes

It is also called *Yang Sheng Jiu* and *Gui Yuan Qi Ju Jiu*. Its modification *Gui Yuan Xian Jiu* in the book *Shi Jian Ben Cao* consists of only *Dang Gui* and *Long Yan Rou,* having the special effect of tonifying the heart and blood.

(4)　*Yuan Rou Bu Xue Jiu*

Ingredients

Long Yan Rou(Arillus Longan)	250 g
Zhi Shou Wu(Radix Polygoni Multiflori Praeparata)	250 g
Ji Xue Teng (Caulis Spatholobi)	250 g
Mi Jiu (millet wine)	1500 g

Process

Cold—steeping

Dosage and Administration

Taken twice daily in the morning and evening, 10—20 ml each time.

Effect

Nourishing blood and vital essence, tonifying the liver, kidney, invigorating the heart, calming the mind, activating blood circulation, dredging the channels and collaterals.

Indications

Deficiency of the heart-blood, consumption of the liver and kidney, sallow complexion, dizziness, blurring of vision, palpitation, insomnia, early-greying of hair, etc.

(5) *Jiao Ai Jiu*

Ingredients

E Jiao (Colla Corii Asini)	30 g
Dang Gui (Radix Angelicae Sinensis)	30 g
Ai Ye (Folium Artemisiae Argyi)	9 g
Sheng Di (Radix Rehmanniae)	15 g
Chuan Xiong (Rhizoma Chuanxiong)	15 g
Bai Shao (Radix Paeoniae Alba)	21 g
Gan Cao (Radix Glycyrrhizae)	9 g
Huang Jiu (millet wine or yellow rice wine)	250 g

Preparation

Pour *Huang Jiu* into an earthen pot, into which 250 g of warm boiled water and the other coarsely ground ingredients except *E Jiao* are then put. Heat the pot over a mild fire until the content boils. Cool the pot, filter the residue out to get the medicated wine, which is then poured into a clean empty earthen pot. Put the small pieces of *E Jiao* into the pot and heat the pot over a mild fire. Keep stirring the content until *E Jiao* is all melted. This medicated wine is thus well-prepared.

Dosage and Administration

For medical treatment, the whole amount is taken on an empty stomach, three times daily in the morning, at noon and in the evening; for health care or adjustment in the convalescence, the dosage is reduced.

Effect

Nourishing the blood, promoting blood circulation, arresting bleeding, regulating menstruation, preventing miscarriage.

Indications

Hypermenorrhea due to deficiency of blood and impairment of *Chong* and *Ren* channels, metrorrhagia, metrastaxis, uterine bleeding during pregnancy, excessive fetal movement, or postpartum continuous bleeding.

Source

The book *Jin Kui Yao Lüe* and the book *Qian Jin Fang*. In the former it is used as a decoction; in the latter, as a medicated wine.

3. Medicated Liquor for Nourishing *Yin*

(1) *Nü Zhen Zi Jiu*

Ingredients

Nü Zhen Zi (Fructus Ligustri Lucidi)	90 g
Mi Jiu (millet wine)	500 g

Process

Cold-steeping

Dosage and Admnistration

Taken on an empty stomach, twice daily in the morning and evening, 20 ml each time.

Effect

Nourishing *Yin*-blood, tonifying the liver and kidney, clearing away heat of deficiency type, strengthening the tendons and bones, darkening hair, improving eyesight.

Indications

Yin deficiency of the liver and kidney, dizziness, blurring of vision, dim eyesight, soreness and weakness of the loins and knees, weakness of the tendons and bones, early-greying of hair, etc.

Notes

The book *Yi Bian* says that this wine also has the action of prolonging life.

(2)　*Er Dong Jiu*

Ingredients

Tian Dong (Radix Asparagi)	60 g
Mai Dong (Radix Ophiopogonis)	60 g
Mi Jiu (millet wine)	500 g

Process

Cold-steeping

Dosage and Administration

Taken on an empty stomach, twice daily in the morning and evening, 20-30 ml each time.

Effect

Nourishing *Yin*, removing heat from the lung, tonifying the kidney, invigorating the stomach, clearing away heart-fire, eliminating fidgeting, promoting the production of body fluid, moisturizing dryness.

Indications

Cough due to lung-dryness, thick sputum, hemoptysis, thirst due to deficiency of body fluid, fidgeting, constipation, etc.

(3)　*Yin Er Xiang Gu Jiu*

Ingredients

Yin Er (Tremella)	30 g
Xiang Gu (Lentinus Edodes)	30 g

Mi Jiu (millet wine)   500 g

Process

Hot—steeping with an adequate amount of crystal sugar

Dosage and Administration

Taken on an empty stomach, three times daily in the morning, at noon and in the evening, 20 ml each time.

Effect

Nourishing *Yin*, replenishing *Qi*, moistening the lung, invigorating the stomach.

Indications

With its mild effect, it is good for middle-age and old people with general debility, especially good for those with the syndrome of *Yin* deficiency and weakened *Qi*. It also serves as an adjuvant treatment for *Yin* deficiency due to lung-heat, cough, hemoptysis, and tumor.

Notes

The extracts from of Bai *Mu Er* and *Xiang Gu* have the action of promoting immunity, resisting cancer and reducing blood-fat.

(4) *Gou Qi Yao Jiu*

Main Ingredients

Gou Qi Zi (Fructus Lycii)

Shu Di Huang (Rhizoma Rehmanniae Praeparata)

Huang Jing (Rhizoma Polygonati)

Bai He (Bulbus Lilii)

Yuan Zhi (Radix Polygalae)

Bai Jiu (Chinese white liquor)

Dosage and Administration

Taken warm, 2-3 times daily, 10-15 ml each time.

Effect

Nourishing the kidney, benefiting the liver.

Indications

Deficiency of the liver and kidney, general debility, emaciation, soreness and weakness of the loins and legs, insomnia, copos in the aged, etc.

This liquor is produced by pharmaceutical factories.

(5) *Yang Shen Gu Ben Jiu*

Ingredients

Xi Yang Shen (Radix Panacis Quinquefolii)	21 g
Tian Dong (Radix Asparagi)	30 g
Mai Dong (Radix Ophiopogonis)	30 g
Sheng Di (Radix Rehmanniae)	30 g
Shu Di (Rhizoma Rehmanniae Praeparata)	30 g
Bai Jiu (Chinese white liquor)	1500 g

Process

Hot-steeping, heat the content through boiling water for a longer time.

Dosage and Administration

Taken on an empty stomach, twice daily in the morning and evening, 10—20 ml each time.

Effect

Nourishing *Yin*, replenishing *Qi*, tonifying vital essence and blood.

Indications

Syndrome due to consumption of *Yin*, deficiency of *Qi* and exhaustion of vital essence, marked by emaciation, listlessness, hectic fever, fidgeting, dry mouth and throat, shortness of breath, dry cough, soreness and weakness of the loins and knees, sallow complexion, early-greying of hair, sterility due to deficiency of essence, etc.

Notes

This prescription is the modification of the prescription of *Ren Shen Gu Ben Wan* recorded in the book *Rui Zhu Tang Jiug Yan Fang*, in which *Ren Shen* is replaced with *Xi Yang Shen* for the purpose of strengthening the action of nourishing *Yin*. The book considers *Ren Shen Gu Ben Wan* to have the effect of keeping hair black, face bright and life longer.

(6) *Chun Shou Jiu*

Ingredients

Tian Dong (Radix Asparagi)	30 g
Mai Dong (Radix Ophiopogonis)	30 g
Shu Di (Rhizoma Rehmanniae Praeparata)	30 g
Sheng Di (Radix Rehmanniae)	30 g
Shan Yao (Rhizoma Dioscoreae)	30 g
Lian Zi Rou (Semen Nelumbinis)	30 g
Da Zao (Fructus Jujubae)	30 g
Jiu (liquor)	2500 g

Process

Hot-steeping

Dosage and Administration

Taken on an empty stomach, twice daily in the morning and evening, 20 ml each time.

Effect

Nourishing *Yin*-blood, invigorating the kidney, strengthening the spleen.

Indications

Syndrome due to deficiency of *Yin*-essence and weakness of

the spleen and kidney, marked by sallow complexion, early-greying of hair, dry mouth and throat, fidgeting, poor appetite, weak limbs, lassitude, etc.

Source

The book *Wan Shi Jia Chuan Yang Sheng Si Yao*

Notes

Compared with *Yang Shen Gu Ben Jiu*, this liquor has the stronger effect of invigorating the kidney and strengthening the spleen but the less strong effect of nourishing *Yin* and replenishing *Qi*.

(7) Gu Jing Jiu

Ingredients

Gou Qi Zi (Fructus Lycii)	120 g
Dang Gui (Radix Angelicae Sinensis)	60 g
Shu Di (Rhizoma Rehmanniae Praeparata)	180 g
Bai Jiu or *Huang Jiu* (Chinese white liquor or yellow rice wine)	3000 g

Process

Hot-steeping. Heat the content through boiling water for a longer time.

Dosage and Administration

Taken on an empty stomach, twice daily in the morning and evening, 20 ml each time.

Effect

Nourishing *Yin*, replenishing vital essence, enriching the blood, tonifying the liver and kidney.

Indications

Syndrome due to deficiency of *Yin*, blood and vital essence, marked by dizziness, blurring of vision, dim eyesight, soreness and weakness of the loins and knees, early-greying of hair, emission, prospermia, male-sterility, etc.

Source

The book *Hui Zhi Tang Jing Yan Fang*

4. Medicated Liquor for Supporting *Yang*

(1) *Xian Ling Pi Jiu*

Ingredients

Yin Yang Huo (Herba Epimedii)	60 g
Bai Jiu or *Huang Jiu* (Chinese white liquor or yellow rice wine)	500 g

Process

Cold-steeping

Dosage and Administration

Taken on an empty stomach, twice daily in the morning and evening, 10—15 ml each time.

Effect

Strengthening *Yang*, invigorating the kidney, tonifying the liver, enhancing the tendons and bones, dispelling wind and dampness.

Indications

Syndrome due to deficiency of the kidney-*Yang*, marked by impotence, female sterility, soreness and weakness of the loins and knees, aversion to cold, lassitude, numbness of the limbs, stiffness of the muscles and tendons, rheumatic pain, etc.

(2) *Ge Jie Jiu*

Ingredients

Ge Jie (Gecko)	1 pair
Huang Jiu (millet or yellow rice wine)	1000 g

Cut *Ge Jie* without head and leg into small pieces and steep the pieces in *Huang Jiu*.

Dosage and Administration

Taken on an empty stomach, twice daily in the morning and evening, 10—20 ml each time.

Effect

Reinforcing the kidney—*Yang*, supplementing the lung—*Qi*, replenishing vital essence and blood, relieving cough and asthma.

Indications

Impotence due to deficiency of the kidney—*Yang*, asthma due to deficiency of the kidney, cough due to deficiency of the lung, asthma and cough due to consumption of deficiency type, weakened *Yang*—*Qi* due to prolonged diseases, lassitude, shortness of breath, etc.

(3) *Lu Rong Jiu*

Ingredients

Lu Rong (Cornu Cervi Pantotrichum)	9 g
Shan Yao (Rhizoma Dioscoreae)	30 g
Bai Jiu (Chinese white liquor)	500 g

Process

Cold—steeping

Dosage and Administration

Taken on an empty stomach, twice daily in the morning and evening, 10—15 ml each time.

Effect

Supplementing the kidney—*Yang*, replenishing vital essence and blood, strengthening the tendons and bones, regulating *Chong* and *Ren* channels.

Indications

Lassitude due to deficiency of Yang and essence, weakness of the limbs, dizziness, blurring of vision, deafness, amnesia, impotence, coldness and dampness of scrotum, emission, enuresis, thin leukorrhea, sterility due to coldness in the womb, etc.

Source

The book *Pu Ji Fang*

(4)　*Fu Fang Lu Rong Chong Cao Jiu*

Ingredients

Lu Rong (Cornu Cervi Pantotrichum)	6 g
Dong Chong Xia Cao (Cordyceps)	30 g
Gou Qi Zi (Fructus Lycii)	30 g
Bai Jiu (Chinese white liquor)	500 g

Process

Cold—steeping

Dosage and Administration

Taken on an empty stomach, twice daily in the morning and evening, 10—15 ml each time.

Effect

Similar to those of *Lu Rong Jiu* in addition to the strong points of tonifying the lung, liver and kidney, relieving asthma and cough, and removing sputum.

Indications

Phlegm—retention, asthma and cough due to deficiency of the lung and kidney. The others are the same as those of *Lu Rong Jiu*.

(5)　*Yang Shen Er Xian Jiu*

Ingredients

Yang Gao Wan (goat testis)	1 pair
Yin Yang Huo (Herba Epimedii)	150 g

Xian Mao (Rhizoma Curculiginis)   150 g
Gou Qi Zi (Fructus Lycii)   150 g
Tu Si Zi (Semen Cuscutae)   150 g
Bai Jiu (Chinese white liquor)   10 kg

Process

Cold-steeping

Dosage and Administration

Taken on an empty stomach, twice daily in the morning and evening, 10 ml each time.

Effect

Enhancing *Yang*, tonifying the kidney, invigorating the liver, strengthening the tendons and bones.

Indications

General debility due to deficiency of *Yang*, deficiency of the liver and kidney, lassitude, aversion to cold, soreness and weakness of the loins and knees, weakness of the muscles and tendons, impotence, cold sperm, steribility due to coldness in the womb, etc.

(6) *San Bian Bu Jiu*

Main Ingredients

Hai Gou Bian (Peniet Testes Callorhini)

Mei Lu Bian (Peniet Testes Cervi)

Guang Gou Bian (Peniet Testes Canini)

Ren Shen (Radix Ginseng)

Lu Rong (Cornu Cervi Pantotrichum)

Da Hai Ma (Hippocampus)

Ge Jie (Gecko)

Shang Rou Gui (Cortex Cinnamomi)

Shang Chen Xiang (Lignum Aquilariae Resinatum)

Fei Yang Qi Shi (Actinolitum)
Wu Hua Long Gu (Os Draconis)
Fu Pen Zi (Fructus Rubi)
Bu Gu Zhi (Fructus Psoraleae)
Tu Si Zi (Semen Cuscutae)
Yin Yang Huo (Herba Epimedii)
He Shou Wu (Radix Polygoni Multiflori)
Sang Piao Xiao (Oötheca Mantidis)
Ba Ji Tian (Radix Morindae Officinalis)
Shan Yu Rou (Fructus Corni)
Dan Pi (Cortex Moutan)
Huang Qi (Radix Astragali)
Niu Xi (Radix Achyranthis Bidentatae)
Qi Guo (Fructus Lycii)
Sheng Di (Radix Rehmanniae)
Shu Di (Rhizoma Rehmanniae Praeparata)
Huang Bai (Cortex Phellodendri)
Chuan Jiao (Pericarpium Zanthoxyli)
Hang Shao (Radix Paeoniae Alba)
Dang Gui (Radix Angelicae Sinensis)
Bai Zhu (Rhizoma Atractylodis Macrocephalae)
Yun Ling (Poria)
Rou Cong Rong (Herba Cistanchis)
Ze Xie (Rhizoma Alismatis)
Chang Pu (Rhizoma Acori Tatarinowii)
Xiao Hui Xiang (Fructus Foeniculi)
Gan Song (Rhizoma Nardostachyos)
Shan Yao (Rhizoma Dioscoreae)
Du Zhong (Cortex Eucommiae)

Yuan Zhi (Radix Polygalae)
Gao Liang Jiu (Chinese white liquor made of sorghum)

Dosage and Administration

Taken orally, twice daily, 30 ml each time.

Effect

Promoting the generation of vital essence, enriching the blood, strengthening the brain, tonifying the kidney.

Indications

General debility, early senility, soreness in the loins and back, dizziness due to anemia, spontaneous sweating, night sweating, pallor, emission due to deficiency of the kidney, neurosism, overtaxation of the brain, palpitation, amnesia, aversion to cold, insomnia, anorexia due to *Qi* deficiency, etc.

Manufacturer

Yantai Pharmaceutical Factory of Traditional Chinese Medicines in Shandong Province

Notes

It is a good tonic of high quality. Regular intake of it can build up health, prevent disease, slow down the process of ageing and prolong life.

(7) *Dong Bei San Bao Jiu*

Main Ingredients

Ren Shen (Radix Ginseng)
Lu Rong (Cornu Cervi Pantotrichum)
Diao Bian (Peniet Testes Martes)

Dosage and Administration

Taken twice daily, 10—30 ml each time.

Effect

Warming the kidney, reinforcing *Yang*, replenishing *Qi*,

strengthening the brain

Indications

Syndrome due to deficiency of the kidney—*Yang*, marked by impotence, premature ejaculation, soreness and weakness of the loins and knees, cold and damp feeling of scrotum.

Manufacturer

Jilin Pharmaceutical Factory of Traditional Chinese Medicines

(8) *Qiong Jiang*

Main Ingredients

Ren Shen (Radix Ginseng)

Lu Rong (Cornu Cervi Pantotrichum)

Long Yan Rou (Arillus Longan)

Chen Pi (Pericarpium Citri Reticulatae)

Gou Ji (Rhizoma Cibotii)

Gou Qi Zi (Fructus Lycii)

Bu Gu Zhi (Fructus Psoraleae)

Huang Jing (Rhizoma Polygonati)

Jin Ying Zi (Fructus Rosae Laevigatae)

Yin Yang Huo (Herba Epimedii)

Dong Chong Xia Cao (Cordyceps)

Huai Niu Xi (Radix Achyranthis Bidentatae)

Ling Zhi (Ganoderma Lucidum seu Japonicum)

Dang Gui (Radix Angelicae Sinensis)

Fo Shou (Fructus Citri Sarcodactylis)

Que Nao (Sparrow brains)

Dosage and Administration

Taken 2—3 times daily, 9—15 ml each time.

Effect

Warming the kidney, reinforcing Yang, nourishing *Qi* and blood.

Indications

General debility, lassitude, soreness and weakness of the loins and limbs, impotence, emission, prospermia, etc.

Manufacturer

Beijing Pharmaceutical Factory of Traditional Chinese Medicines

5. Medicated Liquor for Tonifying both *Qi* and Blood

(1) *Qi Gui Shuang Bu Jiu*

Ingredients

Huang Qi (Radix Astragali)	30 g
Dang Shen (Radix Codonopsis)	30 g
Dang Gui (Radix Angelicae Sinensis)	30 g
Long Yan Rou (Arillus Longan)	30 g
Sang Shen Zi (Fructus Mori)	30 g
Chen Pi (Pericarpium Citri Reticulatae)	9 g
Bai Jiu or *Huang Jiu* (white liquor or millet wine)	1500 g

Process

Hot / cold—steeping

Dosage and Administration

Taken on an empty stomach, twice daily in the morning and evening, 10—20 ml each time.

Effect

Replenishing *Qi*, tonifying the blood, nourishing the heart, strengthening the stomach.

Indications

Listlessness, sallow complexion, lassitude, shortness of

breath, languor, dizziness, blurring of vision, palpitations, amnesia, poor appetite, etc.

(2) *Ba Zhen Jiu*

Ingredients

Ren Shen (Radix Ginseng)	9 g
Fu Ling (Poria)	21 g
Bai Zhu (Rhizoma Atractylodis Macrocephalae)	21 g
Dang Gui (Radix Angelicae Sinensis)	21 g
Bai Shao (Radix Paeoniae Alba)	21 g
Shu Di (Rhizoma Rehmanniae Praeparata)	24 g
Chuan Xiong (Rhizoma Chuanxiong)	12 g
Gan Cao (Radix Glycyrrhizae)	9 g
Sheng Jiang (Rhizoma Zingiberis Recens)	9 g
Da Zao (Fructus Jujubae)	10 dates
Bai Jiu or *Huang Jiu* (white liquor or millet wine)	3000 g

Process

Hot—steeping

Dosage and Administration

Taken on an empty stomach, twice daily in the morning and evening, 10—15 ml each time.

Effect

Tonifying *Qi* and blood, strengthening the spleen, activating blood circulation.

Indications

Similar to that of *Qi Gui Shuang Bu Jiu*, such as deficiency of the spleen and stomach, insufficiency of *Qi* and blood, consumption of the heart and lung, etc.

Notes

Dang Shen (Radix Codonopsis Pilosulae) may be used to replace Ren Shen .the dosage being 30g.

(3) **Shi Quan Da Bu Jiu**

Ingredients

Huang Qi (Radix Astragali)	45 g
Dang Shen (Radix Codonopsis Pilosulae)	45 g
Fu Ling (Poria)	30 g
Bai Zhu (Rhizoma Atractylodis Macrocephalae)	30 g
Shu Di (Rhizoma Rehmanniae Praeparata)	45 g
Dang Gui (Radix Angelicae Sinensis)	30 g
Bai Shao (Radix Paeoniae Alba)	30 g
Chuan Xiong (Rhizoma Chuanxiong)	15 g
Rou Gui (Cortex Cinnamomi)	15 g
Gan Cao (Radix Glycyrrhizae)	15 g
Bai Jiu (Chinese white liquor)	5000 g

Process

Cold / hot–steeping

Dosage and Administration

Taken on an empty stomach, twice daily in the morning and evening, 10–15 ml each time.

Effect

Warm in nature, this liquor has a stonger tonifying effect than Ba Zhen Jiu.

Indications

Syndrome due to deficiency of Qi and blood and with the symptoms of Yin–cold type.

6. **Medicated Liquor for Tonifying Yin and Yang**

(1) Chong Cao Jiu

Ingredients

Dong Chong Xia Cao (Cordyceps)	30 g
Bai Jiu (Chinese white liquor)	500 g

Process

Cold-steeping

Dosage and Administration

Taken on an empty stomach, twice daily in the morning and evening, 10−20 ml each time. The residue is retained and more liquor is added for a second steeping.

Effect

Tonifying not only the kidney-*Yang* but also the lung-*Yin* with the effect of arresting bleeding, eliminating phlegm, and relieving asthma and cough.

Indications

General debility in the convalescence, listlessness, lassitude, poor appetite, or spontaneous sweating and aversion to cold; impotence, emission, soreness and weakness of the loins and knees, or prolonged cough, asthma of deficiency type, hemotysis due to consumptive diseases. This liquor is used either for health care or for an adjuvant treatment.

(2) *Er Xian Jiu*

Ingredients

Xian Mao (Rhizoma Curculiginis)	30 g
Yin Yang Huo (Herba Epimedii)	30 g
Ba Ji Tian (Radix Morindae Officinalis)	30 g
Dang Gui (Radix Angelicae Sinensis)	30 g
Huang Bai (Cortex Phellodendri)	21 g
Zhi Mu (Rhizoma Anemarrhenae)	30 g
Bai Jiu (Chinese white liquor)	2000 g

Process

Cold-steeping

Dosage and Administration

Taken on an empty stomach, three times daily in the morning, at noon and in tne evening, 10-20 ml each time.

Effect

Tonifying the kidney-*Yang*, nourishing the kidney-*Yin*, clearing away kidney-fire, regulating *Chong* and *Ren* channels.

Indications

Climacteric hypertension, climacteric syndrome, irregular menstruation, amenorrhea, other chronic diseases with the symptoms of flaming-up of deficiency-fire due to deficiency of both *Yin* and *Yang*.

(3) Zi Yin Bai Bu Yao Jiu

Ingredients

Shu Di (Rhizoma Rehmanniae Praeparata)	90 g
Sheng Di (Radix Rehmanniae)	90 g
Zhi Shou Wu (Radix Polygoni Multiflori Praeparata)	90 g
Gou Qi Zi (Fructus Lycii)	90 g
Sha Yuan Zi (Semen Astragali Complanati)	90 g
Lu Jiao Jiao (Colla Cornus Cervi)	90 g
Dang Gui (Radix Angelicae Sinensis)	75 g
Hu Tao Rou (Semen Juglandis)	75 g
Long Yan Rou (Arillus Longan)	75 g
Rou Cong Rong (Herba Cistanchis)	60 g
Bai Shao (Radix Paeoniae Alba)	60 g
Ren Shen (Radix Ginseng)	60 g
Niu Xi (Radix Achyranthis Bidentatae)	60 g
Bai Zhu (Rhizoma Atractylodis Macrocephalae)	60 g

Yu Zhu (Rhizoma Polygonati Odorati)	60 g
Gui Ban Jiao (Colla Carapacis et Plastri Testudinis)	60 g
Bai Ju Hua (Flos Chrysanthemi)	60 g
Wu Jia Pi (Cortex Acanthopanacis)	60 g
Huang Qi (Radix Astragali)	45 g
Suo Yang (Herba Cynomorii)	45 g
Du Zhong (Cortex Eucommiae)	45 g
Di Gu Pi (Cortex Lycii Radicis)	45 g
Dan Pi (Cortex Moutan)	45 g
Zhi Mu (Rhizoma Anemarrhenae)	45 g
Huang Bai (Cortex Phellodendri)	30 g
Rou Gui (Cortex Cinnamomi)	30 g

Preparation

Break up all the above into coarse powder and wrap the powder in a silk bag. Put the bag in a jar, into which an appropriate amount of warm liquor (about 25–30 kg) is then poured. Seal the jar and let it stand for 15–20 days to have the herbs steeped. Filter the liquor out for use with the bag remaining in the jar. Add 7.5–10 kg of liquor to the jar for a second steeping.

Dosage and Administration

Taken warm, on an empty stomach, twice daily in the morning and evening, 10–20 ml each time.

Effect

Invigorating *Yin*, reinforcing *Yang*, nourishing blood, replenishing vital essence, supplementing *Qi*, tonifying the Five–*Zang*, strengthening the tendons and bones.

Indications

Syndrome due to deficiency of both *Yin* and *Yang*, Source The book *Lin Shi Huo Ren Lu Hui Bian*

7. Medicated Liquor for Tonifying the Five—Zang

As is stated, medicated liquors introduced above have the effect of benefiting one or more than one organs. Medicated liquor for tonifying the five—organs is also effective for tonifying and regulating *Qi* and blood, *Yin* and *Yang*.

(1) *Fu Ling Jiu*

Ingredients

Fu Ling (Poria)	60 g
Bai Jiu (Chinese white liquor)	500 g

Process

Cold—steeping

Dosage and Administration

Taken on an empty tomach, three times daily, before breakfast, lunch ,and supper or before bed time, 10—20 ml each time.

Effect

Strengthening the spleen, restoring *Qi,* nourishing the heart, calming the mind.

Indications

General debility due to deficiency of the spleen, anorexia, lassitude, muscular numbness, emaciation, palpitation, insomnia, etc.

(2) *Shen Xian Yao Jiu Wan*

Ingredients

Mu Xiang (Radix Aucklandiae)	9 g
Ding Xiang (Flos Caryophylli)	6 g
Tan Xiang (Lignum Santali)	6 g
Qian Cao (Radix Rubiae)	60 g
Sha Ren (Fructus Amomi)	15 g
Hong Qu (Monascus Purpureus Went)	30 g

Preparation

Grind the above ingredients into fine powder and make the powder into boluses with honey, each weighing 9g. 1–3 boluses are steeped in 500g of white liquor

Dosage and Administration

Taken in an appropriate amount each time.

Effect

Strengthening the spleen, checking upward adverse flow of the lung or the stomach–*Qi*, promoting digestion, relieving stuffiness of the chest.

Indications

Weakness of the spleen and stomach, anorexia, fullness in the stomach after meals.

Source

The book *Qing Tai Yi Yuan Pei Fang*

Notes

Qian Cao is used in large dose for the purpose of turning the liquor reddish. In practice, its dose may be reduced.

(3) *Yang Xin An Shen Jiu*

Ingredients

Long Yan Rou (Arillus Longan)	30 g
Suan Zao Ren (Semen Ziziphi Spinosae)	30 g
Fu Shen (Poria cum Ligno Hospite)	30 g
Bai Zi Ren (Semen Biotae)	15 g
Wu Wei Zi (Fructus Schisandrae)	15 g
Mai Dong (Radix Ophiopogonis)	15 g
Bai Jiu (Chinese white liquor)	2000 g

Process

Cold–steeping

Dosage and Administration

Taken three times daily, 10 ml in the morning and at noon, 20 ml before bed time.

Effect

Nourishing the heart, calming the mind, enriching *Yin*, tonifying the blood.

Indications

Palpitation, irritability, insomnia, dreamfulness, lassitude, amnesia, etc., all due to deficiency of *Yin*—blood and weakness of the heart and mind.

(4) Shen Ge Chong Cao Jiu

Ingredients

Ren Shen (Radix Ginseng)	30 g
Ge Jie (Gecko with the head and legs removed)	a pair
Dong Chong Xia Cao (Cordyceps)	30 g
Hu Tao Ren (Semen Juglandis)	30 g
Bai Jiu (Chinese white liquor)	2 kg

Process

Cold—steeping

Dosage and Administration

Taken warm, on an empty stomach, twice daily in the morning and evening, 10—20 ml each time.

Effect

Tonifying the lung and kidney, reinforcing *Yang-Qi*, supplementing vital essence and blood, activating inspiration and relieving asthma.

Indications

Deficiency and weakness of *Yang-Qi*, general debility due to prolonged disease, listlessness, lassitude, amnesia, insomnia, soreness and weakness of the loins and knees, asthma and cough of deficiency type, etc.

(5) *Fu Fang Hai Ma Jiu*

Ingredients

Hai Ma (Hippocampus)	a pair
Ming Xia (shrimp)	30 g
Yin Yang Huo (Herba Epimedii)	15 g
Bai Jiu(Chinese white liquor)	500 g

Process

Hot / cold—steeping

Dosage and Administration

Taken twice daily in the morning and evening, 10—20 ml each time.

Effect

Tonifying the kidney, supporting *Yang*, strengthening the tendons and bones, promoting digestion, regulating *Qi*.

Indications

Impotence due to deficiency of the kidney—*Yang*, listlessness, lassitude, inappetence, shortness of breath, soreness and weakness of the loins and knees, frequent night—urination, etc.

(6) *Shou Wu Qi Ju Jiu*

Ingredients

He Shou Wu (Radix Polygoni Multiflori)	30 g
Gou Qi Zi (Fructus Lycii)	30 g
Ju Hua (Flos Chrysanthemi)	30 g
Dang Gui (Radix Angelicae Sinensis)	21 g
Long Yan Rou(Arillus Longan)	21 g
Hu Ma Ren (Semen Canabis)	30 g
Bai Jiu (Chinese white liquor)	2000 g

Process

Hot / cold-steeping

Dosage and Administration

Taken twice daily in morning and evening, on an empty stomach, 10—20 ml each time.

Effect

Tonifying and nourishing the liver, kidney, vital essence and blood, improving eyesight, calming the mind, slowing down the process of ageing.

Indications

Dizziness, blurring of vision, dim eyesight, listlessness, weakness of the loins and knees, early-greying of hair, emission, morbid leuckorrhea, amnesia, palpitation, all due to deficiency of the liver, kidney, vital essence and blood.

(7) *Bu Xue Shun Qi Yao Jiu*

Ingredients

Tian Dong (Radix Asparagi)	120 g
Mai Dong (Radix Ophiopogonis)	120 g
Sheng Di (Radix Rehmanniae)	250 g
Shu Di (Rhizoma Rehmanniae Praeparata)	250 g
Ren Shen (Radix Ginseng)	60 g
Fu Ling (Poria)	60 g
Gou Qi Zi (Fructus Lycii)	60 g
Sha Ren (Fructus Amomi)	21 g
Mu Xiang (Radix Aucklandiae)	15 g
Chen Xiang (Lignum Aquilariae Resinatum)	9 g

Preparation

Grind the above into coarse powder and put the powder into a silk bag. Put the bag into a porcelain jar with 15 kg of white liquor. Boil the jar in water until the liquor boils and then continue the heating with a mild heat for half an hour until the liquor turns dark. Cool the jar and let it stand for a few days. Finally, remove the liquor for use.

Dosage and Administration

Taken on an empty stomach, twice daily in the morning and evening, 10—20 ml each time.

Effect

Invigorating *Qi*, tonifying blood, nourishing *Yin*, regulating and supplementing the five organs, strengthening the stomach, promoting the flow of *Qi*.

Indications

Listlessness, pale complexion, lassitude, languor with no desire for speaking, early-greying of hair, dizziness, blurring of vision, weakness of the loins and knees, poor appetite, amnesia, palpitation, etc., all due to weakness of the five *Zang* and deficiency of *Qi* and blood.

8. Medicated Liquor for Prolonging Life

This kind of medicated liquor acts in delaying ageing to prolong life usually by harmonizing *Yin* and *Yang*, tonifying *Qi* and the blood, and nourishing the five *Zang* organs. Some of the liquors introduced above are also effective in slowing down the process of becoming senile if taken regularly.

In the following are some of medicated liquors for prolonging life.

(1) *Bai Sui Jiu*

Ingredients

Mi Zhi Huang Qi (honeyed Radix Astragali)	60 g
Fu Shen (Poria cum Ligno Hospite)	60 g

Dang Gui (Radix Angelicae Sinensis)	36 g
Shu Di (Rhizoma Rehmanniae Praeparata)	36 g
Sheng Di (Radix Rehmanniae)	36 g
Dang Shen (Radix Codonopsis)	30 g
Mai Dong (Radix Ophiopogonis)	30 g
Fu Ling (Poria)	30 g
Bai Zhu (Rhizoma Atractylodis Macrocephalae)	30 g
Zao Pi (Fructus Corni)	30 g
Chuan Xiong (Rhizoma Chuanxiong)	30 g
Gui Ban Jiao (Colla Carapacis et Plastri Testudinis)	30 g
Fang Feng (Radix Saposhinkoviae)	30 g
Gou Qi (Fructus Lycii)	30 g
Chen Pi (Pericarpium Citri Reticulatae)	30 g
Wu Wei Zi (Fructus Schisandrae)	24 g
Qiang Huo (Rhizoma seu Radix Notopterygii)	24 g
Rou Gui (Cortex Cinnamomi)	18 g
Hong Zao (Fructus Jujubae)	1000 g
Bing Tang (crystal sugar)	1000 g
Gao Liang Jiu (sorghum liquor)	10 kg

Preparation

Put the above into a porcelain pot and boil the pot in water for a period of time in which a joss stick is burned up (about two hours) or bury the pot in earth and let it stay there for 7 days, the latter method being better. After that filter the liquor out for use.

Dosage and Administration

Taken in an adequate amount each time.

Effect

Tonifying *Qi* and the blood, nourishing *Yin*-essence,

strengthening the kidney—fire, promoting the flow of *Qi*, dispelling wind, reinforcing the five—*Zang* organs, blackening hair, brightening the face, prolonging life.

Indications

Deafness, decline of eyesight, grey hair, pale complexion, disorders in the aged, middle—aged and weak.

Source

The book *Yao Fang Za Lu*

Notes

The book says, "The prescription was called *Zhou Gong Bai Sui Jiu*, which had been obtained in the north of China. Because of taking this medicated liquor, no one among the three generations of Zhou's died before 70, and Zhou Weng himself reached the age of over 100 by taking this liquor for 40 years."

(2) Yan Shou Jiu Xian Jiu

Ingredients

Ren Shen (Radix Ginseng)	60 g
Chao Bai Zhu (parched Rhizoma Atractylodis Macrocephalae)	60 g
Fu Ling (Poria)	60 g
Chao Gan Cao (Parched Radix Glycyrrhizae)	60 g
Dang Gui (Radix Angelicae Sinensis)	60 g
Chuan Xiong (Rhizoma Chuanxiong)	60 g
Shu Di (Rhizoma Rehmanniae Praeparata)	60 g
Chao Bai Shao (Radix Paeoniae Alba parched with liquor)	60 g
Gou Qi Zi (Fructus Lycii)	250 g
Sheng Jiang (Rhizoma Zingiberis Recens)	60 g
Da Zao (Fructus Jujubae with the core removed)	30 dates

Bai Jiu (high-quality white liquor)	17.5 kg

Process

Hot-steeping

Dosage and Administration

Taken in an adequate amount at any time.

Effect

Tonifying *Qi* and the blood, invigorating the liver and kidney.

Indications

Deficiency of *Qi* and blood, weakness of the liver and kidney.

Source

The book *Ming Yi Xuan Yao Ji Shi Qi Fang*

Notes

The book says, this liquor has the effect of "treating all disorders due to deficiency and consumption and restoring one's youthful vigor". It is, in fact, made up of *Ba Zhen Tang* plus *Gou Qi Zi*. *Gou Qi Zi* itself steeped in liquor has the action of restoring *Qi*, brightening complexion, etc. Large dose of it makes this liquor more potent and more effective than *Ba Zhen Jiu*, with the additional effect of prolonging life and resisting senility.

(3)　*Liao Bai Ji Yan Shou Jiu*

Ingredients

Huang Jing (Rhizoma Polygonati)	60 g
Tian Dong (Radix Asparagi)	45 g
Song Ye (Folium Pini)	90 g
Cang Zhu (Rhizoma Atractylodis)	60 g
Gou Qi Zi (Fructus Lycii)	75 g
Bai Jiu (Chinese white liquor)	5 kg

Dosage and Administration

Taken twice daily in the morning and evening, 10-20 ml each time.

Effect

Nourishing the kidney, moistening the lung, replenishing the liver, tonifying the spleen, enriching *Yin*-essence, invigorating the heart-*Qi*, improving eyesight, removing wind and dampness, strengthening the tendons and bones.

Indications

Lassitude, decline of appetite, dizziness, dim-eyesight, stiff muscles and joints, restlessness, insomnia, early-greying of hair, etc., all due to weakness of all the *Zang*-organs and deficiency of *Yin*-essence.

Source

The book *Zhong Zang Jing*

Notes

This is a milder medicated liquor for prolonging life.

(4)　*Jing Shen Yao Jiu*

Ingredients

Ren Shen (Radix Ginseng)	15 g
Sheng Di (Radix Rehmanniae)	15 g
Gou Qi Zi (Fructus Lycii)	15 g
Yin Yang Huo (Herba Epimedii)	9 g
Sha Yuan Zi (Semen Astragali Complanati)	9 g
Mu Ding Xiang (Fructus Eugenia Caryophyllata)	9 g
Chen Xiang (Lignum Aquilariae Resinatum)	3 g
Yuan Zhi Rou (Radix Polygalae)	3 g

Li Zhi He (Semen Litchi)	7 pieces
Gao Liang Jiu (sorghum liquor)	1 kg

Process

Cold-steeping for 45 days

Dosage and Administration

Once daily. take 10 ml by sipping.

Effect

Replenishing *Qi*, reinforcing, *Yang*, nourishing *Yin*, invigorating the liver and kidney, strengthening the spleen and stomach, calming the mind, improving intelligence, dispelling cold, relieving pain, restoring energy of the aged and middle-aged, slowing down the process of ageing.

Notes

This medicated liquor was developed by the famous contemporary TCM-physician Wu Zhaoxian, introduced in the Sichuan Journal of TCM by his student.

9. Medicated Liquor for Preventing Diseases

Here is a brief introduction to several medicated liquors which are commonly used for prevention, as an adjuvant, or in the convalescence. Medicated liquor specifically for treating diseases is not included.

(1) *Ju Zha Yi Xin Jiu*

Ingredients

Ju Hua (Flos Chrysanthemi)	30 g
Shan Zha (Fructus Crataegi)	45 g
Bai Jiu (Chinese white liquor)	500 g

Process

Cold-steeping

Dosage and Administration

Taken three times daily, 10—20 ml each time.

Effect

Calming the liver, improving eyesight, expelling wind, removing heat, strengthening the stomach, promoting digestion, dissipating stasis. Modern research has proved that *Ju Hua* has the action of resisting thrombus; *Shan Zha* has the action of reducing blood-fat and strengthening the stomach; both of them have the action of lowering blood pressure, increasing the amount of blood flow in the coronary arteries. resisting myocardial ischemia and slowing down the process of ageing. This liquor is suitable for the prevention and adjuvant treatment of coronary heart disease. Regular intake of it will have the effect of prolonging life.

Indications

Hypertension, hyperlipemia, atherosclerosis.

(2) *Jian Xin Ling Jiu*

Ingredients

Huang Qi (Radix Astragali)	30 g
Dan Shen (Radix Salviae Miltiorrhizae)	30 g
Chuan Xiong (Rhizoma Chuanxiong)	12 g
Gui Zhi (Ramulus Cinnamomi)	6 g
Bai Jiu (Chinese white liquor)	500 g

Process

Cold-steeping

Dosage and Administration

Taken three times daily, 10—20 ml each time.

Effect

Replenishing *Qi,* activating blood circulation, inducing the flow of *Yang,* strengthening resistance to fatigue and myocardial ischemia, enhancing hypoxia tolerance.

Indications

It is suitable for the prevention, adjuvant treatment and adjustment in the convalescence of coronary heart disease and ischemic cerebrovascular disease.

Notes

This is developed by the Affiliated Hospital of Shandong College of Traditional Chinese Medicine

(3)　*Tu Su Jiu*

Ingredients

Ma Huang (Herba Ephedrae)

Chuan Jiao (Pericarpium Zanthoxyli)

Xi Xin (Herba Asari)

Fang Feng (Radix Saposhinkoviae)

Cang Zhu (Rhizoma Atractylodis)

Gan Jiang (Rhizoma Zingiberis)

Rou Gui (Cortex Cinnamomi)

Jie Geng (Radix Platycodi)

Preparation

Grind the above ingredients in their equal quantity into coarse powder. Put the powder into a silk bag. Steep the bag in an adequate amount of white liquor within a container. Seal the container and let it stand for three days. Then filter the liquor out for use.

Dosage and Administration

Taken in an adequate amount based on the concentration of the medicines and one's capacity for liquor, initially in small dosage.

Effect

Expelling wind, dispersing cold, warming the middle-Jiao to strengthening the spleen.

Indications

Prevention and treatment of common cold due to wind-cold and stomachache due to cold.

Source

The book *Jing Yue Quan Shu* (Jing Yue's Complete Works)

Notes

This is a medicated liquor traditionally used in China for preventing infectious epidemic diseases. There are many prescriptions for this liquor, some of which contain toxic or excessively potent drugs. They are not introduced here. But it must be pointed out that they must be taken with great care.

(4) *Du Huo Ji Sheng Jiu*

Ingredients

Sheng Di (Radix Rehmanniae)	9 g
Bai Shao (Radix Paeoniae Alba)	9 g
Gui Xin (Ramulus Cinnamomi)	9 g
Fu Ling (Poria)	9 g
Du Zhong (Cortex Eucommiae)	9 g
Niu Xi (Radix Achyranthis Bidentatae)	9 g
Sang Ji Sheng (Ramulus Loranthi)	15 g
Du Huo (Radix Angelicae Pubescentis)	6 g
Qin Jiao (Radix Gentianae Macrophyllae)	6 g
Chuan Xiong (Rhizoma Chuanxiong)	6 g
Ren Shen (Radix Ginseng)	6 g
Fang Feng (Radix Saposhinkoviae)	6 g
Xi Xin (Herba Asari)	3 g
Dang Gui (Radix Angelicae Sinensis)	3 g

| *Gan Cao* (Radix Glycyrrhizae) | 3 g |
| *Bai Jiu* (Chinese white liquor) | 1000 g |

Process

Cold-steeping

Dosage and Administration

Taken 1-2 times daily, 20-30 ml each time.

Effect

Tonifying the liver and kidney, replenishing *Qi* and blood, dispelling wind and dampness, relieving rheumatic pain.

Indications

Rheumatic or rheumatoid arthritis, chronic pain of the loins and legs, sciatica, etc., all due to weakness of the liver and kidney and deficiency of *Qi* and blood.

It is suitable for the treatment or adjustment in the convalescence of the syndromes of wind, cold and dampness due to weakness of the liver and kidney and deficiency of *Qi* and blood.

Source

The book *Wan Bing Hui Chun*

Notes

This is a medicated liquor having the effect of strengthening the body resistance to eliminate pathogenic factors. The dosages of its ingredients and the process of making it are established by some later physicians.

(5) *Shen Rong Jiu*

Ingredients

Ren Shen (Radix Ginseng)	60 g
Lu Rong (Cornu Cervi Pantotrichum)	30 g
Dang Gui (Radix Angelicae Sinensis)	6 g

Qin Jiao (Radix Gentianae Macrophyllae)	6 g
Hong Hua (Flos Carthami)	6 g
Gou Qi Zi (Fructus Lycii)	6 g
Fang Feng (Radix Saposhinkoviae)	3 g
Bie Jia (Carapax Trionycis)	3 g
Bi Xie (Rhizoma Dioscroreae Hypoglaucae)	3 g
Qiang Huo (Rhizoma seu Radix Notopterygii)	3 g
Chuan Niu Xi (Radix Achyranthis Bidentatae)	3 g
Du Huo (Radix Angelicae Pubescentis)	3 g
Du Zhong (Radix Eucommiae)	3 g
Bai Zhu (Rhizoma Atractylodis Macrocephalae)	3 g
Yu Zhu (Rhizoma Polygonati Odorati)	3 g
Ding Xiang (Flos Caryophylli)	2.4 g

Preparation

Put the ingredients and 10 kg of white liquor which has been stored for many years into a container. Seal the container and let it stand for several years. Then filter out the liquor, to which 120 g of crystal sugar and 1 kg of white liquor are added. This medicated liquor is thus well-prepared.

Dosage and Administration

Taken twice daily, 10–20 ml each time.

Effect

First, replenishing *Qi* and warming *Yang;* second, tonifying the liver and kidney, nourishing *Yin*-essence, strengthening the loins and knees, dispelling wind, removing dampness, and activating blood circulation.

Indications

It is suitable for the adjuvant treatment and adjustment in the convalescence of all the disorders due to the invasion of wind, cold or damp evils in the cases of deficiency of *Qi* and blood and weakness of the liver and kidney.

Source

The book *Qing Tai Yi Yuan Pei Fang*

Notes

The book says, "This liquor may be used to treat hemiplegia, facial paralysis, numbness of the extremeties, weakness of the legs, pain of the muscles and joints, all disorders due to evil wind and *Qi* (36 types of winds and 72 types of *Qi*), all pains due to cold or dampness, impairment due to consumption or overstrain, deficiency of the kidney—*Yang*, dysfunction of the digestive system such as indigestion, dysphagia, nausea, vomiting, hiccup, masses due to *Qi* stasis, diarrhea, fullness sensation and cold—pain in the abdomen, impotence, deficiency of blood in female, reddish leukorrhea, sterility, in short, all the disorders due to deficiency and consumption in both male and female. Regular intake of it will enrich one's *Qi* and blood, keep all diseases off enhance longevity and enable the old to be full of vigor."

It may be prepared through cold—steeping, there is no need to be limited to "let it stand for several years".

2.4 Soft Extract for Health Care

Soft extract is a thick, semifluid preparation. It is made in this way: Decoct herbal medicines in water. Remove the residue to get the decoction. Concentrate the decoction to syrupy consistency with addition of sugar or honey. Being a traditional extract dosage form of Chinese medicines for oral administration. it has seen a long history in our country. For instance , in the Spring and Autumn Period (770—475 B.C.)and the Warring States

(475—221 B.C.), prescriptions of soft extract were recorded in the medical book *Wu Shi Er Bing Fang;* in the Tang Dynasty, prescriptions of soft extract for tonification and longevity, such as *Huang Jing Gao, Lu Kang Gao* and *Xian Fang Ning Ling Gao,* were recorded in the books *Qian Jin Yao Fang* and *Qian Jin Yi Fang.* Through the later ages, many kinds of soft extract were developed for health—preserving and disease—curing. Take for example *Qiong Yu Gao* recorded in the book *Hong Shi Ji Yan Fang* in the Song Dynasty. It was not only popular among the people but also appreciated by the palace physicians. Nowadays, it is still regarded as an effective patent medicine. In South China, soft extract is regarded as a good tonic to be taken in winter. Soft extract made by quite a number of pharmacies is also well—received.

Soft extract has been used to prevent and treat various kinds of diseases as well as to preserve health and resist senility. Being characterized by its special and wonderful effects, mild and long—term potency, convenience in storage, carrying and application, simplicity in preparation, and low consumption of drug materials, it is a good, ecomical and practical medicine for health care, which is suitable for strengthening the body, restoring *Qi,* eliminating diseases and resisting senility to prolong life.

Soft extract is usually made up of many ingredients. (But there are also those which are composed of only one ingredient.)The composition and application of a soft extract are both based on differentiation of all the factors concerned. It functions either in strengthening and adjusting the whole body to consolidate the constitution and slow down the process of ageing through regulating *Yin* and *Yang,* enriching *Qi* and blood, nourishing the Five—*Zang* organs, and supplementing vital essence and marrow, or in building up the body through eliminating evil factors to prevent certain diseases and restoring health in the convalescence. Thus soft extract is of many kinds, each of which has its own effect and indications, andis selected through analysis of the factors concerned to treat different individuals.

Soft extract is usually taken with warm boiled water. However, some are taken with warm millet wine to meet the patient's condition; some are sucked in the mouth to treat throat disorders; some for tonification are taken on an empty stomach; some for nourishing the liver to calm the the mind are taken before bedtime; some are taken half an hour before meals to treat diseases in the lower—*Jiao;* some are taken half an hour after meals to treat diseases in the upper—*Jiao*.

The dosage of soft extract is determined according to the nature of the ingredients, the disease condition and the patient's constitution. Mild—natured soft extract without toxicity, especially those made of edible medicines, may be taken in larger dosage. Soft extract containing too potent or toxic ingredients should be taken in small dosage, especially in the beginning, with its dosage increased or reduced according to the reaction after it is taken. Larger dosage is taken to treat patients with strong constitution, critical or severe diseases. Smaller dosage is taken by those who are weak, old, do not suffer from any disease, or suffer from mild or chronic diseases. The dosages of the following prescriptions are the general ones for adults, which may be modified to a certain extent, increasing or reducing.

Following are the usual methods of making at home soft extract for health care.

Preparation of Materials

Get ready materials such as the medicines, cane sugar or honey ordered in the prescription. Remove dust and impurities from the herbal medicines and process them according to the conventions (Crush them into coarse powder if necessary). White, granulated or crystal sugar is usually used, brown suger being used in rare occasions. Sugar is processed through parching or melting. By parching is meant to put the sugar into a bronze pot and parch it till it is melted, the color becoming yellowish, bubbles and whitish smoke appearing. In the course of parching, frequent stirring is needed to make the sugar heated evenly. By melting we mean to process the sugar into an invert one. The steps are as follows: 10 kg of sugar and 5—6 kg of water are boiled together for half an hour or so; an adequate amount of 10% tartaric acid is then evenly added while stirring; heat is maintained, the process requiring two hours of mild boiling. By doing so, the cane sugar is made to transform into glucose or fructose. Honey of high quality is selected and refined in the following way:Heat honey in a pot until it is melted; remove the foam to allow nearly all the water in the honey to evaporate; when the color becomes brown and large bubbles appear, water, equal in amount to 10% of the heated honey, is carefully added; heat is maintained until the content boils; pour the content out of the pot while still hot and filter it with a silk sifter to remove the impurities. The honey should be refined to the point where it is neither under done nor overdone. Generally, it is suitable to refine 500 g of honey into 400 g.

Concentration of Decoction

Decoct the medicines in water for a few hours after they are steeped for a period from a few hours to half a day to get the docoction. Do the same another 2 times. Mix all the decoction with the juice squeezed out from the residue and let the mixture stand still to settle the particles. The mixture is filtered with layers of gauze and heated again in the pot over a strong fire until boiling. Remove foam on the surface and continue the heat with mild fire to keep the content simmering and continue the evaporation slowly, continual stirring being needed lest sticking occur and the content be burnt owing to overheating. It is suitable to heat the content until when some of it is pushed up with a stick, it drops down in the form of laminae. In summer the content may be made a little thicker, while in winter a little thinner.

Preparation of Soft Extract

Mix the processed sugar or honey evenly with the concentrated decoction by continuous stirring. Preparation of soft extract is thus finished. Or while the sugar is nearly to be prepared, add a certain amount of decoction reserved before hand to dilute the sugar. Pour the thin sugar content out and filter it with a sifter. Mix the filtered sugar content with the concentrated decoction in a pot and decoct the mixture with mild heat until it is properly condensed. In every step, an earthenware, bronze or aluminium pot not an iron one is used.

Storage

Soft extract is stored in a glass, enamel, pottery or porcelain container, which is airtight and kept in a cool, dark place.

In the following are introduced various kinds of soft extract for health care. Most of them are from ancient or modern literature. But the dosages of medicines, the preparations and the analyses of effects are enriched by the author's modern knowledge and experience. Prescriptions without sources indicated are the proved ones established by the author.

2.4.1 Soft Extract for Invigorating *Qi*

1. Ren Shen Gao

Ingredients

Ren Shen (Radix Ginseng)	250 g

Preparation

Ren Shen is crushed into coarse powder and decocted three times. The decoctions is then condensed, and the refined honey is finally added to get the extract.

Dosage and Administration

Taken twice daily, in the morning and evening, 15 g each time.

Effect

Enriching the primordial *Qi*, strengthening the spleen, enhancing mental power, resisting senility.

Indications

Syndromes due to deficiency of *Qi*, infirmity with age.

Source

The book *Jing Yue Quan Shu*

2. Dai Shen Gao

Ingredients

Dang Shen (Radix Codonopsis)	250 g
Huang Qi (Radix Astragali)	250 g
Bai Zhu (Rhizoma Atractylodis Macrocephalae)	250 g
Long Yan Rou (Arillus Longan)	250 g

Preparation

All the above is decocted, the decoction is condensed, and 250 g of processed sugar is added, the extract being well-prepared.

Dosage and Administration

Taken twice daily in the morning and evening, 15 g each time.

Effect

Replenishing *Qi*, strengthening the spleen, nourishing the heart.

Indications

Syndromes due to deficiency of *Qi*, general debility in the aged, *Qi* deficiency of the heart and spleen in particular.

Source

The book *Zhong Yao Cheng Fang Pei Ben*

3. Yi Qi Kai Wei Gao

Ingredients

Ren Shen (Radix Ginseng)	30 g
Fu Ling (Poria)	250 g
Huang Qi (Radix Astragali)	250 g
Chao Mai Ya (parched Fructus Hordei Germinatus)	250 g
Shan Zha (Fructus Crataegi)	250 g
Sha Ren (Fructus Amomi)	15 g

Preparation

All the above is decocted, the decoction is condensed, an adequate amount of refined honey is then added to get the extract.

Dosage and Administration

Taken twice daily in the morning and evening, 15 g each time.

Effect

Replenishing *Qi*, strengthening the spleen and removing undigested food, as well as promoting the flow of *Qi* and activating the functional activities of the stomach.

Indications

General debility, *Qi* deficiency, weakness of the spleen and stomach, poor appetite.

Notes

This extract can exert both its tonifying and resolving actions at the same time, avoiding the disadvantage of affecting the function of the stomach due to mere tonification.

2.4.2 Soft Extract for Nourishing the Blood

1. *Sang Shen Gao*

Ingredients

Sang Shen (Fructus Mori)   1000 g

Preparation

Pound and squeeze Sang shen to get its juice, which is condensed into soft extract. Or an adequate amount of refined honey is added to the concentrated juice to form the extract.

Dosage and Administration

Taken 2—3 times daily, 30 g each time.

Effect

Nourishing the blood and *Yin,* darkening hair, moistening the large intestine.

Indications

Early—greying of hair, constipation due to dryness in the intestines, deficiency of *Yin*—blood in the middle—aged and the aged.

Source

The book *Su Wen Bing Ji Qi Yi Bao Ming Ji*

2. *Qi Yuan Gao*

Ingredients

Gou Qi Zi (Fructus Lycii)	500 g
Long Yan Rou (Arillus Longan)	500 g

Preparation

The above is decocted, the decoction is condensed into extract. Or an adequate amount of refined honey is added to the concentrated decoction to form the extract.

Dosage and Administration

Taken 2—3 times daily, 15—30 g each time.

Effect

Supplementing the vital essence and blood, nourishing the heart, calming the mind, invigorating the liver and kidney.

Indications

Insufficiency of the heart-blood, weakness of the liver and kidney.

Source

The book *She Sheng Mi Zhi*

Notes

The book points out that this extract can calm the mind, nourish the blood, strengthen the tendons and bones, moisten the muscles and skin and brighten complexion. It seems to have the action of resisting senility and improving one's looks. The two medicines are edible, so this extract is a mild tonic and may by taken regularly.

3. Shou Wu Bu Xue Gao

Ingredients

He Shou Wu (Radix Polygoni Multiflori)	250 g
Da Zao (Fructus Jujubae)	500 g
Sang Shen Zi (Fructus Mori)	500 g

| *Long Yan Rou* (Arillus Longan) | 500 g |
| *Hei Zhi Ma* (Semen Sesami Nigrum) | 500 g |

Preparation

All the above is decocted, the decoction is condensed, and an adequate amount of refined honey is added to get the extract.

Dosage and Administration

Taken 2—3 times daily, 15—30 g each time.

Effect

Mainly nourishing the blood, secondly invigorating *Qi* and *Yin,* enhancing the heart and spleen, darkening hair, moistening the large intestine.

Indications

Insufficiency of *Yin*—blood, early—greying of hair, dysphoria, constipation due to dryness in the intestines.

Notes

This extract is a mild tonic for enriching *Yin*—blood. It is likely to have the action of moistening the muscles and skin, brightening complexion and resisting senility.

4. Dang Gui Bu Xue Gao

Ingredients

Dang Gui (Radix Angelicae Sinensis)

Chuan Xiong (Rhizoma Chuanxiong)

Huang Qi (Radix Astragali)

Gan Cao (Radix Glycyrrhizae)

Dang Shen (Radix Codonopsis)

Bai Shao (Radix Paeoniae Alba)

E Jiao (Colla Corii Asini)

Fu Ling (Poria)

Shu Di (Rhizoma Rehmanniae Praeparata)

Dosage and Administration
Taken according to the instructions
Effect
Nourishing the blood, replenishing *Qi*.
Indications
General debility, sallow complexion, dizziness. blurring of vision, deficiency of blood in the convalescence, consumption of blood after giving birth, etc.
Manufacturer
Zhonglian Pharmaceutical Factory in Wuhan City

2.4.3 Soft Extract for Nourishing *Yin*

1. *Er Dong Gao*
Ingredients
Tian Dong (Radix Asparagi)	500 g
Mai Dong (Radix Ophiopogonis)	500 g

Preparation
The two herbs are decocted, the decoction is condensed, and an adequate amount of refined honey is finally added to get the extract.
Dosage and Administration
Taken 2–3 times daily, 15 g each time.
Effect
Nourishing *Yin*, moistening the lung, expelling fire.
Indications
Consumption of body fluid due to *Yin* deficiency, cough due to phlegm-heat, lung-dryness due to *Yin* deficiency in the middle-aged and the elderly.
Source

The book *Zhang Shi Yi Tong*

2. Er Zhi Gao

Ingredients

Nu Zhen Zi (Fructus Ligustri Lucidi)	500 g
Han Lian Cao (Herba Ecliptae)	500 g

Preparation

The above is decocted, the decoction is condensed, and an adequate amount of refined honey is added to the condensed decoction to form the extract.

Dosage and Administration

Taken 2–3 times daily, 15 g each time.

Effect

Nourishing *Yin*, invigorating the kidney, enhancing the liver.

Indications

Syndrome due to *Yin* deficiency of the liver and kidney, marked by dizziness, tinnitus, insomnia, dreamfulness, early-greying of hair, soreness of the loins and knees, emission, and night sweating, as well as hemorrhage due to *Yin* deficiency.

Source

The book *Yang Shi Jia Cang Fang Jie*

Notes

In the book the prescription is for pill dosage form.

3. Yang Yin Gao

Ingredients

Sha Shen (Radix Adenophorae Strictae)	250 g
Yu Zhu (Rhizoma Polygonati Odorati)	250 g
Mai Dong (Radix Ophopogonis)	250 g
Hua Fen (Pollen)	250 g
Bai He (Bulbus Lilii)	250 g

Preparation

The above is decocted in water, the decoction is condensed, mix the condensed decoction evenly with an adequate amount of refined honey, the extract being formed.

Dosage and Administration

Taken 2—3 times daily, 15 g each time.

Effect

Nourishing *Yin*, promoting the production of body fluid, moistening and strengthening the lung and stomach, calming the mind to relieve restlessness.

Indications

Dry mouth and throat, dry cough with scanty expectoration, restlessness, palpitation, all due to overconsumption of body fluid caused by *Yin* deficiency of the lung and stomach.

2.4.4 Soft Extract for Supporting *Yang*

1. *Suo Yang Gao*

Ingredients

Suo Yang (Herba Cynomorii)   1500 g

Preparation

Suo Yang is decocted in water and the decoction is condensed. The condensed decoction is evenly mixed with 250 g of refined honey and the extract is thus well-prepared.

Dosage and Administration

Taken orally, twice daily, 30 g each time.

Effect

Reinforcing the kidney—*Yang*, supplementing the essence and blood, moistening the intestines.

Indications

Insufficiency of the kidney—*Yang*, consumption and deficiency of the vital essence and blood, constipation due to overconsumption of body fluid caused by dryness in the intestines.

Source

The book *Ben Cao Qie Yao*

2. Cong Rong Er Xian Gao

Ingredients

Rou Cong Rong (Herba Cistanchis)	500 g
Yin Yang Huo (Herba Epimedii)	500 g
Xian Mao (Rhizoma Curculiginis)	250 g

Preparation

The above is decocted in water and the decoction is condensed. The condensed decoction is evenly mixed with an adequate amount of processed granulated sugar with the extract being formed.

Dosage and Administration

Taken orally, twice daily in the morning and evening, 15 g each time.

Effect

Reinforcing the kidney—*Yang*, strengthening the tendons and bones, eliminating cold—dampness.

Indications

Impotence, weakness of the loins and knees, flaccidity of the extremities, all due to insufficiency of the kidney—*Yang*; disorders due to wind, cold and dampness and numbness of the limbs.

Notes

Because it is dry and heat—natured, patients without the syndrome due to *Yang* deficiency should not take this medicine regularly.

3. *Ge Jie Dang Shen Gao*

Ingredients

Ge Jie (Gecko)

Dang Shen (Radix Codonopsis)

Dosage Form

Soft extract, 250 g in each bottle.

Dosage and Administration

Taken with warm boiled water, twice daily, 10 g each time.

Effect

Invigorating the kidney, supporting *Yang*, tonifying the lung, strengthening the spleen, relieving cough, arresting asthma.

Indications

Asthenia due to various causes; chronic cough, anemia sallow complexion and indigestion due to deficiency of the kidney—*Yang* and the lung—*Yin*.

Manufacturer

Nanning Pharmaceutical Factory of Traditional Chinese Medicines in Guangxi

2.4.5 Soft Extract for Tonifying Both *Qi* and Blood

1. *Liang Yi Gao*

Ingredients

Ren Shen (Radix Ginseng)	120 g
Shu Di (Rhiaoma Rehmanniae Praeparata)	500 g

Preparation

The above is decocted in water, the decoction is condensed, the condensed decoction is mixed evenly with an adequate amount of refined honey or crystal sugar, and the extract is thus well-prepared.

Dosage and Admnistration

Taken orally, twice daily in the morning and evening, 15 g each time.

Effect

Invigorating the primordial *Qi,* nourishing *Yin*—blood.

Indications

Insufficiency of vital essence and *Qi* in the interior, deficiency of *Yin* —blood.

Source

The book *Jing Yue Quan Shu*

Notes

This is a mild extract for tonifying *Qi* and blood. It may be taken regularly. *Ren Shen* may be replaced with 250 g of *Dang Shen* (Radix Codonopsis Pilosulae).

2. *Shi Quan Da Bu Gao*

Ingredients

Dang Shen (Radix Codonopsis)	500 g
Mi Zhi Huang Qi (honeyed Radix Astragali)	500 g
Chao Bai Zhu (parched Rhizoma Atractylodis Macrocephalae)	500 g
Chao Bai Shao (parched Radix Paeoniae Alba)	500 g
Fu Ling (Poria)	500 g
Shu Di Huang (Rhizoma Rehmanniae Praeparata)	750 g
Dang Gui (Radix Angelicae Sinensis)	750 g
Chuan Xiong (Rhizoma Chuanxiong)	250 g
Rou Gui (Cortex Cinnamomi)	250 g
Mi Zhi Gan Cao (Radix Glycyrrhizae Praeparata)	250 g

Preparation

All the above is decocted in water and the decoction is condensed. 530 g of granulated sugar is dissolved in water and heated and filtered, and then evenly mixed with 1000 g of the condensed decoction into soft extract.

Dosage and Administration

Dissolved in boiling water and taken before a meal, twice daily, 15 g each time.

Effect

Warming and tonifying the primordial *Qi*

Indications

Syndromes due to deficiency of *Qi* and blood

Source

The book *Jiang Su Sheng Yao Pin Biao Zhun*

3. Yang Shen Shuang Bu Gao

Ingredients

Xi Yang Shen (Radix Panacis Quinquefolii)	30 g
Shan Yao (Rhizoma Dioscoreae)	500 g
Gou Qi Zi (Fructus Lycii)	500 g
Sang Shen Zi (Fructus Mori)	750 g
Da Zao (Fructus Jujubae)	750 g
Long Yao Rou (Arillus Longan)	750 g

Preparation

All the above is decocted in water, the decoction is condensed, an adequate amount of refined honey or crystal sugar is mixed with the condensed decoction into soft extract.

Dosage and Administration

Taken orally, twice daily, 30 g each time.

Effect

Nourishing the blood, enriching *Yin*, mildly tonifying the heart, spleen, liver and kidey.

Indications

Syndromes due to deficiency of *Qi*, insufficiency of blood and consumption of *Yin*.

Notes

All the herbs except *Xi Yang Shen* are edible. As *Xi Yang Shen* is rare and expensive, it may be replaced with *Tai Zi Shen* (Radix Pseudostellariae), of which the dosage is ten times that of *Xi Yang Shen*.

2.4.6 Soft Extract for Tonifying the Five-*Zang* Organs

1. *Gou Qi Gao*

Ingredients

Gou Qi Zi (Fructus Lycii) 500 g

Preparation

Gou Qi Zi is decocted in water and the decoction is condensed into soft extract. Or an adequate amount of refined honey is mixed with the condensed decoction into soft extract.

Dosage and Administration

Taken orally, twice daily in the morning and evening, 15-30g each time.

Effect

Tonifying the liver and kidney, nourishing *Yin*, moistening the lung, improving eyesight.

Indications

Such disorders due to *Yin* deficiency of the liver and kidney as dizziness, blurring of vision, hypopsia, soreness and weakness of the loins and knees, as well as cough due to *Yin* deficiency.

Source

The book *Shou Shi Bao Yuan*

2. Cang Zhu Gao

Ingredients

Cang Zhu (Rhizoma Atractylodis)	500 g
Fu Ling (Poria)	500 g

Preparation

The above is decocted in water, the decoction is condensed, an adequate amount of refined honey or granulated sugar is evenly mixed with the condensed decoction into soft extract.

Dosage and Administration

Taken orally, 2—3 times daily, 15—30 g each time.

Effect

Strengthening the spleen and stomach, replenishing *Qi*.

Indications

Such disorders due to impairment of the heart and spleen caused by overstrain in the middle—aged and the aged and due to weakness of the spleen and stomach as poor appetite, decline of vigor, amnesia, insomnia, and edema, soreness and heavy feeling of the legs and feet.

Source

The book *Wei Sheng Za Xing Fang*

Notes

Cang Zhu Gao recorded in the book is prepared in the routine way, forming this extract.

3. Fu Ling Gao

Ingredients

Fu Ling (Poria)	1000 g
Song Zhi (Colophonium)	500 g

Song Zi Ren (Semen Pini)	250 g
Bai Zi Ren (Semen Biotae)	250 g

Preparation

Fu Ling is steamed and dried seven times. *Song Zhi* is refined. Then all the ingredients are ground into powder, which is sifted and mixed with 1000 g of honey. The mixture is put into a bronze container with water and decocted over a mild fire for a day and night into soft extract.

Dosage and Administration

Taken three times daily, 15—30 g each time.

Effect

Nourishing the heart, calming the mind, strengthening the body.

Indications

Such disorders due to deficiency of the heart—Qi and heart—blood as disturbed mind, palpitation, insomnia, amnesia.

Source

The book *Tai Ping Sheng Hui Fang*

Notes

This prescription has the same ingredients as *Xian Fang Ning Ling Gao* recorded in the book *Qian Jin Yi Fang*. In the book *Tai Ping Sheng Hui Fang* there is a sentence to describe this extract: "Take this extract regularly rather than in too large a dosage. Regular intake of it may have the effect of building up health, improving eyesight, recovering one's youthful vigour, turning grey hair into black, regenerating teeth and prolonging life."

4. *Run Fei Gao*

Ingredients

Nan Sha Shen (Radix Adenophorae)	50 g

Mai Dong (Radix Ophiopogonis)	50 g
Tian Dong (Radix Asparagi)	50 g
Hua Fen (Pollen)	50 g
Pi Pa Ye (Folium Eriobotryae)	50 g
Xing Ren (Semen Armeniacae Amarum)	50 g
He Tao Ren (Semen Juglandis)	50 g
Bing Tang (crystal sugar)	50 g
Chuan Bei Mu (Bulbus Fritillariae Cirrhosae)	120 g
Ju Bing (orange in the form of cake)	250 g

Preparation

Remove the hair of *Pi Pa Ye* and grind *Chuan Bei Mu* and *Bing Tang* into powder separately. The ingredients except *Chuan Bei Mu* and *Bing Tang* are decocted in water and the decoction is concentrated. The thick decoction is mixed with the powder of *Chuan Bei Mu* and *Bing Tang* and 6000 g of honey into soft extract.

Dosage and Administration

Taken orally, twice daily, 15 g each time.

Effect

Nourishing the lung—*Yin*, relieving cough, reducing phlegm.

Indications

Disorders due to dryness in the lung caused by *Yin* deficiency, such as dry mouth and throat, unproductive cough or cough with little but sticky sputum.

Source

The book *Jiang Su Sheng Yao Pin Biao Zhun*

2.4.7 Other Soft Extract for Tonifying the Body and Prolonging Life

1. *Qiong Yü Gao*

Ingredients

Ren Shen (Radix Ginseng)	75 g
Sheng Di (Radix Rehmanniae)	800 g
Fu Ling (Poria)	153 g
Bai Mi (Mel)	500 g

Preparation

Bai Mi is refined, the other ingredients are ground into powder and decocted in water, the decoction is condensed and mixed with the refined honey into soft extract.

Dosage and Administration

Taken orally, 2–3 times daily, 15 g each time.

Effect

Invigorating *Qi* and *Yin*, promoting the production of vital essence and blood, nourishing the kidney, enhancing the lung, strengthening the spleen and stomach, tonifying the heart.

Indications

Unproductive cough due to deficiency and consumption, dry throat, hemoptysis.

Source

The book *Hong Shi Ji Yan Fang* compiled by Hong Zun in the Song Dynasty.

Notes

The dosage and ingredients have been modified according to the original prescription in the book. For instance, such ingredients as *Chen Xiang* (Lignum Aquilariae Resinatum) and *Hu Po*

(Succinum) are sometimes added. Taken by the middle—aged and the aged, this extract will exert the effect of restoring Qi, strengthening the body resistance, consolidating constitution, expelling phlegm and slowing down the process of ageing.

This prescription is characterized by strict composition, benefiting all the organs, invigorating both Qi and Yin, and nourishing but not affecting functioning activity of the stomach. Therefore, it may be administered regularly and has a place in the palace medicine of the Qing Dynasty.

Recent research has shown that this extract has the action of increasing the count of T lymphocytes and reducing the content of serum IgA obviously in the old, both the count and content are almost the same as those in the control group of young persons. This action of improving the immunologic function in the aged may be considered as the mechanism for *Qiong Yu Gao* to strengthen the body resistance, consolidate constitution, eliminate diseases and prolong life.

2. *Yi Shou Yang Zhen Gao*

Ingredients

Sheng Di Huang (Rhizoma Rehmanniae Praeparata)	8000 g
Ren Shen (Radix Ginseng)	750 g
Fu Ling (Poria)	1500 g
Mi (Mel)	5000 g
Tian Dong (Radix Asparagi)	250 g
Mai Dong (Radix Ophiopogonis)	250 g
Di Gu Pi (Cortex Lycii)	250 g

Preparation

All the above except *Mi* is ground into powder, then mixed

with *Mi* thoroughly and put into a porcelain jar. The jar is sealed, placed in a bronze pot and boiled in water for three days and nights, warm water being added to keep the surface of the water in the pot just below the edge of the jar. Then the jar is sealed with wax paper and laid in a well for a day and night. Finally place the jar in the pot again and boil it in water for another day and night to let the water in the jar evaporate.

Dosage and Administration

Taken after being mixed with warm liquor, 2–3 times daily, 1–2 spoons each time.

Effect and Indications

The same as those of *Qiong Yü Gao*

Notes

The dosages of medicines and the preparation are from *Nei Jing Pian* of the book *Dong Yi Bao Jian* This extract has three ingredients more than *Qiong Yü Gao*: *Tian Dong*, *Mai Dong* and *Di Gu Pi*, this enhancing its effect of nourishing *Yin*.

3. He Che Gao

Ingredients

Dang Shen (Radix Codonopsis)	60 g
Sheng Di (Radix Rehmanniae)	60 g
Gou Qi Zi (Fructus Lycii)	60 g
Dang Gui (Radix Angelicae Sinensis)	60 g
Zi He Che (Placenta Hominis)	one

Preparation

All the above is decocted thoroughly, the concentrated decoction is mixed with refined honey into soft extract.

Dosage and Administration

Taken in the morning, after being mixed with millet wine,

3—5 spoons each time.

Effect

Enriching *Qi*, nourishing the blood, supporting *Yang*, replenishing *Yin*, supplementing marrow, tonifying the liver and kidney.

Indications

General debility and senilism due to insufficiency of *Qi*, blood, *Yin* and *Yang*.

Source

It has another name *Hun Yuan Gao*, and is recorded the book *Qing Tai Yi Yuan Pei Fang*.

Notes

The book says, this extract can be used "to treat men and women with syndromes due to various kinds of deficiency and injuries, such as the five kinds of strains and the seven kinds of impairments, susceptibility to diseases and intolerance of strain due to weakness of the primordial *Qi* from congenital factors, impotence and sterility due to deficiency of the kidney, habitual abortion due to cold of deficiency type in the uterus". Regular intake of it may restore the youthful vigour in the old. The book also points out that during the time when this extract is taken, anger, sexual life, Chinese white liquor and all kinds of meat are all avoided.

4. Gui Lu Er Xian Gao

Ingredients

Lu Jiao (Cornu Cervi)	500 g
Gui Ban (Carapax et Plastrum Testudinis)	250 g
Gou Qi Zi (Fructus Lycii)	100 g
Ren Shen (Radix Ginseng)	50 g

Preparation

The first two ingredients are sawed up, scraped clean, steeped in water and decocted over mulberry-leaf fire into a gum. The last two ingredients are decocted in water, the decoction is mixed with the gum into the soft extract.

Dosage and Administration

Taken in the morning, after being mixed with wine, 9 g each time.

Effect

Warming *Yang*, benefiting *Yin*, nourishing the liver and kidney, potently invigorating *Qi*, blood, essence and marrow.

Indications

Consmptive diseases, exhaustion of essence, nocturnal emission, emaciation, languor, blurred vision, etc.

Source

The book *Xian Chuan Si Shi Jiu Fang*. The above-mentioned dosage, preparation and administration are all based on the book *Yi Fang Ji Jie*.

Notes

Regular intake of this extract may prolong one's life, making him live as long as a tortoise does. So it is known as *Xian Gao* (an extract having the effect of making one live as long as a supernatural being).

5. Hong Yu Gao

Ingredients

Yu Zhu (Rhizoma Polygonati Odorati)	90 g
Ren Shen (Radix Ginseng)	90 g
Wu Wei Zi (Fructus Schisandrae)	60 g
Gui Ban Jiao (Colla Carapacis et Plastri Testudinis)	60 g
Dang Gui (Radix Angelicae Sinensis)	60 g

Da Sheng Di (Radix Rehmanniae)	60 g
Fu Ling (Poria)	60 g
Gou Qi Zi (Fructus Lycii)	60 g
Chuan Niu Xi (Radix Achyranthis Bidentatae)	30 g
Bai Lian Xu (Stamen Nelumbinis)	15 g
Zhu Sha (Cinnabaris)	3 g

Preparation

All the above is decocted in water, the decoction is condensed, and the condensed decoction is mixed with an adequate amount of refined honey into soft extract.

Dosage and Administration

Taken orally, 2—3 times daily, 15 g each time.

Effect

Supplementing the vital essence and marrow, consolidating *Qi*, nourishing the blood, regulating the five *Zang* organs, enhancing the nine orifices, benefiting health greatly.

Indications

Senility due to deficiency and impairments in the middle—aged and the aged

Source

The book *Ji Yan Liang Fang* in the Qing Dynasty

Notes

This prescription is based on, but has more ingredients than, that of *Qiong Yu Gao,* which enhances its effect of tonifying the liver and kidney, nourishing *Yin*—blood and calming the mind. It is advisable for the middle—aged and the aged to take it regularly. As *Zhu Sha* is toxic, it is better to omit it or to replace it with other ingredients having the action of nourishing the heart to calm the mind.

6. Jia Jian Fu Yuan He Zhong Gao

Ingredients

Dang Shen (Radix Codonopsis)	45 g
Bai Zhu (Rhizoma Atractylodis Macrocephalae baked in earth)	30 g
Fu Ling (Poria)	30 g
Dang Gui (Radix Angelicae Sinensis baked in earth)	30 g
Xu Duan (Radix Dipsaci parched with liquor)	30 g
Huang Qi (Radix Astragali)	30 g
Chao Gu Ya (parched Fructus Oryzae Germinatus)	30 g
Ji Nei Jin (Endothelium Corneum Gigeriae Galli roasted)	30 g
Zhi Ban Xia (Rhizoma Pinelliae Praeparata)	24 g
Sheng Jiang (Rhizoma Zingiberis)	24 g
Zhi Xiang Fu (Rhizoma Cyperi Praeparata)	18 g
Shu Di (Rhizoma Rehmanniae Praeparata)	18 g
Sha Ren (Fructus Amomi)	12 g
Pei Lan Cao (Herba Eupatorii)	12 g
Hong Zao Rou (Fructus Jujubae with the core removed)	20 dates

Preparation

All the above is decocted in water thoroughly, the decoction is condensed, the condensed decoction is mixed with an adequate amount of crystal sugar into soft extract.

Dosage and Administration

Taken with boiled water, 9 g each time.

Effect

Strengthening the spleen, replenishing *Qi*, nourishing the blood, promoting digestion to eliminate retained food and tonifying the liver and kidney as well.

Indications

General debility due to prolonged illness, weakness of the spleen and stomach, poor appetite, distension in the abdomen, retching, hiccup, indigestion, etc.

Source

The book *Ci Xi Guang Xu Yi Fang Xuan Yi*

Notes

This prescription was established specially for the sake of Cixi Empress Dowager in the Qing Dynasty.

7. *Jia Jian Fu Yuan Yi Yin Gao*

Ingredients

Dang Shen (Radix Codonopsis)	60 g
Chao Bai Zhu (parched Rhizoma Atractylodis Macrocephalae)	30 g
Fu Ling (Poria)	30 g
Shan Yao (Rhizoma Dioscoreae)	30 g
Dang Gui (Radix Angelicae Sinensis baked in earth)	30 g
Nü Zhen Zi (Fructus Ligustri Lucidi)	30 g
Bai Shao (Radix Paeoniae Alba parched with vinegar)	24 g
Dan Pi (Cortex Moutan)	18 g
Zhi Xiang Fu (Rhizoma Cyperi Praeparata)	18 g
Lu Jiao Jiao (Colla Cornus Cervi melted)	15 g
Sha Ren (Fructus Amomi)	12 g
Yin Chai Hu (Radix Stellariae)	9 g

Preparation

All the above except *Lu Jiao Jiao* is decocted in water thoroughly, the decoction is concentrated, first mixed evenly with the melted *Lu Jiao Jiao* and then with an adequate amount of refined honey into soft extract.

Dosage and Adminis tration

Taken with boiled water, 12 g each time.

Effect

This prescription is, in fact, the modification of *Xiao Yao San* with the main ingredients of *Si Jun Zi Tang*. Besides its main effect, it also has the action of strengthening the spleen, replenishing *Qi*, regulating the liver and spleen to promote the flow of *Qi*, warming the kidney, invigorating *Yin* and nourishing the blood.

Indications

Consumptive diseases due to stagnation of the liver—*Qi*

Source

The book *Ci Xi Guang Xu Yi Fang Xuan Yi*

Notes

Mild and reliable in nature, this extract has tonifying effect without affecting functioning activity of the stomach, it was once prepared for Cixi Empress Dowager in the Qing Dynasty.

2.4.8 Soft Extract for Health Care Used to Prevent and Treat Diseases

1. *Ju Hua Yan Ling Gao*

Ingredients

Xian Ju Hua (Flos Chrysan themi), fresh and in an adequate amount

Preparation

Xian Ju Hua is decocted in water thoroughly, the decoction is concentrated and mixed with small amount of refined honey into soft extract.

Dosage and Administration

Taken with boiled water, 9—12 g each time.

Effect

Dispelling wind, clearing away heat, calming the liver, improving eyesight.

Indications

Dizziness, blurring of vision, headache and conjunctival congestion due to hyperfunction of the liver—*Yang* and wind—heat pathogen.

Source

The book *Ci Xi Guang Xu Yi Fang Xuan Yi*

Notes

This prescription was established specially for Cixi Empress Dowager. It has been found out through modern pharmacological and clinical studies that this extract may be used to treat hypertension, coronary heart disease, etc., showing that *Ju Hua* does have the action of eliminating diseases and prolonging life through its effect of preventing and treating such kind of diseases in the middle—aged and the aged, and that there is something in the old saying : "*Ju Hua* can prolong one's life."

2. *Ming Mu Yan Ling Gao*

Ingredients

Shuang Sang Ye (Folium Mori)	30 g
Ju Hua (Flos Chrysanthemi)	30 g

Preparation

The above is decocted in water thoroughly, the decoction is concentrated and mixed with small amount of refined honey into soft extract.

Dosage and Administration

Taken with boiled water, 9 g each time.

Effect and Indications

Similar to those of *Ju Hua Yan Ling Gao*

Source

The book *Ci Xi Guang Xu Yi Fang Xuan Yi*

Notes

According to the book, this is an extract specially used to treat eye disease of Cixi Empress Dowager.

3. *Jia Zhu Li Li Gao*

Ingredients

Huang Li (pear)	100 pears
Xian Zhu Ye (fresh Herba Lophatheri)	100 pieces
Xian Lu Gen (fresh Rhizoma Phragmitis)	30 pieces
Lao Shu Ju Hong (ExocarpiumCitri Grandis)	20 pieces
Bi Qi (Bulbus Eleocharis Tuberosae)	50 pieces
Zhu Li (Succus Bambusae)	adeqate amount

Preparation

The same as the above

Effect

Nourishing *Yin* to promote the production of body fluid, moistening the lung to arrest cough, clearing away heat to eliminate phlegm.

Indications

Phthisical cough due to dryness in the lung caused by *Yin* deficiency

Source

The book *Ci Xi Guang Xu Yi Fang Xuan Yi*

Notes

This extract was once used to treat Emperor Guangxu for his cough.

4. Li Yan Gao

Ingredients

Mai Dong (Radix Ophiopogonis)	100 g
Pang Da Hai (Semen Sterculiae Lychnophorae)	100 g
Tian Hua Fen (Radix Trichosanthis)	100 g
Huang Li (pear)	1000 g
Xian Qing Guo (fresh Fructus Canarii)	500 g
Jie Geng (Radix Platycodi)	50 g
Mu Hu Die (Semen Oroxyli)	50 g
Gan Cao (Radix Glycyrrhizae)	30 g
Shuang Hua (Flos Lonicerae)	75 g
Shi Shuang (Mannosum Kaki)	30 g

Preparation

All the above except *Shi Shuang* is decocted in water, the decoction is condensed and mixed first with *Shi Shuang* and then with an adequate amount of refined honey into soft extract.

Dosage and Administration

Taken with boiled water or sucked in the mouth, three times daily, 9—15 g each time.

Effect

Clearing away heat, replenishing *Yin*, promoting the production of body fluid, relieving sore-throat.

Indications

Sore throat, dry mouth and throat, hoarseness, etc.

Notes

This can play a part in voice-protecting for teachers and actors or actresses.

5. Shou Wu Ju Zha Gao

Ingredients

He Shou Wu (Radix Polygoni Multiflori)	500 g
Ju Hua (Flos Chrysanthemi)	500 g
Sheng Shan Zha (Fructus Crataegi)	500 g

Preparation

The above is decocted in water, the decoction is condensed and mixed with an adequate amount of refined honey into soft extract.

Dosage and Administration

Taken three times daily, 10—15 g each time.

Effect

Nourishing the liver and kidney, calming the liver to improve eyesight, activating blood circulation.

Indications

Hypertension, hyperlipemia, coronary heart disease.

Notes

It is used for prevention, in the convalescence, or as an adjuvant.

6. Yi Qi Huo Xue Gao

Ingredients

Huang Qi (Radix Astragali)	500 g
Dan Shen (Radix Salviae Miltiorrhizae)	500 g
Huang Jing (Rhizoma Polygonati)	250 g
Yu Jin (Radix Curcumae)	250 g
Sheng Shan Zha (Fructus Crataegi)	250 g

Preparation

The above is decocted in water, the decoction is condensed and mixed with an adequate amount of refined honey into soft extract.

Dosage and Administration

Taken three times daily, 15 g each time.

Effect

Replenishing *Qi*, promoting the circulation of blood.

Indications

All the disorders due to deficiency of *Qi* and stagnation of blood, such as coronary heart disease, ischemic cerebrovascular accident and its sequelae, chronic obstructive pulmonary emphysema, and chronic pulmonary heart disease in the remission stage.

7. Lao Guan Cao Gao

Ingredients

Lao Guan Cao (Herba Erodii seu Geranii)	500 g
Dang Gui (Radix Angelicae Sinensis)	125 g
Bai Xian Pi (Cortex Dictamni)	62.5 g
Chuan Xiong (Rhizoma Chuanxiong)	62.5 g
Hong Hua (Flos Carthami)	31 g

Preparation

All the above is decocted in water thoroughly, the decoction is condensed and mixed with an adequate amount of refined honey into soft extract.

Dosage and Administration

Taken 2–3 times, 9–15 g each time.

Effect

Expelling wind–dampness, promoting blood circulation to remove obstruction in the channels.

Indications

Pain due to pathogenic wind-dampness, stiffness of the muscles and tendons, spasm and numbness of the limbs, traumatic injury, itchy skin, etc.

Source

The book *Qing Tai Yi Yuan Pei Fang*

2.5 Chinese Herbal Tea for Health Care

Chinese herbal tea is a tea dosage form of Chinese herbs. It is of two types. One, known as *Dai Cha Yin* in the form of coarse powder with or without tea leaves, is steeped in boiling water and then taken orally as tea is made and drunk. It fulfils the purpose of personally maintaining one's own health, and its action and administration will be introduced later in this section. The other, in the form of lumps of coarse powder mixed with flour paste or medicated leaven, is also steeped in boiling water and then taken. *Wu Shi Cha* is an example of this type. Usually produced by pharmaceutical factories, it is not discussed in this section.

China is the home of tea and has seen several thousand years of cultivating and drinking tea. Tea is a fine beverage and has the action of relieving thirst and restlessness, resolving phlegm, promoting digestion, inducing diuresis, eliminating toxic substances and refreshing oneself. Thus tea has enjoyed long popularity.

In the long practice of tea drinking, people found out that tea mixed with suitable medicines had the potency to prevent and treat diseases and that some medicines might be substituted for tea and infused with boiling water for oral use. Hence, *Dai Cha Yin* (herbal tea used to prevent and treat diseases or to maintain one's health and prolong life) came into being. The medical book

Wai Tai Mi Yao compiled by *Wang Tao* early in the Tang Dynasty 1,200 years ago first dealt with *Dai Cha Yin*, of which many prescriptions were recorded in a number of medical books of later generations. For instance, in the palace medical file of the Qing Dynasty, there are numerous prescriptions of herbal teas widely used to treat diseases and build up health. This is characteristic of the palace medicine of the Qing Dynasty. In the recent years, herbal teas for prolonging life and reducing weight as well as the miraculous herbal tea of the palace medicine of the Qing Dynasty have been put to clinical use .This shows that taking herbal teas has become a widely-used way of maintaining one's own health.

Herbal teas have many unique merits: small in dosage and saving drug material, taken just after being infused with boiling water and saving fuel (without the need to be decocted over fire), easier to prepare and more suitable for long-standing administration than decoction, prescribed either for drug therapy and dietetic therapy or for prevention and treatment of diseases or for health care. All these are enjoyed by both the old and the young. Therefore, herbal tea has become a fine remedy for health care.

Dai Cha Yin is widely administered. It is used for the treatment of mild cases, for the adjustment of chronic diseases, for the adjuvant treatment and recuperation of serious diseases, for the protection of health and for the retardation of senility. In addition, regular intake of *Dai Cha Yin* will be rewarded by the prevention and treatment of the disorders in the oral cavity, throat, esophagus, stomach and intestines, as the tea can act directly on the lining of the above organs.

Dai Cha Yin is characterized by its medicine administration and prescription composition. Medicines administered in it are usually mild-natured, and sweet and mild tasting, such as fruits, vegetables, sugar and honey which are edible and easy to obtain. Drugs too bitter in taste and hard in quality, drugs whose active principles are difficult to steep out, and animal products or highly pot ent drugs are rarely chosen. As to its prescription composition, the principle followed is "few" and "little". That is, the ingredients of a prescription of *Dai Cha Yin* are a few, usually between 5—7; the amount of each ingredient is minute, generally not over 10 g, and the dose of a whole prescription is small. In spite of the above characteristic, a *Dai Cha Yin*'s composition and the compatibility of its ingredients are both strictly based on overall analysis and differentiation of all the factors concerned.

The preparation of *Dai Cha Yin* is simple. That which should be paid attention to is as follows: to select high-quality and clean herbs, to remove any dust and impurities in them if necessary, not to use contaminated or spoiled herbs, to break up the herbs into coarse powder not containing too much fine powder which will make the tea turbid, to put the powder into filter pouches so that one pouch may be administered each time, to dry the powder so that it may be well stored and to keep it dry in order to protect it from worms and mould.

Dai Cha Yin is prepared and taken as follows: It is steeped in boiling water in a cup, vacuum-cup, a tea-pot or a thermos bottle just as if making tea, and taken as tea, boiling water added if necessary. Alternatively, it may be decocted in water for a moment and drunk.

Appropriate *Dai Cha Yin* should be prescribed according to the differentiation of an individual's constitution, disease state and age as well as the particular season in order to achieve good curative effects in the prevention and treatment of diseases and in the retardation of senility. It should be remembered that *Dai Cha Yin,* being small in dose, mild in nature and slow in drug potency, is just an adjuvant used to treat some diseases. It should not be the sole treatment for emergency and severe cases lest the opportunity to cure them be missed. When *Dai Cha Yin* is used for health care and longevity, the effects will be ensured only by its long-term regular administration.

Following are the various kinds of herbal teas for health care. Those with the sources indicated are all from the documents consulted, some of which are briefly introduced and their doses, preparations, administrations and actions have been modified slightly by the author's own clinical experience and modern knowledge, some of which have no dosage noted, which may be determined by the readers according to individual need with the dosage of each ingredient limited to between 1.5–6 g. Those without sources indicated are the proved ones composed by the author himself.

2.5.1 Herbal Tea for Invigorating *Qi* and Enriching Blood

1. *Shen Qi Dai Cha Yin*

Ingredients

Ren Shen (Radix Ginseng)	3 g
Huang Qi (Radix Astragali)	9 g
Da Zao (Fructus Jujubae)	5 dates
Chen Pi (Pericarpium Citri Reticulatae)	1.5 g

Preparation and Administration

The above is infused with boiling water and taken as tea.

Effect

Invigorating primordial *Qi* without causing any stagnation, strengthening the spleen and stomach, delaying senility.

Indications

Regular in take of it is suitable for those who are weak due to the deficiency of *Qi*.

Notes

Ren Shen may be substituted by *Dang Shen* (Radix Codonopsis).

2. Wu Bao Cha Tang

Source

The book *Ren Shou Lu*

Ingredients (each in an adequate amount)

Shu Mi Mian (broomcorn millet flour)

Zhi Ma (Semen Sesami)

Niu Ru (milk)

Shan Yao (Rhizoma Dioscoreae)

Niu Gu Sui (ox marrow)

Preparation and Administration

Grind *Zhi Ma* and *Shan Yao* into powder. Dissolve *Niu Gu Sui* in sesame oil. Parch *Shu Mi Mian*. Mix the above processed ingredients evenly with *Niu Ru* and *Wu Bao Cha Tang* is thus prepared. An appropriate amount is infused with boiling water and taken every morning.

Effect

Invigorating *Qi,* strengthening the spleen, replenishing vital essence, enriching the blood, nourishing the liver and kidney.

Indications

Taking it regularly is included in dietetic therapy and fit for those infirm with age.

3. Guan Yin Mian Cha

Source

The book *Ren Shou Lu*

Ingredients

Chao Hei Zhi Ma (parched Semen Sesami)	500 g
Ou Fen (lotus root starch)	500 g
Nian Huang Mi (glutinous yellow rice)	500 g
Bai Tang (white sugar)	500 g
Chao Shan Yao (parched Rhizoma Dioscoreae)	500 g

Preparation and Administration

The above is ground into fine powder, of which an appropriate amount is infused with boiling water for oral use.

Effect

Replenishing *Qi*, strengthening the spleen invigorating vital essence, enriching the blood, nourishing the liver and kidney.

Indications

Suitable for those weak and senile

4. Wu Xiang Nai Cha

Source

The book *Ren Shou Lu*

Ingredients

Niu Ru (milk)

Bai Sha Tang (white granulated sugar)

Feng Mi (Mel)

Xing Ren (Semen Armeniacae Amarum)

Zhi Ma (Semen Sesame)

Preparation and Administration

Xing Ren and *Zhi Ma* are broken up into coarse powder,

which is mixed evenly with *Bai Sha Tang* and *Feng Mi*. *Niu Ru* is heated and poured into the mixture and the delicious *Wu Xiang Nai Cha* is thus well prepared. It is taken every day.

Effect

Replenishing *Qi*, Supplementing vital essence, enriching the blood, moistening the lung, relaxing the bowels and nourishing the liver and kidney.

Indications

It is especially applicable to those who are infirm with age and have the symptoms of cough and constipation.

5. *Zhu Dong Dai Cha Yin*

Source

The book *Chuan Ya Nei Wai Pian*

Ingredients

Bai Zhu (Rhizoma Atractylodis Macrocephalae)	4.5 g
Mai Dong (Radix Ophiopogonis with pith removed)	3 g

Preparation and Administration

The above is decocted in water in summer and taken as tea.

Effect

Invigorating *Qi*, strengthening the spleen, nourishing *Yin*, moistening the heart and lung.

Indications

It is suitable for those with syndromes due to deficiency of the spleen—*Qi* or *Yin* deficiency of the heart and lung.

Notes

It is called *Dai Cha Tang* in the book.

6. *Sang Long Dai Cha Yin*

Ingredients

Sang Shen Zi (Fructus Mori)　　　　　　　　15 g
Long Yan Rou (Arillus Longan)　　　　　　　15 g

Preparation and Administration

The above is infused with boiling water and drunk as tea.

Effect

This herbal tea acts mainly in enriching the blood in addition to replenishing Yin, invigorating Qi, nourishing the heart, tranquilizing the mind, promoting the production of body fluid, moistening the intestines.

Indications

Deficiency of the vital essence and blood, dizziness, tinnitus, insomnia, amnesia, severe palpitation, anorexia, weariness, early-greying of hair, constipation due to dry feces.

7.　Yi Qi Sheng Jin Dai Cha Yin

Ingredients

Ren Shen (Radix Ginseng)

Xian Shi Hu (fresh Herba Dendrobii)

Mai Dong (Radix Ophiopogonis)

Xian Qing Guo (fresh Fructus Canarii)

Lao Mi (long-stored rice)

Effect

Replenishing Qi, nourishing Yin, promoting the production of body fluid, removing heat, relieving sore-throat.

Indications

Deficiency of Qi and Yin, consumption and lack of body fluid, dry mouth, dry and sore throat.

Notes

According to the description in the book Qing Dai Gong Ting Yi Hua, empress dowager Ci Xi was once treated with this herbal tea.

8. *Bu Xue He Wei Dai Cha Yin*

Ingredients

Dang Gui Shen (Radix Angelicae Sinensis)
　　　　　(middle part is used)
Chuan Xiong (Rhizoma Chuanxiong)
Bai Shao (Radix Paeoniae Alba)
Sheng Di (Radix Rehmanniae)
Guang Mu Xiang (Radix Saussureae Lappae)
Zhi Shi (Fructus Aurantii Immaturus)
Cang Zhu (Rhizoma Atractylodis)
Jiao San Xian (parched Massa Fermentata Medicinalis)
　　　　　(parched Fructus Crataegi)
　　　　　(parched Fructus Hordei Germinatus)

Effect

Enriching the blood

Indications

Dysfunction of the spleen and stomach, deficiency of *Yin*-blood.

Notes

This herbal tea was originally called as *He Wei Dai Cha Yin*. It is, in fact, composed of the prescription *Si Wu Tang* and herbs with the action of activating the flow of *Qi*, or removing food retention and promoting digestion. Only when the spleen and stomach function well, can the food be transformed into *Qi* and blood. The efficacy of this herbal tea lies in its promotion of these functions. According to the description in the book *Qing Dai Gong Ting Yi Hua*, Zhen, an imperial concubine of emperor Guang Xu, was once treated with this herbal tea.

2.5.2 Herbal Tea for Nourishing *Yin* and Supporting *Yang*

1. *Yu Shi Dai Cha Yin*

Ingredients

Yu Zhu (Rhizoma Polygonati Odorati)	6 g
Shi Hu (Herba Dendrobii)	6 g

Preparation and Administration

The above is infused with boiling water and taken as tea.

Effect

Nourishing *Yin* moistening dryness, promoting the production of body fluid.

Indications

Syndrome due to *Yin* deficiency of the lung and stomach, marked by dry and heat cough, phthisical cough due to *Yin* deficiency, dry mouth and tongue due to the consumption of body fluid, weakness and soreness of the loins and knees, blurred vision as well as diabetes due to *Yin* deficiency.

2. *Er Shen Er Dong Dai Cha Yin*

Ingredients

Sha Shen (Radix Adenophorae)	6 g
Xuan Shen (Radix Scrophulariae)	6 g
Mai Dong (Radix Ophiopogonis)	6 g
Tian Dong (Radix Asparagi)	6 g

Effect

Nourishing *Yin*, promoting the production of body fluid, clearing away heat and removing fire.

Indications

Yin impairment of the lung and stomach, marked by dry

mouth and throat, dry cough with little sputum, phthisical cough with blood, and anorexia; *Yin* impairment due to febrile disease, marked by restlessness, insomnia, flaring-up of fire of deficiency type, congestion of eye, sore throat and constipation caused by dry feces.

Notes

Those with constitution of *Yin*-deficiency type can take the above two herbal teas.

3. Shen Ling Dai Cha Yin

Ingredients

Sha Shen (Radix Adenophorae)
Fu Ling (Poria)
Tian Dong (Radix Asparagi)

Effect

Nourishing *Yin* first and supporting the spleen second.

Indications

Syndrome due to *Yin* deficiency of the lung, the stomach and the kidney, and complicated by the deficiency of the spleen.

Notes

It was recorded in the book *Qing Dai Gong Ting Yi Hua* that a concubine called Ding of the emperor Qian Long in the Qing Dynasty had taken this herbal tea.

4. Xian Ling Pi Cha

Ingredients

Yin Yang Huo (Herba Epimedii)	9 g
Rou Cong Rong (Herba Cistanchis)	6 g

Preparation and Administration

The above is infused with boiling water and taken as tea.

Effect

Supplementing kidney-*Yang*, strengthening the tendons and bones, replenishing the vital essence and blood.

Indications

Impotence, infertility, weakness of the loins and knees, cold pain, hypertension and coronary heart disease, all due to deficiency of the kidney-*Yang*.

5. Fu Fang Du Zhong Cha

Ingredients

Du Zhong (Cortex Eucommiae)	9 g
Sang Ji Sheng (Ramulus Taxilli seu Visci)	9 g
Huai Niu Xi (Radix Achyranthis Bidentatae)	9 g

Preparation and Administration

The above is infused with boiling water and taken as tea.

Effect

Tonifying the liver and kidney, strengthening the tendons and bones.

Indications

Lumbago and weakness of the feet and knees due to deficiency of the kidney, hypertension with symptoms due to deficiency of the liver and kidney.

6. Xin Er Xian Dai Cha Yin

Ingredients

Xian Mao (Rhizoma Curculiginis)	4.5 g
Yin Yang Huo (Herba Epimedii)	6 g
Du Zhong (Cortex Eucommiae)	6 g
Xuan Shen (Radix Scrophulariae)	6 g
Nü Zhen Zi (Fructrus Ligustri Lucidi)	6 g
Gou Qi Zi (Fructus Lycii)	6 g

Preparation and Administration

The above is infused with boiling water and taken as tea.

Effect

Tonifying the liver and kidney, warming *Yang*, nourishing *Yin*, removing fire.

Indications

Syndrome due to deficiency of both *Yin* and *Yang* and both the liver and kidney, or complicated by flaring-up of fire of deficiency type, and hypertension and coronary heart disease with symptoms due to the above syndrome.

Notes

The establishment of this prescription, whose composition follows that of the prescription of *Er Xian Tang*, is armed at regulating both *Yin* and *Yang*. When this prescription is prescribed, the dosage of its herbs with the action of supporting *Yang* and those nourishing *Yin* should be modified according to the different deficient conditions of *Yin* and *Yang*.

7. Fu Fang Gou Qi Cha

Ingredients

Gou Qi Zi (Fructus Lycii)	6 g
Bai He (Bulbus Lilii)	6 g
He Shou Wu (Radix Polygoni Multiflori)	6 g
Huang Jing (Rhizoma Polygonati)	6 g
Yin Yang Huo (Herba Epimedii)	6 g

Preparation and Administration

The above is infused with boiling water and taken as tea.

Effect

Mildly reinforcing *Qi*, blood, *Yin* and *Yang* with the five *Zang* organs benefited, retarding senility, building up constitution, prolonging life.

Indications

It is suitable for those weak, middle-aged or aged to take regularly.

2.5.3 Herbal Tea for Regulating the Function of the Spleen and Stomach to Promote]Digestion

1. *He Wei Dai Cha Yin*

Source

The book *Qing Dai Gong Ting Yi Hua*

Ingredients

Sheng Bai Zhu (Rhizoma Atractylodis Macrocephalae)

Cang Zhu (Rhizoma Atractylodis)

Fu Ling (Poria)

Chen Pi (Pericarpium Citri Reticulatae)

Jin Shi Hu (Herba Dendrobii)

Gu Ya (Fructus Oryzae Germinatus)

Jian Qu (Massa Medicata Fermentata)

Guang Sha Ren (Fructus Amomi)

Effect

Strengthening the spleen and stomach, nourishing *Yin,* promoting digestion.

Indications

Syndrome due to weakness of the spleen and stomach and complicated by *Yin* deficiency of the stomach, marked by anorexia and food retention.

Notes

It is recorded in the book *Qing Dai Gong Ting Yi Hua* that this prescription was one of those for regulation and invigoration once used to treat the emperor *Guang Xu* after his illness.

2. Er Shen Dai Cha Yin

Ingredients

Fu Shen (Poria cum Ligno Hospite)

Shen Qu (Massa Fermentata Medicinalis)

Effect

Strengthening the spleen, calming the mind, regulating the stomach to promote digestion.

Indications

Deficiency of the spleen, anorexia, indigestion, uneasiness.

Notes

According to the book *Qing Dai Gong Ting Yi Hua*, Yu, a concubine of the emperor Jia Qing in the Qing Dynasty was once treated with this herbal tea after her illness.

3. Wu Xian Dai Cha Yin

Ingredients

Shen Qu (Massa Fermentata Medicinalis)	6 g
Chao Shan Zha (parched Fructus Crataegi)	6 g
Chao Mai Ya (parched Fructus Hordei Germinatus)	6 g
Chao Gu Ya (parched Fructus Oryzae Germinatus)	6 g
Sha Ren (Fructus Amomi)	3 g

Preparation and Administration

The above is infused with boiling water and taken as tea.

Effect

First, promoting digestion and removing any stagnation and food retention; second, activating the flow of *Qi* and regulating the function of the stomach.

Indications

Food retention, distention and fullness in the stomach and abdomen, and belching with disagreeable odour of undigested food.

4. Gan Lu Cha

Source

The book *Yao Ji Xue*

Ingredients

Wu Yao (Radix Linderae)	24 g
Chao Hou Po (parched Cortex Magnoliae Officinalis)	24 g
Chao Zhi Shi (parched Fructus Aurantii)	24 g
Chao Shan Zha (parched Fructus Crataegi)	24 g
Chen Pi (Pericarpium Citri Reticulatae)	120 g
Chao Shen Qu (parched Massa Fermentata Medicinalis)	45 g
Chao Gu Ya (parched Fructus Oryzae Germinatus)	30 g
Hong Cha (black tea)	90 g

Preparation

The above is ground into coarse powder, mixed evenly and put into pouches, 9 g in each.

Administration

One pouch and one piece of *Sheng Jiang* (Rhizoma Zingiberis Recens) are decocted or steeped in boiling water for oral use.

Effect

Regulating the flow of *Qi*, promoting digestion and removing stagnation.

Indications

Food retention, *Qi* stagnation, distending and depressing sensation in the stomach and abdomen, anorexia and non-acclimatization.

2.5.4 Herbal Tea for Tranquilizing the Mind

1. An Shen Dai Cha Yin

Source

The book *Ci Xi Guang Xu Yi Fang Xuan Yi*

Ingredients

Duan Long Chi (forged Os Draconis)	9 g
Shi Chang Pu (Rhizoma Acori Graminei)	3 g

Preparation and Administration

The above is decocted in water and taken as tea.

Effect

Relieving convulsions, inducing resuscitation, calming the mind.

Indications

Palpitation, susceptibility to fright.

Notes

It is recorded in the book *Ci Xi Guang Xu Yi Fang Xuan Yi* that this herbal tea was once used to treat the emperor Guang Xu's disease affecting the Heart Channel.

2. Yuan Rou Er Ren Cha

Ingredients

Long Yan Rou (Arillus Longan)	12 g
Chao Suan Zao Ren (parched Semen Ziziphi Spinosae)	12 g
Chao Bai Zi Ren (parched Semen Platycladi)	6 g

Preparation and Administration

The above is infused in boiling water and taken as tea.

Effect

Nourishing the heart to calm the mind.

Indications

Palpitation, insomnia and amnesia, all due to deficiency of the heart—*Qi* and heart—blood.

3. Qing Xin Dai Cha Yin

Ingredients

Lian Zi Xin (Plumula Nelumbinis)	3 g
Deng Xin (Medulla Junci)	3 g
Zhu Ye (Herba Lophatheri)	3 g
Chao Suan Zao Ren (Parched Semen Ziziphi Spinosae)	9 g

Preparation and Administration

The above is infused with boiling water and taken as tea.

Effect

Removing heart—fire, nourishing the heart to calm the mind.

Indications

Palpitation and insomnia due to *Yin* deficiency of the heart and flaring heart—fire, hypertension with the above symptoms.

2.5.5 Herbal Tea for Preventing and Treating Common Diseases

1. Ju Zha Dai Cha Yin

Ingredients

Ju Hua (Flos Chrysanthemi)	12 g
Sheng Shan Zha (fresh Fructus Crataegi)	12 g

Preparation and Administration

The above is infused in boiling water and taken as tea.

Effect

Lowering blood pressure, reducing blood—fat, resisting

myocardial ischemia.

Indications

Hypertension, hyperlipemia, coronary heart disease.

2. *Shou Wu Jue Ming Cha*

He Shou Wu (Radix Polygoni Multiflori)	12 g
Jue Ming Zi (Semen Cassiae)	12 g

Preparation and Administration

The above is infused in boiling water and taken as tea.

Effect

Reducing blood-fat, resisting atherosclerosis and myocardial ischemia.

Indications

Hyperlipemia, atherosclerosis and coronary heart disease accompanied by constipation.

3. *Fu Fang Yu Mi Xu Cha*

Ingredients

Yu Mi Xu (Stigma Maydis)	30 g
Che Qian Zi (Semen Plantaginis)	15 g
Ze Xie (Rhizoma Alismatis)	12 g

Preparation and Administration

The above is infused with boiling water and taken as tea.

Effect

Inducing diuresis, lowering blood pressure, blood sugar concentration and blood-fat level.

Indications

Nephritic edema, ascites due to cirrhosis, hypertension.

4. *Jian Fei Dai Cha Yin*

Ingredients

Wu Long Cha (tea of Wulong type)	6 g

He Ye (Folium Nelumbinis)	0 g
Ze Xie (Rhizoma Alismatis)	12 g
Sheng Shan Zha (Fructus Crataegi)	12 g
Yi Yi Ren (Semen Coicis)	12 g
Chen Pi (Pericarpium Citri Reticulatae)	3 g

Preparation and Administration

The above is infused with boiling water and taken as tea.

Effect

Reducing blood-fat, inducing diuresis, cutting down one's weight.

Indications

Those who suffer from simple obesity or hyperlipemia should take it regularly.

5. *Xiao Fei Jian Shen Cha*

Main Ingredients

Tian Qi (Radix Notoginseng)

Shan Cha (Camellia)

Bai Pi Gen (Rhizoma Imperatae)

Dosage Form

Tea put in pouches, 4-4.8 g in each.

Dosage and Administration

Taken hot after being steeped in boiling water for a moment, 1 pouch each time, three times daily, the tea of one pouch is infused with boiling water 2-3 times.

Effect

Regulating metabolism, promoting lipodieresis, reducing blood-fat, activating blood circulation.

Indications

Simple obesity, cardio-cerebral diseases, or disorders in the aged.

6. *Fu Fang Luo Bu Ma Cha*

Ingredients

Luo Bu Ma Ye (Folium Apocyni Veneti)	3 g
Gou Teng (Ramulus Uncariae cum Uncis)	15 g
Dan Pi (Cortex Moutan)	6 g

Preparation and Administration

The above is infused with boiling water and taken as tea.

Effect

Lowering blood pressure.

Indications

Hypertension, especially that due to hyperactivity of the liver-Yang.

7. *Huang Yu Shi Dai Cha Yin*

Ingredients

Huang Qi (Radix Astragali)	15 g
Yu Mi Xu (Stigma Maydis)	30 g
Shi Wei (Folium Pyrrosiae)	21 g

Preparation and Administration

The above is infused with boiling water and taken as tea.

Effect

Invigorating *Qi*, promoting diuresis. Patients with proteinuria due to nephritis will have the protein and edema reduced to a certain extent if they take it regularly.

8. *He Pei Fang Shu Cha*

Ingredients

Xian He Ye (fresh Folium Nelumbinis)	one piece
Pei Lan (Herba Eupatorii)	6 g
Huo Xiang (Herba Agastachis)	6 g

Ju Hua (Flos Chrysanthemi)   6 g
Jin Yin Hua (Flos Lonicerae)   6 g

Preparation and Administration

The above is infused with boiling water and taken as tea.

Effect

Clearing away summer—heat and summer—dampness.

Usage

Prevention of heatstroke.

9. Wen Zhong Cha

Ingredients

Gan Jiang (Rhizoma Zingiberis)   6 g
Liang Jiang (Rhizoma Alpiniae Officinarum)   3 g
Chen Pi (Pericarpium Citri Reticulatae)   3 g
Wu Zhu Yu (Fructus Evodiae)   1.5 g
Ding Xiang (Flos Caryophylli)   1.5 g

Preparation and Administration

The above is infused with boiling water and taken as tea.

Effect

Warming the middle—*Jiao,* dispelling cold, relieving pain.

Indications

Pain in the stomach and abdomen, hiccup, vomiting, all due to stomach—cold.

10.   Jian Wei Cha

Ingredients

Xu Chang Qing (Radix Cynanchi Paniculati)   9 g
Mai Dong (Radix Ophiopogonis)   9 g
Sheng Gan Cao (Radix Glycyrrhizae)   6 g
Ju Hong (Exocarpium Citri Reticulatae)   4.5 g
Mei Gui Hua (Flos Rosae Rugosae)   1.5 g

Preparation and Administration

The above is infused with boiling water and taken as tea.

Notes

According to the report written by Gao Shujun and issued in the ninth issue of the Journal of New Traditional Chinese Medicine, 1981, this herbal tea was administered to treat superficial and atrophic antral gastritis with the total effective rate reaching 90.98%, and the obvious effective rate 44.26%.

11. Qing Jie Cha

Ingredients

Jin Yin Hua (Flos Lonicerae)	12 g
Ju Hua (Flos Chrysanthemi)	12 g
Bo He (Herba Menthae)	6 g
Sheng Gan Cao (Radix Glycyrrhizae)	6 g
Huang Lian (Rhizoma Coptidis)	3 g
Zhu Ye (Herba Lophatheri)	3 g

Preparation and Asmonistration

The above is infused with boiling water and taken as tea.

Effect

Removing heat and toxic substances

Indications

Prevention and treatment of furuncle, boil, congestion and swelling and pain of the eyes, all due to toxic heat.

2. 6 Medicated Gruel for Health Care

Medicated gruel for health care refers to a thin porridge prepared by cooking selected Chinese drugs having the action of protecting health together with rice or millet and certain condiments under the guidance of the theories of TCM .It is used to treat diseases. Taking medicated gruel, an important method of protecting health, is included in dietotherapy.

Medicated gruel is a good dosage form with a long history and distinctive features. It is characterized by amassment of the advantages of medication, dietotherapy and tonification with both drugs and food, by embodiment of the superiority of the synergy of rice or millet and drugs, by exertion of the essential action of invigorating the spleen, nourishing the stomach and building up the body, and by being easy to administer.

In the practice of long life, the Chinese people have developed the habit of taking gruel, which has a history of several thousand years in China. Furthermore, they have long since used medicated gruel prepared by cooking rice or millet and Chinese drugs to treat diseases, the earliest records of which may be traced to the book *Shi Ji Bian Que Cang Gong Lie Zhuan* written by Si Maqian in the Han Dynasty and 14 Kinds of Medical Books unearthed from the Han Tombs at Mawangdui, Hunan Province. Zhang Zhongjing, a famous physician in the Han Dynasty, also gave much elucidation on the administration of medicated gruel. During the Tang and Song Dynasties, there was a great development in medicated gruel therapy, which was widely used at that time by physicians and common people to treat and prevent diseases. In the Yuan Dynasty, the publications of the book *Yin Shan Zheng Yao* written by Hu Sihui and the book *Shou Qin Yang Lao Xin Shu* written by Zhou Xuan made contributions to the development of health preservation with medicated gruel. Since the Ming and Qing Dynasties, medicated gruel therapy has further developed and become a systematic therapy for curing diseases, strengthening health and prolonging life.

Medicated gruel can be used as a means to prevent diseases and as an adjuvant for acute diseases. It may be administered either for recuperation in patients newly recovered from illness or in women having just given birth, or for self-nourishment in patients suffering from chronic diseases. Taking it is indeed a good way for middle-aged and elderly people to keep fit. Medicated gruel may be prepared by cooking rice or millet with crude or finely powdered drugs, original juice of drugs or decoction of drugs. When medicated gruel is to be prescribed, attention should be paid to the selection of an appropriate one through differentiating the syndrome, to the reasonable administration of it, to the seasonal and local factors, to the proper make-up of it, to the method of cooking it, to the choice of spices and container, to the need of dietetic restraint, to the determination of treatment course, etc.

Different medicated gruels are composed of different ingredients and have such different actions as invigorating *Qi*, enriching blood, restoring *Yang* and nourishing *Yin*. An indicated gruel may be chosen according to its action.

1. *Ren Shen Zhou*

Source

The book *Shi Jian Ben Cao*

Ingredients

Ren Shen (Radix Ginseng) powdered	3 g
Bing Tang (crystal sugar)	small amount
Jing Mi (Semen Oryzae Sativae)	100 g

Preparation

Cook the powder of *Ren Shen* and *Jing Mi* into gruel

in a clay pot. When the gruel is about to be well done, add the crystal suger to it.

Effect

Invigorating primordial *Qi*, tonifying the five-*Zang* organs, preventing ageing.

Indications

All the disorders due to the deficiency of *Qi*, blood and body fluids, such as weak physiques in the aged, deficiency and weakness of the five-*Zang* organs, emaciation due to long-lasting diseases, poor appetite, chronic diarrhea, palpitation, shortness of breath, insomnia, amnesia, sexual hypofunction, etc.

Administration

Taken on an empty stomach in the morning in autumn or winter.

Caution

This gruel should not be prepared in an iron vessel. In the course of treatment, radish and tea are to be avoided.

Notes

3 g of *Ren Shen* in the prescription may be substituted by 15 g of *Dang Shen* (Radix Codonopsis).

2. Bu Xu Zheng Qi Zhou

Source

The book *Sheng Ji Zong Lu*

Ingredients

Zhi Huang Qi (Radix Astragali Praeparata)	30—60 g
Ren Shen (Radix Ginseng)	3—5 g
Bai Tang (white sugar)	small amount
Jing Mi (Semen Oryzae Sativae)	100—150 g

Preparation

Cut *Ren Shen* and *Huang Qi* into thin slices, which are steeped in cold water in a clay pot for half an hour. Bring the content to the boil with strong heat, then maintain the boil on a lower heat until a concentrated decoction may be got. Filter the decoction out and cook the drugs in the same way for the second deccotion. Mix the two deccotions and divide the mixture into two portions. Put either portion, *Jing Mi* and an appropriate amount of water into a pot and heat the pot in the morning or evening. At the time when the gruel is nearly ready, add *Bai Tang* to it.

Effect

Invigorating vital−*Qi*, curing consumptive diseases, strengthening the spleen and stomach, preventing senility.

Indications

Syndrome due to the deficiency of *Qi* and blood, marked by internal injury due to overstrain, weak physiques in the elderly, spontaneous sweating due to debility, poor appetite, general edema due to deficiency of *Qi*, etc.

Administration

Take the gruel in the morning or evening A course of treatment involves 3−−5 days, Between two courses there should be an interval of 2−−3 days.

Caution

In the course of treatment, radish and tea are to be avoided.

Notes

Ren Shen may be ground into fine powder, which is put into the gruel and cooked.

3. Da Zao Zhou

Source

The book *Sheng Ji Zong Lu*

Ingredients

Da Zao (Fructus Jujubae)	10—15 dates
Jing Mi (Semen Oryzae Sativae)	100 g

Preparation

Cook the two ingredients into gruel in regular way.

Effect

Invigorating *Qi* and blood, strengthening the spleen and stomach.

Indications

Poor appetite due to deficiency of the stomach in the elderly, loose stools due to deficiency of the spleen, *Qi* and blood, thrombocytopenia, anemia, chronic hepatitis, allergic purpura, malnutrition, and body weakness after illness.

Administration

Taken as light refreshments or as a food at breakfast or supper.

Caution

This gruel is contraindicated for obese middleaged and elderly people with the syndrome of abundant phlegm-dampness.

4. Shen Ling Zhou

Source

The book *Sheng Ji Zong Lu*

Ingredients

Ren Shen (Radix Ginseng)	3—5 g
Bai Fu Ling (Poria)	15—20 g
Sheng Jiang (Rhizoma Zingiberis Recens)	3—5 g

Jing Mi (Semen Oryzae Sativae)   100 g

Preparation

Cut *Ren Shen* and *Sheng Jiang* into slices and pound *Fu Ling* into particles. Decoct the slices and particles in water for the decoction. Cook the decoction and *Jing Mi* into gruel.

Effect

Restoring and invigorating *Qi*, nourishing the spleen and stomach.

Indications

Weak physiques due to deficiency of *Qi*, *Qi* deficiency of the spleen and stomach listlessness, poor appetite, regurgitation, vomiting, loose stools, etc.

Administration

This gruel should be eaten warm on an empty stomach in the morning and evening intermittently all the year round.

Notes

15 g of *Dang Shen* (Radix Codonopsis) may be used to substitute for *Ren Shen*.

5. Shan Yao Zhou

Source

The book *Sa Qian Zhai Jing Yan Fang*

Ingredients

Shan Yao (Rhizoma Dioscoreae)   45—60 g
Jing Mi (Semen Oryzae Sativae)   100—150 g

Preparation

Clean *Shan Yao* and cut it into slices. Cook the slices and *Jing Mi* into gruel.

Effect

Invigorating the spleen and stomach, nourishing the lung

and kidney.

Indications

Hypofunction of the spleen and stomach, chronic diarrhea, cough and asthma due to overstrain, poor appetite, listlessness, diabetes, chronic nephritis, etc.

Administration

This gruel may be eaten hot in the morning and evening all the year round.

Notes

If *Xian Shan Yao* (fresh Rhizoma Dioscoreae) is used, its dose should be 100—120 g.

6. Bai Bian Dou Zhou

Source

The book *Yan Nian Mi Zhi*

Ingredients

Chao Bai Bian Dou (Parched Semen Dolichoris Album)   60 g

Jing Mi (Semen Oryzae Sativae)   100 g

Preparation

Cook the two into gruel with *Bai Bian Dou* well done.

Effect

Invigorating the spleen and stomach, clearing away summer-heat, arresting diarrhea.

Indications

Defeciency of the spleen and stomach, poor appetite, vomiting, chronic diarrhea, dysentery due to summer-dampness, restlessness and thirst in summer, etc.

Administration

Taken at breakfast and supper in summer and autumn.

Notes

If *Xian Bai Bian Dou* (fresh Semen Dolichoris Album) is used, its dose should be 120 g.

7. Huang Qi Zhou

Source

The book *Leng Lu Yi Hua*

Ingredients

Sheng Huang Qi (Radix Astragali)	30—60 g
Jing Mi (Semen Oryzae Sativae)	100 g
Chen Pi (Pericarpium Citri Reticulatae) (powdered)	1 g
Hong Tang (brown sugar)	small amount

Preparation

Decoct *Huang Qi* in water to get concentrated decoction, which is cooked together with *Jing Mi* and *Hong Tang*. At the time when the gruel is about to be well prepared, add the powder of *Chen Pi* to it.

Effect

Invigorating primordial *Qi*, strengthening the spleen and stomach, inducing diuresis to alleviate edema.

Indications

Disorders due to the deficiency of *Qi* and blood, such as internal injury due to overstrain, chronic diarrhea, spontaneous sweating due to weak physique, senile edema, chronic hepatitis, chronic nephritis, unhealing ulcer, etc.

Administration

Taken hot at breakfast and supper.

Caution

This gruel is contraindicated for patients with the syndrome of *Yin* deficiency.

8. Luo Hua Sheng Zhou

Source

The book *Zhou Pu*

Ingredients

Luo Hua Sheng (Semen Arachidis Hypogaeae with the red coat)	45 g
Jing Mi (Semen Oryzae Sativae)	100 g
Bing Tang (crystal sugar)	proper amount
Huai Shan Yao (Rhizoma Dioscoreae)	30 g

Preparation

Wash *Hua Sheng* clean and break it up. Cut *Shan Yao* into slices. Cook the broken *Hua Sheng*, *Jing Mi* and the sliced *Shan Yao* together. Before the gruel is well prepared, add *Bing Tang* to it.

Effect

Strengthening the spleen to induce appetite and promote digestion, moistening the lung to arrest cough, nourishing blood to activate lactation.

Indications

Unproductive cough due to dryness of the lung, regurgitation due to deficiency of the spleen, anemia, postpartum hypolactation, etc.

Administration

This gruel may be eaten over a long period.

Caution

15 g of *Bai He* may be used instead of *Shan Yao*. In the process of cooking, the red skin of peanut should be retained. Over-intake of this gruel is contra-indicated in patients suffering

from diarrhea.

9. *Zhu Yu Er Bao Zhou*

Source

The book *Yi Xue Zhong Zhong Can Xi Lu*

Ingredients

Shan Yao (Rhizoma Dioscoreae)	60 g
Sheng Yi Yi Ren (Semen Coicis)	60 g
Shi Bing (dried persimmon)	30 g

Preparation

Cook *Yi Yi Ren* until it is well done. Pound *Shan Yao* and cut *Shi Bing* until they become small pieces, which are cooked together with the well-done *Yi Yi Ren* into gruel.

Effect

Invigorating the lung, strengthening the spleen, nourishing the stomach.

Indications

Disorders due to *Qi* deficiency of the spleen and lung, such as internal heat due to deficiency of *Yin*, phthisical or dry cough, loose stool, poor appetite, etc.

Administration

This gruel is mainly used for the recuperation of patients with chronic diseases. It is to be taken twice daily. One course of treatment involves 5—7 days.

Notes

In this gruel *Shan Yao* is used as a substitute for *Jing Mi* (Semen Oryzae Sativae).

10. *Nuo Mi E Jiao Zhou*

Source

The book *Shi Yi Xin Jian*

Ingredients

E Jiao (Colla Corii Asini)	30 g
Nuo Mi (Semen Oryzae Glutinosae)	100 g
Hong Tang (brown sugar)	small amount

Preparation

Cook *Nuo Mi*. Before it is well done, add to it *E Jiao* which has been pounded into small pieces. Continue cooking and keep stirring the content for 2—3 minutes and then add the brown sugar, thus obtaining the gruel.

Effect

Nourishing *Yin*, supplementing blood, enriching blood to arrest bleeding, preventing miscarriage, replenishing the lung.

Indications

Deficiency of blood, cough due to consumptive diseases, long-lasting cough with hemoptysis, haematemesis and epistaxis, hematochezia and hypomenorrhea due to deficiency of blood, metrostaxis, threatened abortion, vaginal bleeding during pregnancy, etc.

Administration

This gruel can be eaten intermittently. One course of treatment involves 3 days.

Caution

Too frequent intake of this gruel by those with the syndrome of deficiency of the spleen and stomach is not advisable.

11. Long Yan Rou Zhou

Source

The book *Lao Lao Heng Yan*

Ingredients

Long Yan Rou (Arillus Longan)	15 g

Hong Zao (Fructus Jujubae)	3—5 g
Jing Mi (Semen Oryzae Sativae)	100 g
Bai Tang (white sugar)	small amount

Preparation

Cook the ingredients into gruel, to which a small amount of white sugar may be added for the sake of those who prefer sweet food.

Effect

Tonifying the heart, relieving mental strain, benefiting the spleen, nourishing blood.

Indications

Disorders due to deficiency of the heart-blood, such as palpitation, insomnia, poor memory, anemia, and diarrhea due to deficiency of the spleen, edema, weak physique, neurosism, etc.

Administration

Taken hot and in limited amount each time.

Caution

This gruel is contraindicated for those being ill with common cold of wind-cold type marked by aversion to cold, fever and thick greasy tongue coating.

12. Xian Ren Zhou

Source

The book *Zun Sheng Ba Jian*

Ingredients

He Shou Wu (Radix Polygoni Multiflori)	30—60 g
Jing Mi (Semen Oryzae Sativae)	100 g
Hong Zao (Fructus Jujubae)	3—5 dates
Hong Tang (brown sugar)	small amount

Preparation

Decoct *He Shou Wu* to get concentrated decoction, which is put into a clay pot and cooked together with *Jing Mi* and *Hong Zao*. Add *Hong Tang* when the gruel is nearly done and continue the cooking for 1—2 minutes.

Effect

Invigorating *Qi* and blood, replenishing the liver and kidney.

Indications

Deficiency of the liver and kidney, early-greying of hair, dizziness and tinnitus due to deficiency of blood, soreness and weakness of the loins and knees, constipation, hypertension, coronary heart disease, hyperlipemia, neurosism, etc.

Administration

One course of treatment involves 7—10 days. Between every two courses there should be a five-day interval. In the course of treatment this gruel is to be taken twice daily.

Caution

This gruel should not be prepared in an iron pot. It is contraindicated for those suffering from diarrhea. In the course of treatment, scallion and garlic are to be avoided.

13. *Ru Zhou*

Source

The book *Qu Xian Shen Yin*

Ingredients

Niu Ru (cows milk) an appropriate amount
Da Mi (rice)   100 g
Bai Tang (white sugar)   small amount

Preparation

Cook the rice till it is nearly half done and skim the soup over it. Add the milk and sugar and cook the content into gruel.

Effect

Restoring *Qi* to cure consumptive diseases, strengthening the spleen and stomach.

Indications

All the consumptive diseases, deficiency of *Qi* and blood, emaciation after an illness or childbirth, senile weakness, malnutrition in infants, etc.

Administration

Eaten hot on an empty stomach in the morning and evening

Caution

Yang Ru (milk from ewe) may be used instead of *Niu Ru*. If this gruel is prepared for infants, *Ren Ru* (human milk) should be used. In summer, the milk must be kept fresh.

14. *Hai Shen Zhou*

Source

The book *Lao Lao Heng Yan*

Ingredients

Hai Shen (sea cucumber) an appropriate amount

Jing Mi (Semen Oryzae Sativae)   100 g

Preparation

Soak *Hai Shen* with water to soften and clean it, cut it into pieces and boil it thoroughly. And then cook it together with *Jing Mi* into gruel.

Effect

Tonifying the kidney, replenishing vital essence, nourishing blood.

Indications

Deficiency of vital essence and blood, weak constitution,

sexual hypofunction, seminal emission, frequent urination, neurosism, etc.

Administration

This gruel may be regularly taken on an empty stomach in the morning. The course of treatment may be longer or shorter. It is determined according to the need.

Caution

Nuo Mi (Semen Oryzae Glutinosae) may be used instead of *Jing Mi*.

15. *Sang Shen Zhou*

Source

The book *Zhou Pu*

Ingredients

Sang Shen (Fructus Mori)	20—30 g
Nuo Mi (Semen Oryzae Glutinosae)	100 g
Bing Tang (crystal sugar)	small amount

Preparation

Steep *Sang Shen* in water for a few minutes and then clean it. Cook it together with *Nuo Mi* into gruel in a clay pot. Before the gruel is well prepared, *Bing Tang* is added.

Effect

Tonifying the liver and kidney, nourishing blood, improving eyesight.

Indications

Yin deficiency of the liver and kidney, dizziness, blurred vision or hypopsia, soreness and weakness of the loins and knees, early—greying of hair, constipation due to dryness in the intestines, etc.

Administration

Eaten regularly on an empty stomach

Caution

This gruel is contraindicated for those suffering from diarrhea and may not be prepared in an iron pot. If *Xian Sang Shen* (fresh Fructus Mori) is used instead of the dried, the dosage should be 30—60 g.

16. Ji Zhi Zhou

Source

The book *Zhong Guo Peng Ren*

Ingredients

Mu Ji (a hen)	weighing 1500—2000 g
Jing Mi (Semen Oryzae Sativae)	100 g

Preparation

Clean the hen and boil it in water to get the concentrated soup. Divide the soup into several portions, in each of which one of the several portions of *Jing Mi* is cooked into gruel.

Effect

Nourishing the five—*Zang* organs, invigorating *Qi* and the blood.

Administration

Taken hot

Caution

This gruel should be avoided by patients with fever.

17. Tu Si Zi Zhou

Source

The book *Zhou Pu*

Ingredients

Tu Si Zi (Semen Cuscutae)	30—60 g
Jing Mi (Semen Oryzae Sativae)	100 g

Bai Tang (white sugar) an appropriate amount

Preparation

Clean *Tu Si Zi* and pound it into small pieces, which is decocted in water for the decoction. Cook the decoction and *Jing Mi* into gruel. When the gruel is about to be well done, the sugar is added.

Effect

Tonifying the kidney to replenish vital essence, nourishing the liver to improve eyesight.

Indications

Deficiency of the liver and kidney, soreness and weakness of the loins and knees, impotence, seminal emission, premature ejaculation, dizziness, tinnitus, frequent urination, etc.

Administration

Taken in the morning and evening and for a long time

Caution

If *Xian Tu Si Zi* (fresh Semen Cuscutae) is used instead of the dried, the dosage should be 69—100 g.

18. *Cong Rong Yang Rou Zhou*

Source

The book *Ben Cao Gang Mu*

Ingredients

Rou Cong Rong (Herba Cistanchis)	10—15 g
Jing Yang Rou (fine mutton)	100 g
Jing Mi (Semen Oryzae Sativae)	100 g
Xi Yan (refined salt)	small amount
Cong Bai (Bulbus Allii Fistulosi)	2 pieces
Sheng Jiang (Rhizoma Zingiberis Recens)	3 slices

Preparation

Wash *Rou Cong Rong* and *Jing Yang Rou* clean and cut them into small pieces separately. Decoct *Rou Cong Rong* in a clay pot for the decoction. Cook the decoction together with *Jing Yang Rou* and *Jing Mi*. After the content boils, *Xi Yan, Cong Bai* and *Sheng Jiang* are added and heat is continued until the gruel is done.

Effect

Invigorating the kidney—*Yang*; strengthening the spleen and stomach, loosening the bowels to relieve constipation.

Indications

Deficiency of the kidney—*Yang*, impotence, seminal emission, premature ejaculation cold—pain in the loins and knees, infertility due to coldness of the womb, emaciation and weakness of the body, internal injury due to overstrain, insufficiency of the spleen—*Yang*, constipation in the elderly due to deficiency of *Yang*. etc.

Administration

Winter is the proper season for this gruel to be taken. One course of treatment involves 5—7 days.

Caution

This gruel is avoided in summer and by those suffering from diarrhea or sexual hyperfunction. It must not be prepared in an iron pot.

19. Hu Tao Zhou

Source

The book *Hai Shang Ji Yan Fang* (Hai Shang Ji's Empirical Recipes)

Ingredients

Hu Tao Ren (Semen Juglandis)   10—15 g

Jing Mi (Semen Oryzae Sativae)	100 g

Preparation

Smash *Hu Tao Ren* and cook it together with *Jing Mi* into gruel.

Effect

Tonifying the kidney, reinforcing the lung, moistening the intestines.

Indications

Pain in the waist and weakness of the legs due to deficiency of the kidney, unrelieved cough and shortness of breath due to deficiency of the lung, chronic constipation, debility after recovering from a disease, urinary calculus, etc.

Administration

Taken as usual

Caution

This gruel is contraindicated for old people who discharge thin stools.

20. Li Zhi Zhou

Source

The book *Quan Zhou Ben Cao*

Ingredients

Gan Li Zhi (dried Fructus Litchi)	5–7 fruits
Jing Mi (Semen Oryzae Sativae)	100 g

Preparation

Remove the shells of *Gan Li Zhi* to get the pulp, which is cooked in water together with *Jing Mi* into gruel.

Effect

Warming *Yang*, invigorating *Qi*, promoting the production of body fluid, nourishing the blood.

Indications

Diarrhea in the aged due to deficiency of *Yang*, diarrhea before dawn, halitosis, etc.

Administration

This gruel is to be eaten at supper. Taking it for 3—5 days is considered as one course of treatment.

Caution

Those with the syndrome of hyperactivity of fire due to deficiency of *Yin* should avoid this gruel. *Nuo Mi* (Semen Oryzae Glutinosae)can be used to substitute for *Jing Mi*.

21. Li Zi Zhou

Source

The book *Ben Cao Gang Mu*

Ingredients

Li Zi (chestnuts)	10—15 nuts
Jing Mi (Semen Oryzae Sativae)	100 g

Preparation

Remove the shells of *Li Zi* and cook it together with *Jing Mi* into gruel.

Effect

Tonifying the kidney, strengthening the muscles and tendons, invigorating the spleen and stomach.

Indications

Infirmity with age, pain of the loins due to deficiency of the kidney, weakness of the legs, diarrhea due to deficiency of the spleen, etc.

Administration

Taken at breakfast and supper all the year round

Caution

30 g of *Li Fen* (powder of chestnut) may be used to substitute for 10—15 chestnuts and *Nuo Mi* (Semen Oryzae Glutinosae) may be used to replace *Jing Mi*.

22. Que Er Yao Zhou

Source

The book *Tai Ping Sheng Hui Fang*

Ingredients

Ma Que (sparrow)	5 sparrows
Tu Si Zi (Semen Cuscutae)	30—45 g
Fu Pen Zi (Fructus Rubi)	10—15 g
Gou Qi Zi (Fructus Lycii)	20—30 g
Jing Mi (Semen Oryzae Sativae)	100 g
Xi Yan (fine salt)	small amount
Cong Bai (Bulbus Allii Fistulosi)	2 pieces
Sheng Jiang (Rhizoma Zingiberis Recens)	3 slices

Preparation

Tu Si Zi, *Fu Pen Zi* and *Gou Qi Zi* are decocted in a clay pot to get the decoction. The *Ma Que* whose feathers and viscera have been removed are cleaned and bake—stirred with wine. Finally the prepared *Ma Que*, the decoction and *Jing Mi* are cooked together in an appropriate amount of water into gruel. When the gruel is about to be well done, *Xi Yan*, *Cong Bai* and *Sheng Jiang* are added.

Effect

Strengthening *Yang*, replenishing vital essence and the blood, tonifying the liver and kidney, warming the loins and knees.

Indications

Deficiency of the kidney—*Qi*, cold—soreness of the loins and knees, impotence, premature ejaculation, seminal emission, dizziness, tinnitus, profuse and clear urine, irregular leukorrhea, etc.

Administration

This gruel is to be taken in winter. One course of treatment involves 3—5 days.

Caution

This gruel should be avoided by those with the symptom of fever or sexual hyperfunction.

23. Lu Jiao Jiao Zhou

Source

The book *Ben Cao Gang Mu*

Ingredients

Lu Jiao Jiao (Colla Cornus Cervi)	15—20 g
Jing Mi (Semen Oryzae Sativae)	100 g
Sheng Jiang (Rhizoma Zingiberis Recens)	3 slices

Preparation

Cook *Jing Mi* alone in water. When the content boils, *Lu Jiao Jiao* and *Sheng Jiang* are added. Continue the cooking until the gruel is well prepared.

Effect

Tonifying the kidney—*Yang*, replenishing vital essence and the blood.

Indications

Deficiency of the kidney—*Qi*, emaciation due to consumptive diseases, impotence, seminal emission, premature ejaculation, infertility due to cold womb, metrorrhagia, metrostaxis, irregular leukorrhea, etc.

Administration

This gruel is to be taken in winter. One course of treatment involves 3—5 days.

Caution

This gruel should not be prescribed in summer and it is contraindicated for those with the syndrome of hyperactivity of fire due to deficiency of *Yin* or with the symptom of fever.

24. Gou Qi Yang Shen Zhou

Source

The book *Yin Shan Zheng Yao*

Ingredients

Gou Qi Ye (Folium Lycii)	250 g
Xian Yang Shen (fresh sheep kidney)	a whole one
Yang Rou (mutton)	100 g
Jing Mi (Semen Oryzae Sativae)	100—150 g
Cong Bai (Bulbus Allii Fistulosi)	2 pieces
Xi Yan (fine salt)	small amount

Preparation

Wash *Xian Yang Shen* clean, remove the membrane in it and cut it into small pieces. Wash *Yang Rou* clean and cut it into small pieces, too. Decoct *Gou Qi Ye* in water for the decoction. Cook the decoction, the small pieces of *Yang Shen* and *Yang Rou*, *Jing Mi* and *Cong Bai* together into gruel. Before the gruel is well prepared, *Xi Yan* is added.

Effect

Replenishing the kidney—*Yin,* tonifying the kidney—*Qi,* reinforcing the kidney—*Yang* .

Indications

Internal injury due to the kidney deficiency, soreness

and weakness of the loins and knees, dizziness, tinnitus, sexual hypofunction, deficiency of *Yang* in the elderly, etc.

Administration

Taken in winter

Caution

This gruel is contraindicated for those whose constitutions are of *Yang*-excess type. *Gou Qi Zi* (Semen Lycii) may be used to replace *Gou Qi Ye*.

25. *Shan Yu Rou Zhou*

Source

The book *Zhou Pu*

Ingredients

Shan Yu Rou (Fructus Corni)	15—20 g
Jing Mi (Semen Oryzae Sativae)	100 g
Bai Tang (white sugar)	an appropriate amount

Preparation

Wash *Shan Yu Rou* clean and remove its pits and cook it together with *Jing Mi* in a clay pot into gruel. When the gruel is about to be well prepared, *Bai Tang* is added.

Effect

Tonifying the liver and kidney, controlling nocturnal emission, astringing sweating.

Indications

Deficiency of the liver and kidney, dizziness, blurred vision, tinnitus, soreness of the loins, incessant sweating due to debility, seminal emission, enuresis, etc.

Administration

Taking this gruel for 3—5 days is considered one course of treatment.

Caution

This gruel should not be taken again once the disease is cured. It is contraindicated for those suffering from a fever or dribbling urination.

26. Yu Zhu Zhou

Source

The book *Zhou Pu*

Ingredients

Yu Zhu (Rhizoma Polygonati Odorati)	15—20 g
Jing Mi (Semen Oryzae Sativae)	100 g
Bing Tang (crystal sugar)	small amount

Preparation

Yu Zhu is decocted in water and the decoction is concentrated The concentrated decoction is mixed with *Jing Mi* and cooked in an appropriate amount of water into thin gruel. Before the gruel is well cooked *Bing Tang* is added, the cooking being continued for another 1—2 minutes.

Effect

Nourishing *Yin*, moistening the lung, promoting the production of body fluid to relieve cough.

Indications

Deficiency of the lung—*Yin*, dry cough with less or no sputum due to dryness of the lung, or restlessness and thirst occurred after recovering from febrile diseases, and fever due to deficiency of *Yin*. Taking this gruel may be treated as an accessory therapy for various heart diseases and cardiac functional insufficiency.

Administration

It is taken in the morning and evening. One course of treatment involves 5—7 days.

Caution

This gruel is contraindicated for those with the syndrome of phlegm retained and *Qi* stagnated in the stomach or with the symptom of indigestion. If *Xian Yu Zhu* (fresh Rhizoma Polygonati Odorati)is used instead of the dried the dosage should be 30—60 g.

27.　*Tian Men Dong Zhou*

Source

The book *Yin Shi Bian Lu*

Ingredients

Tian Dong (Radix Asparagi)	15—20 g
Jing Mi (Semen Oryzae Sativae)	90—100 g
Bing Tang (crystal sugar)	small amount

Preparation

Decoct *Tian Men Dong* in water for the concentrated decoction, which is cooked with *Jing Mi* into gruel. When the gruel is almost done, *Bing Tang* is added.

Effect

Nourishing *Yin*, moistening the lung, promoting the production of body fluid to relieve cough.

Indications

Deficiency of the kidney—*Yin*, excess heat in the interior due to deficiency of *Yin*, dry mouth due to absence of body fluid, or deficiency of the lung—*Yin*, dry cough with little sputum, afternoon low fever, night sweating, etc.

Administration

3-5 days are involved in one course of treatment. There should be a 3-day-interval between every two courses.

Caution

This gruel is contraindicated for those who are suffering from diarrhea due to cold of deficiency type or who have been attacked by exogenous wind-cold.

28. Sha Shen Zhou

Source

The book *Zhou Pu*

Ingredients

Sha Shen (Radix Adenophorae)	15-30 g
Jing Mi (Semen Oryzae Sativae)	100 g

Bing Tang (crystal sugar) an appropriate amount

Preparation

Decoct *Sha Shen* in water for the decoction, which is cooked with *Jing Mi* into gruel. When the gruel is nearly done, *Bing Tang* is added.

Effect

Moistening the lung, nourishing the stomach, removing phlegm to arrest cough.

Indications

Dry cough with little sputum due to dryness of the lung, or long-standing unproductive cough due to deficiency of the lung-*Qi* and *Yin* deficiency of the lung and stomach, dry throat, or thirst due to the exhaustion of body fluid by febrile diseases.

Administration

Taken as usual.

Caution

This gruel should be cooked thin. It is contraindicated for

those with the symptom of cough due to wind—cold.

29. Bai He Fen Zhou

Source

The book *Ben Cao Gang Mu*

Ingredients

Bai He Fen (Bulbus Lilii) in the form of powder	30 g
Jing Mi (Semen Oryzae Sativae)	100 g
Bing Tang (crystal sugar)	an appropiate amount

Preparation

Cook *Bai He Fen* and *Jing Mi* together into gruel. When the gruel is about to be done, add *Bing Tang*.

Effect

Moistening the lung to relieve cough, nourishing the heart to calm the mind.

Indications

Senile chronic bronchitis, cough due to heat or dryness in the lung, residual fever in the late stage of febrile diseases, neurosism, menopausal syndrome, etc.

Administration

Taken as usual.

Caution

This gruel is contraindicated for those with the symptom of cough due to wind—cold or with the syndrome of cold of deficiency type in the spleen and stomach. If *Xian Bai He* (fresh Bulbus Lilii) is used, the dosage should be 60 g.

30. Lian Zi Fen Zhou

Source

The book *Tai Ping Sheng Hui Fang*

Ingredients

Lian Zi Fen (Semen Nelumbinis) in the form of powder	15–20 g
Jing Mi (Semen Oryzae Savitae)	100 g

Preparation

Cook *Lian Zi* until it is done. Peel it and dry it and grind it into powder, which is then cooked together with *Jing Mi* into gruel.

Effect

Nourishing the heart to calm the mind, replenishing the kidney, tonifying the spleen, preventing ageing.

Indications

Infirmity with age, insomnia or dream-disturbed sleep, chronic diarrhea, frequent urination at night, etc.

Caution

Contraindicated for those with the symptom of fever due to cold or the symptom of constipation.

31. *Suan Zao Ren Zhou*

Source

The book *Tai Ping Sheng Hui Fang*

Ingredients

Suan Zao Ren (Semen Ziziphi Spinosae)	30–40 g
Jing Mi (Semen Oryzae Sativae)	100 g

Preparation

Crush *Suan Zao Ren* and decoct it in water for the concentrated decoction. Cook *Jing Mi* in an appropriate amount of water. When *Jing Mi* is half done, add the decoction to it and continue the cooking until the gruel is well prepared.

Effect

Nourishing the liver, relieving mental stress, calming the mind, arresting sweating.

Indications

Neurosism, senile insomnia, severe palpitation, spontaneous sweating, night sweating, etc.

Administration

Taken hot at supper.

Notes

Either prepared or unprepared *Suan Zao Ren* may be used.

32. Shan Zha Zhou

Source

The book *Zhou Pu*

Ingredients

Shan Zha (Fructus Crataegi)	30—40 g
Jing Mi (Semen Oryzae Sativae)	100 g
Sha Tang (granulated sugar)	10 g

Preparation

Decoct *Shan Zha* in a clay pot for the concentrated decoction, which is then cooked together with *Jing Mi* and *Sha Tang* into gruel.

Effect

Strengthening the spleen and stomach, promoting digestion, dispersing blood stasis.

Regular intake of this gruel by the aged may have the effect of preventing diseases and strengthening the body.

Indications

Retention of food, abdominal pain, diarrhea, postpartum pain caused by stasis of blood, lochiorrhea, dysmenorrhea, infantile indigestion, hypertension, coronary heart disease, hyperlipemia, etc.

Administration

This gruel is eaten as light refreshments at breakfast, lunch and supper. One course of treatment involves 7–10 days.

Caution

This gruel is contraindicated for those with the syndrome of deficiency of the spleen and stomach; it should not be taken on an empty stomach. If *Xian Shan Zha* (fresh Fructus Crataegi) is used, the dosage should be 60 g.

33. *Yi Yi Ren Zhou*

Source

The book *Guang Ji Fang*

Ingredients

Yi Yi Ren Fen (Semen Coicis) in the form of powder	30–60 g
Jing Mi (Semen Oryzae Sativae)	100 g

Preparation

Wash *Yi Yi Ren*, dry it in the sun, and then grind it into fine powder, which is cooked with *Jing Mi* into gruel.

Effect

Strengthening the spleen and stomach, inducing diuresis, resisting tumour.

If the aged and the middle-aged eat it regularly, they may enjoy the effect of preventing diseases, building up the body, retarding ageing and prolonging life.

Indications

Senile edema, spasm of the muscles and tendons, and numbness and pain due to wind-dampness.

Taking this gruel may serve as an accessory therapy for preventing and treating carcinoma of stomach, carcinoma of intestine and cervical carcinoma.

Administration

Eaten hot at breakfast and supper.

2.7 Medicated Cake for Health Care

Cake is a kind of common food made by steaming or baking the paste of powdered rice, wheat or bean. It is popular among the Chinese people since it is soft and easy to digest. The book *Ben Cao Gang Mu* (Compendium of Materia Medica) has described the cake made of *Jing Mi* (Semen Oryzae Sativae) like this: " It has the action of nourishing the spleen, stomach and intestines, invigorating *Qi* and regulating the middle—*Jiao*." As for medicated cake, it is made in the following way: Grind traditional Chinese medicines with the action of health—preserving into fine powder, which is mixed with one of the powders of rice, wheat or bean. Add white sugar and cooking oil to the mixture, which is made into pastes. Steam or bake the pastes until they are done.

Medicated cake is a delicious food. Furthermore it may serve as a product for health care in dietotherapy because it contains herbal medicines with the action of preventing and treating diseases, protecting health, retarding ageing and prolonging life.

Medicated cakes are usually used to help treat senile and infantile patients with chronic disorders of the spleen and stomach or help recuperate patients in convalescence as well as those used for preventing and treating other diseases. According to the ancient literature, some of them have the action of tonifying the spleen, replenishing the kidney and slowing down the process of ageing and they are especially suitable for the aged to take regularly. Taking medicated cakes is a convenient, practical and self-health-preserving method, for most medicines contained in them are mild in nature and the making of them at home is easy. The medicated cakes introduced below, in which alteration of ingredients or dosage may occur, are mostly selected from relevant literature. The introduction and analyses concerned have been enriched with the author's modern knowledge and experience. The prescriptions without the sources indicated are the proved ones created by the author.

1. Yang Chun Bai Xue Gao

Source

The book *Shou Shi Bao Yuan* written by Gong Tingxian, a medical official of the Institute of Imperial Physicians in the Ming Dynasty

Ingredients

Bai Fu Ling (Poria)	150 g
Huai Shan Yao (Rhizoma Dioscoreae)	150 g
Qian Shi Ren (Semen Euryales)	150 g
Lian Zi Rou (Semen Nelumbinis)	150 g
Chen Cang Mi (long-stored rice)	300 g
Nuo Mi (Semen Oryzae Glutinosae)	300 g
Bai Sha Tang (white granulated sugar)	900 g

Preparation

Bai Fu Ling with its skin removed is ground together with *Huai Shan Yao*, *Qian Shi Ren* and *Lian Zi Rou* (Semen Nelumbinis with the plumule and skin removed) into fine powder. Steam the powder, *Chen Cang Mi* and *Nuo Mi* together until they are well done. Mix the well-done ingredients with *Bai Sha Tang* thoroughly and knead the mixture with water into a paste. Make the paste into cakes with a mould. Dry the cakes in the sun and then store them for use.

Administration

Eaten freely by men, women or children.

Effect

Strengthening the spleen, nourishing the stomach, replenishing the kidney, tonifying the heart.

Indications

General debility, dysfunction of the spleen and stomach, listlessness and poor appetite.

Notes

This cake is most suitable for the aged. If it is used to treat various kinds of consumptive diseases, very good curative effects will be achieved.

2. *Mi Chuan Er Xian Gao*

Source

The book *Fu Shou Jing Gang* and the book *Ji Yang Gang Mu* both of which are classics of the Ming Dynasty.

Ingredients

Ren Shen (Radix Ginseng)	250 g
Shan Yao (Rhizoma Dioscoreae)	250 g
Bai Fu Ling (Poria)	250 g
Qian Shi Ren (Semen Euryales)	250 g
Lian Zi Rou (Semen Nelumbinis with the plumule and skin removed)	250 g
Nuo Mi (Semen Oryzae Glutinosae)	750 g
Jing Mi (Semen Oryzae Sativae)	1750 g

Feng Mi (Mel)	250 g
Bai Tang (white sugar)	250 g

Preparation

Grind *Ren Shen, Shan Yao, Bai Fu Ling, Qian Shi Ren, Lian Zi Rou, Nuo Mi* and *Jing Mi* into fine powder and stir the powder evenly. Dissolve *Feng Mi* and *Bai Tang* in water and mix them with the powder thoroughly into a desirable mixture. Steam the mixture into Chinese chessman—like pieces and bake the pieces on mild fire. The baked pieces are *Mi Chuan Er Xian Gao*.

Administration

Mi Chuan Er Xian Gao may be eaten as a light refreshments. It may also be made into powder, which is stored in a porcelain pot. Every morning, a large spoonful of the powder is infused with boiled water and eaten.

Effect

Strengthening the teeth, blackening the hair, invigorating both *Yin* and *Yang*, replenishing the kidney—*Yin*, nourishing the spleen and stomach.

Indications

Same as those of *Yang Chun Bai Xue Gao*.

Notes

Compared with *Yang Chun Bai Xue Gao*, this cake contains one more ingredient—*Ren Shen*, which enhances its effect of invigorating primordial *Qi* and strengthens its tonifying action.

3. *Jiu Xian Wang Dao Gao*

Source

The book *Wan Bing Hui Chun* written by Gong Tingxian in the Ming Dynasty and the book *Chuan Ya Nei Wai Pian* written by Zhao Xuemin in the Qing Dynasty

Ingredients

Lian Zi Rou (Semen Nelumbinis with the plumule and skin removed)	120 g
Chao Shan Yao (parched Rhizoma Dioscoreae)	120 g
Bai Fu Ling (Poria)	120 g
Yi Ren (Semen Coicis)	120 g
Chao Mai Ya (parched Fructus Hordei Germinatus)	60 g
Chao Bai Bian Dou (parched Semen Dolichoris Album)	60 g
Qian Shi (Semen Euryales)	60 g
Shi Shuang (Pruina Kaki)	30 g
Bai Tang (white sugar)	600 g
Nuo Mi (Semen Oryzae Glutinosae)	2500 g

Preparation

Grind all the ingredients together into powder except *Nuo Mi* which is ground separately. Mix the two kinds of powder with an appropriate amount of water into paste. Steam the paste until it is done. Cut the steamed paste into pieces and dry the pieces in the sun.

Administration

Eaten with rice soup, and at will.

Effect

Tranquilizing the mind, strengthening primordial *Qi*, invigorating the spleen and stomach, activating appetite, restoring *Qi*, promoting the regeneration of tissues, removing dampness and heat.

Indications

It is advisable for those who are old or have weak constitutions to eat this kind of cakes regularly, for this will build up their health and prolong their lives.

Notes

Compared with *Yang Chun Bai Xue Gao*, this kind of cakes contain four more ingredients: *Yi Ren, Mai Ya, Bai Bian Dou* and *Shi Shuang*, which not only enhances its action of invigorating the spleen and inducing appetite but also causes it to have the action of promoting digestion, dispelling dampness, clearing away heat and benefiting the production of body fluid, avoiding stagnation of *Qi*—a side effect often caused by mere tonification.

4. Ba Xian Bai Yun Gao

Source

The book *Ming Yi Xuan Yao Ji Shi Qi Fang*

Ingredients

Gan Shan Yao (dried Rhizoma Dioscoreae)	120 g
Lian Zi Rou (Semen Nelumbinis with the plumule and skin removed)	120 g
Bai Fu Ling (Poria)	120 g
Qian Shi Rou (Semen Euryales with the plumule and skin removed)	120 g
Yi Yi Ren (Semen Coicis)	120 g
Bai Shao Yao (Radix Paeoniae Alba)	60 g
Bai Zhu (Rhizoma Atractylodis Macrocephalae)	60 g
Sha Ren (Fructus Amomi)	30 g
Shang Bai Mi Fan (cooked fine rice)	1500 g
Nuo Mi (Semen Oryzae Glutinosae)	750 g
Bai Sha Tang Shuang (frost of white granulated sugar)	1250 g

Preparation

Grind the first 8 ingredients into fine powder and mix the

powder with *Shang Bai Mi Fan* and *Nuo Mi* into a well-stirred mixture, to which *Bai Sha Tang Shuang* is then added. Steam the mixture containing all the ingredients into cakes.

Administration

Eaten at will.

Effect

Having the miraculous action of keeping health, invigorating primordial *Qi* and regulating physiological functions.

Notes

Cakes of this kind contain four more herbal medicines than *Yang Chun Bai Xue Gao*: *Yi Yi Ren*, *Bai Shao*, *Bai Zhu* and *Sha Ren*, which not only enhances its effect of invigorating the spleen and stomach but also its action of removing dampness, promoting the circulation of *Qi*, enriching blood, astringing *Yin* and nourishing the liver. Though having tonifying action, they are not greasy in nature, being a good medicated cake for tonification.

5. *Ba Xian Zao Chao Gao*

Source

The book *Ji Yang Gang Mu*

Ingredients

Chao Bai Zhu (parched Rhizoma Atractylodis Macrocephalae)	120 g
Shan Yao (Rhizoma Dioscoreae)	120 g
Zhi Shi (Fructus Aurantii Immaturus)	60 g
Bai Fu Ling (Poria)	60 g
Chao Chen Pi (parched Pericarpium Citri Reticulatae)	60 g
Lian Zi Rou (Semen Nelumbinis with the plumule and skin removed)	60 g

Shan Zha (Fructus Crataegi with the core removed)	60 g
Ren Shen (Radix Ginseng)	30 g
Bai Mi (fine rice)	2750 g
Nuo Mi (Semen Oryzae Glutinosae)	750 g
Feng Mi (honey)	1500 g

Preparation

Grind the first eight ingredients into fine powder and then grind *Bai Mi* and *Nuo Mi* too. Mix the two powders and *Feng Mi* thoroughly and make the mixture into a paste. Cut the paste into small pieces and steam the pieces until they are done. Bake the steamed pieces dry and store them in a clay pot. These pieces are the cakes.

Administration

The cakes may be eaten now and then, 3–5 pieces each time.

Effect

Regulating the function of the spleen and stomach, treating incessant diarrhea, being of great benefit to the aged.

Indications

Cakes of this kind may be eaten regularly by middle-aged and old people with the symptom of anorexia due to Qi-deficiency of the spleen.

Notes

The cakes contain four(*Bai Zhu, Zhi Shi, Chen Pi* and *Shan Zha*)more and one(*Qian Shi*) less medicines than *Mi Chuan Er Xian Gao*, Which enhances its action of promoting the flow of Qi, improving appetite and benefiting digestion, and causes it to be a fine medicated cake which, not greasy in nature, has tonifying action but does not induce any stagnation.

6. *Ba Zhen Gao*

Source

The book *Qing Tai Yi Tuan Pei Fang*

Ingredients

Yi Mi (Semen Coicis)	90 g
Qian Shi (Semen Euryales)	90 g
Bian Dou (Semen Dolichoris Album)	90 g
Jian Lian (Semen Nelumbinis with the plumule and skin removed)	90 g
Shan Yao (Rhizoma Dioscoreae)	90 g
Dang Shen (Radix Codonopsis)	60 g
Fu Ling (Poria)	60 g
Bai Zhu (Rhizoma Atractylodis Macrocephalae)	30 g
Bai Tang (white sugar)	240 g
Bai Mi Fen (Powder of white rice)	an appropriate amount

Preparation

Grind the above ingredients except the last one into fine powder. Mix the powder with *Bai Mi Fen* into a mixture. Make the mixture into cakes.

Administration

Eaten at will, 2–3 times each day.

Effect

Taking a leading role in mildly strengthening and nourishing the spleen and stomach with miraculous curative effects.

Indications

Ba Zhen Gao is indicated for those whose constitutions and spleen−*Qi* are weak. Eating it may be treated as an accessory therapy for some diseases.

Caution

Regular intake of *Ba Zhen Gao* tends to result in stagnation of the stomach—*Qi*, as it does not contain medicines with the action of regulating the flow of *Qi* or promoting digestion.

Notes

Cakes of this kind contain four(*Dang Shen. Bai Zhu, Bian Dou* and *Yi Mi*)more medicines than *Yang Chun Bai Xue Gao*, which enhances its action of replenishing *Qi*, strengthening the spleen and removing dampness, and causes it to be a fine medicated cake for invigorating the spleen and stomach.

Being neither cold nor hot in nature and with unfailing effects, *Ba Zhen Gao* was once appreciated in the palace of the Qing Dynasty, in which the emperors Qianlong and Guangxu and the empress dowager Cixi all liked to eat it.

Shandong College of TCM inherited the experience which had been accumulated in using medicated cakes to protect health since the Ming and Qing Dynasties, absorbed the achievements of modern scientific researches and has developed *Ba Zhen Shi Pin* (eight-treasure food). *Ba Zhen Shi Pin* is made up of both food substances and medicines such as *Shan Yao, Lian Zi Rou, Shan Zha,* etc., embodying the principle that tonifying the body should be combined with promoting digestion. It has the action of strengthening the spleen, regulating the stomach, promoting digestion, tonifying the kidney, nourishing the heart, replenishing the lung, removing stagnation of *Qi*, eliminating food retention, dispelling dampness and calming the mind. Observations have shown that *Ba Zhen Shi Pin* does have the action of promoting children's growth and appetite. Laboratory experiments have also proved that it has the action of promoting the growth of young animals, raising the level of hemoglobin, strengthening the body, regulating digestive function, and greatly improving the conditions of the animals with the syndrome of deficiency of the spleen. This indicates again that medicated cakes for health care do have the action of tonifying the body and protecting health.

7. Jian Pi Yang Xin Gao

Ingredients

Fu Shen (Poria cum Ligno Hospite)	60 g
Lian Zi Rou (Semen Nelumbinis with the plumule and skin removed)	60 g
Shan Yao (Rhizoma Dioscoreae)	60 g
Bai He (Bulbus Lilii)	60 g
Long Yan Rou (Arillus Longan)	60 g
Bai Tang (white sugar)	150 g
Nuo Mi Fen (powdered Semen Oryzae Glutinosae)	1000 g

Preparation

Grind the first five ingredients into fine powder. Mix the powder with *Bai Tang* and *Nuo Mi Fen* thoroughly. Steam the mixture into cakes, which may be baked dry for storage.

Administration

Eaten at will and regularly.

Effect

Strengthening the spleen, replenishing Qi, nourishing the heart, calming the mind, tonifying the kidney, enriching blood, being a good food used in dietetic therapy for strengthening both the heart and spleen.

Indications

Deficiency of Qi and blood in the heart and spleen, listlessness, poor appetite, bad memory, insomnia, palpitation, shortness of breath, sallow complexion, etc.

Notes

Compared with the above-mentioned medicated cakes, cakes of this kind have the stronger action of nourishing the heart to calm the mind.

8. He Zhong Xiao Shi Gao

Ingredients

Fu Ling (Poria)	45 g
Bai Bian Dou (Semen Dolichoris Album)	45 g
Lian Zi Rou (Semen Nelumbinis with the plumule and skin removed)	45 g
Shan Yao (Rhizoma Dioscoreae)	45 g
Chao Shan Zha (parched Fructus Crataegi)	45 g
Chao Mai Ya (parched Fructus Hordei Germinatus)	45 g
Chao Gu Ya (parched Fructus Oryzae Germinatus)	45 g
Sha Ren (Fructus Amomi)	9 g
Bai Tang (white sugar)	150 g
Mi Fen (powder of rice)	1000 g

Preparation

Grind the first eight ingredients into fine powder. Mix the powder with *Bai Tang* and *Mi Fen* thoroughly and steam the mixture into cakes. The cakes may be cut into pieces, which are then baked dry.

Administration

Eaten at will and regularly.

Effect

Invigorating the spleen and stomach, replenishing *Qi*, regulating the stomach to promote digestion, activating the flow of *Qi*.

Indications

Deficiency of the spleen and stomach, poor appetite, abdominal distention, stuffiness and fullness in the epigastrium and abdomen, and food retention.

Notes

Cakes of this kind have both tonifying and resolving effects and their tonifying effect will not cause any stagnation.

2.8　Medicated Pancake for Health Care

Medicated pancake is also a kind of conventional drug form in traditional Chinese medicine, and it is of either internal or external administration. Taking medicated pancake orally is a common form of dietary treatment with medicated food, which is often used for health care. In this section we will describe medicated pancake.

Medicated pancake is made of traditional Chinese drugs with health-protecting action and in the form of fine powder, and wheat flour, bean flour or rice flour sometimes plus dates or sugar and edible oil. It may be made by steaming, baking or frying. As the pancake is easy to make, convenient to take, more delicious and actually effective, taking it may be a good method of health-self-protection, especially in the aged and children, as well as in those suffering from general debility. Medicated pancake for health care is, in general, mild in drug nature and slow in drug action, meaning that only constant administration of it will obtain excellent effect. No or few drugs with potent action or toxicity are used in it. If these drugs are found in the prescription, the dosage should be controlled and it must be processed according to the fixed rule. Moreover, the intake of the pancake containing the above-mentioned drugs should be strictly limited to avoid toxic and side effects.

Here are some of the pancakes which have the action or preventing diseases, building up health, prolonging life and combating ageing. The prescriptions with sources indicated are from relevant literature. In these prescriptions, alteration of ingredients or dosage may occur and the analyses of their effects have been enriched with the author's knowledge and experience. The prescriptions without sources indicated are the proved ones created by the authors.

1. *Tian Dong Bing Zi*

Source

The book *Tai Ping Sheng Hui Fang* (Peaceful Holy Benevolent Prescriptions)

Ingredients

Tian Dong (Radix Asparagi)   500 g

Bai Mi (Mel)   100 g

Hu Ma Mo (Semen Sesami in the form of fine powder) 200 g

Hei Dou Huang Mo (Clycine max(L.)Merr. seeds in the form of fine powder) an adequate amount

Preparation

Pound *Tian Dong* to get 150g of its juice and decoct the juice until 50g of it remains. Put *Bai Mi* and Hu Ma Mo, which has been slightly parched, into the juice and stir the mixture evenly. Add an appropriate amount of *Hei Dou Huang Mo* to the mixture and make the the final mixture into pancakes, each of which is 9 cm in diameter and 1.5 cm in thickness. Steam and then bake in a pan or roast the pancakes until they are done.

Dosage and Administration

Take one each time, 3 times a day. When taken, it should be chewed well, and may be swallowed with warm liquor.

Effect

Nourishing *Yin*—essence, supplementing the lung and kidney, making teeth strong and hair black.

The book says, "If one takes this kind of pancakes regularly, he will have his hair changed from grey into black, new teeth generated after the old ones have been lost, his strength greatly increased, and his life prolonged."

Indications

Impairments due to deficiency, infirmity with age, emaciation, hemiplegia, and other disorders due to *Yin*—deficiency of the lung and kidney and the lack of vital essence and *Qi*.

Notes

Both *Tian Men Dong* and *Hu Ma* are antiageing agents. That is why prolonged time of administration of this pancakes will produce the effect of antiageing and longevity enhancement.

2. *Huang Jing Bing*

Source

The book *Tai Ping Sheng Hui Fang*

Ingredients

Huang Jing (Rhizoma Polygonati) an adequate amount

Hei Dou Huang Mo (Clycine max(L.)Merr. seeds in the form of fine powder) an adequate amount

Preparation

Decoct *Huang Jing* In water for the decoction and condense the decoction into a jelly. Mix the jelly with *Hei Dou Huang Mo* which has been parched, and make the mixture into pancakes all of a coin size. Finally steam or bake the pancakes until they are done.

Dosage and Administration

Take two of them daily. The in take is to be gradually increased.

Effect

Invigorating vital essence, benefiting the bone marrow, nourishing *Yin*, replenishing *Qi*, strengthening the tendons and bones.

The book says, "If the aged take this kind of pancakes for a hundred days, they will enjoy their effect; if for a year, they will have their strength doubled, being as strong as the youth."

Indications

Lack of vital essence and bone marrow, *Qi*–weakness due to deficiency of *Yin*, fatigue, inability of the limbs, hemoptysis due to impairment of the lung, etc.

Notes

This kind of pancakes has been long since known to have the action of promoting longevity and delaying ageing. Recent investigations have already shown that it can increase the blood flow in the coronary arteries and the trophic blood flow in myocardium, prevent atherosclerosis, lower blood pressure and the level of blood sugar, which is the reason why it has the action of slowing down the process of ageing and promoting longevity.

3. Zhuang Yang Nuan Xia Yao Bing

Source

The writing *Lao Lao Yu Bian* written by Xu Chunfu in the Ming Dynasty

Ingredients

Pao Fu Zi (Radix Aconiti Lateralis Preparata)   30 g

Shen Qu (Massa Fermentata Medicinalis)	90 g
Pao Gan Jiang (Rhizoma Zingiberis Praeparata)	90 g
Zao (Fructus Jujubae)	30 dates
Gui Xin (Cortex Cinnamomi)	30 g
Wu Wei Zi (Fructus Schisandrae)	30 g
Tu Si Zi (Semen Cuscutae)	30 g
Rou Cong Rong (Herba Cistanchis)	30 g
Shu Jiao (Pericarpium Zanthoxyli)	15 g
Yang Sui (sheep marrow)	90 g
Su (butter)	60 g
Mi (Mel)	120 g
Huang Yang Ru (milk)	1.5 litres
Bai Mian (flour)	500 g

Preparation

Peel *Pao Fu Zi*. Remove the skin and core of *Zao*. Steep *Rou Cong Rong* for one day and night, remove its shrunken skin and fry it dry. Parch *Shu Jiao* a little until it becomes slightly yellowish. Grind the processed *Pao Fu Zi, Tu Si Zi, Rou Cong Rong* and *Shu Jiao* together with *Shen Qu, Pao Gan Jiang, Gui Xin, Wu Wei Zi* into fine powder. Mix the powder with *Bai Mian, Su, Yang Sui, Mi* and *Yang Ru* into a mixture, to which *Zao* is then added. Cook the mixture and put it in a basin with a tight cover. Immediately after the basin has been left in a ventilated place for half a day, remove the content and prepare and cook it again. Then make the content into pancakes. Finally roast them in a stove until they are done.

Dosage and Administration

Take the pancakes on an empty stomach, one daily.

Effect

Warming the kidney—*Yang*, dispelling *Yin*—cold, supplementing vital essence and the marrow.

Indications

Deficiency of the kidey—*Yang*, decline of fire in the gate of life, weakness and impairment due to insufficiency of vital essence and marrow, impotence, emission, frequent urination ay night, lassitude of the loins and knees, aversion to cold, cold limbs, etc.

Notes

The writing *Lao Lao Yu Bian* introduces this kind of pancakes like this: "It has the action of treating various kinds of impairments caused by overstrain, night emission and frequent urination."

Fu Zi is of hot nature and toxicity. It must be processed before being used and overuse of it is avoided. The pancakes containing it should be small in size and shouldn't be taken in excess amount.

4. *Qi Yi Bing*

Source

The book *Yi Xue Zhong Zhong Can Xi Lu*

Ingredients

Sheng Qian Shi (Semen Euryales)	180 g
Sheng Ji Nei jin (Endothelium Corneum Gigeriae Galli)	90 g
Bai Mian (flour)	250 g

Bai Sha Tang (Sacharum), an adequate amount

Preparation

First grind *Sheng Qian Shi* and strain the powder. Then grind and strain *Sheng Ji Nei Jin*, and infuse the powder with boiling water and steep the powder in the water for about a half day. Take out the steeped *Ji Nei Jin* and mix it with the fine powders of *Qian Shi*, *Bai Mian* and *Bai Sha Tang* into a mixture. Make the mixture into pancakes with the water in which *Ji Nei Jin* has been steeped. Finally bake the pancakes in a pan until they become yellowish.

Dosage and Administration

To be taken at will.

Effect

Strengthening the kidney, stop nocturnal emission, invigorating the spleen to promote digestion.

Indications

Deficiency of *Qi* in the aged, marked by failure to cough up sputum, retention of phlegm, stagnation of *Qi*, fullness in the chest and hypochondriac pain, and hernia.

These pancakes are effective for those ill with the syndrome of deficiency of vital energy and cough producing sputum, and remarkably benefit middle-aged and ole people.

5. *Yi Pi Bing*

Source

The book *Yi Xue Zhong Zhong Can Xi Lu*

Ingredients

Bai Zhu (Rhizoma Atractylodis Macrocephalae)	120 g
Ji Nei Jin (Endothelium Corneum Gigeriae Galli)	60 g
Gan Jiang (Rhizoma Zingiberis)	60 g
Shu Zao Rou (Fructus Jujubae)	250 g

Preparation

Grind *Bai Zhu* into powder and bake the powder until it is done. Do the same with *Ji Nei Jin*. Smash *Gan Jiang*. Pound all the above and *Shu Zao Rou* into something like a paste and make the paste into small pancakes. Finally fry the pancakes dry on char fire.

Dosage and Administration

Pancakes of this kind are to be eaten as a snack. When eaten they must be chewed well.

Effect

Strengthening the spleen, warming the stomach, replenishing *Qi*, nourishing blood, promoting digestion.

This is a universal medicated food with mild action of warming and tonifying the middle—*Jiao*.

Indications

Syndrome due to weakness of the spleen and stomach accompanied by cold, marked by anorexia, pain in the hypochondriac and abdominal region, frequent and sudden diarrhea, indigestion, which are aggravated by cold or fatigue.

The book *Yi Xue Zhong Zhong Can Xi Lu* says, "*Yi Pi Bing* may be used to treat the syndrome due to dampness—cold accumulated in the spleen and stomach, marked by poor appetite, frequent diarrhea and indigestion."

Notes

When there hasn't appeared cold manifestation, *Gan Jiang* should be used in smaller amount or even omitted. *Da Zao* with its stones removed is cooked into *Shu Zao Rou*.

6. Yi Shou Bing

Ingredients

Fu Ling (Poria)	30 g
Shan Yao (Rhizoma Dioscoreae)	30 g
He Shou Wu (Radix Polygoni Multiflori)	30 g
Lian Zi Rou (Semen Nelumbinis)	30 g

Gou Qi Zi (Fructus Lycii)	30 g
Bai Mian (flour)	500 g
Bai Tang (Sacharum)	an adequate amount

Preparation

Grind the first 5 ingredients into fine powder. Mix the powder, *Bai Mian* and *Bai Tang* evenly with water into a paste. Make the paste into pancakes and bake the pancakes in the form of biscuit in an oven until they are done.

Dosage and Administration

The pancakes are for one-week use.

Effect

Invigorating both the spleen and the kidney, supplementing *Qi* and vital essence.

Indications

Early senility, weakness of the body, deficiency of both the spleen and the kidney.

Notes

Fu Ling, Shou Wu and *Gou Qi* in the pancakes are all the ideal drugs with the action of slowing down the process of ageing and prolonging life. So pancakes of this kind are not only fit for middle-aged and old people to take regularly but also suitable for those who are weak due to deficiency of both the spleen and the kidney to build up their health.

7. *Jiu Xian Bao Jian Bing*

Ingredients

Fu Ling (Poria)	30 g
Shan Yao (Rhizoma Dioscoreae)	30 g
Yi Mi (Semen Coicis)	30 g
Qian Shi (Semen Eutyales)	30 g

Bai He (Bulbus Lilii)	30 g
Chao Shan Zha (parched Fructus Grataegi)	30 g
Chao Mai Ya (parched Fructus Hordei Germinatus)	30 g
Sha Ren (Fructus Amomi)	9 g
Chao Hei Zhi Ma (Semen Sesami Nigrum)	30 g
Mian Fen (flour)	1000
Bai Tang (white sugar)	an adequate amount

Preparation

Grind the first eight ingredients into fine powder. Mix the powder with *Chao Hei Zhi Ma* and *Bai Tang* into an even mixture. Make the mixture with water into a dough. Form the dough into small pancakes like biscuits. Bake or roast the pancakes until they are done.

Dosage and Administration

To be eaten at will.

Effect

Replenishing the heart and spleen, tonifying the liver and kidney, stopping nocturnal emission, calming the mind, nourishing the five *Zang*—organs, Strengthening the stomach, activating the flow of *Qi*, promoting digestion.

Notes

Because all the herbal medicines in the pancakes can be taken either as drugs or as food, pancakes of this kind have become a mild tonifying food for health care in dietary therapy, and are extensively suitable for people of all ages and both sexes.

2.9　Externally-applied Plaster for Health Care

The plaster, which was known as thin application in the ancient times, has been long since a traditional Chinese preparation for external application. Plasters processed in a special way are applied to the skin, which, through the action of the drugs, may prevent and treat diseases and preserve health. The use of plasters has a long history in China. In the Jin Dynasty, Ge Hong, a physician, recorded in his book *Zhou Hou Bei Ji Fang* plasters made with oil and various pharmaceutical preparations. In the Tang and Song Dynasties, plasters were widely used. In the Ming Dynasty, Gong Tingxian, a physician, stated in his works *Shou Shi Bao Yuan* that frequent application of the plaster *Qian Jin Feng Qi Gao* received the effect of "rejuvenation" and "turning young". In the Qing Dynasty, Wu Shangxian, a physician, collected a lot of prescriptions of various plasters in his book *Li Yue Pian Wen* and the imperial physicians then also used to use plasters to keep the emperors and their mothers healthy and treat their diseases.

Plasters do have wide uses. For instance, diseases grouped under internal medicine, gynecology and pediatrics may be treated with plasters according to the rule "Internal diseases can be treated externally.". When plasters are used to treat surgical and traumatological diseases, they will exert their effects of relieving inflammation, alleviating pain, promoting blood circulation, subduing swelling, arresting bleeding and inducing tissue regeneration.

Applied to relevant tonifying acupoints, plasters for health care are able to prevent diseases, preserve health, delay ageing, and prolong life. Since they are convenient to use, and their actions are mild and lasting with reliable results, the application of them appear to be an appropriate method of self-preserving health.

The book *Li Yue Pian Wen* says that the principle of the external treatment is the same as that of the internal, the drugs used in the external therapy are just those in the internal. The difference between the internal and external therapies is just the difference in the way of applying the same drugs. Disease-treating and health-preserving actions which are produced by plasters externally applied are known to be in accordance with both the nature of the drugs and the medical theories of the internal treatment. So far as the drugs of plasters for health care are concerned, they are largely classified as the ones that contribute to warming the meridian to expel cold, invigorating *Yang* to reinforce primordial *Qi*, supplementing the spleen and kidney, promoting the flow of *Qi*, relieving stasis and dredging the meridian passages. Placed on acupoints such as Shenque(RN8), Qihai(RN6), Guanyuan(RN4)and Shenshu(BL23), the plasters may send off their actions through the skin and muscles to the organs via the meridians, so as to strengthen *Yang*, stop nocturnal emission build up primordial *Qi*, dredge the channels, and promote the circulation of *Qi* and blood. As a result, it is evident that the plasters have the effects of building up health, preventing diseases and holding ageing. Observations have shown that drugs with the action of warming the kidney and restoring *Yang* such as *Ding Xiang* (Flos Caryophylli)and *Rou Gui* (Cortex Cinnamomi), when put on the acupoint Shenque(RN8)to treat chronic bronchitis, can not only reduce the symptoms but also improve immunity of the body, increasing the immunological function of cells and resulting in the prevention of coryza and the improvement of appetite. Thus, plasters have a definite role to play in preserving health.

Plasters are of several types, and the type for health care is, in general, included in the "Black one." It is prepared from active components which are derived from drugs fried in edible vegetable oil. The extracted components should be first freed from the residue and then condensed at high temperatures. When minium is added to the concentrate, a chemical reaction occurs, forming lead plaster. Sesame oil, a kind of vegetable oil, has been considered as the best one that can be used in preparing plasters. Minium generally called "yellow lead" is a fine orange—red or orange powder, which is made of lead. Its main element is lead tetraoxide. The basic procedure for the preparation of plasters of the black—type is as follows:

Frying Materials

Heat the sesame oil in an adequate amount in a pot, and add the drugs to it while stirring conti-nuously. The drugs of loose nature are not placed in the pot until the other drugs have been fried into scorch—yellow, and the floating drugs should be pressed below the oil by means of a dipper. The fire is kept gentle and the temperature of oil may go up to 200 — 220 ℃ (not exceeding 240℃). Heat the pot until the drugs in it are dark—brown and their inside has turned scorched—yellow; and when the temperature of oil drops below 200℃, the oil will be freed from the residue of the drugs and used as medicated oil.

Refining Oil

Heat the medicated oil by intense fire until its temperature rises up to 320℃ −330℃ and then adopt moderate fire with continual stirring to maintain its temperature within this range. The oil is regarded as being available if its fumes turn from black to white, its foam comes from the pot walls towards the center and the oil is refined up to the state in which "a drop of oil dripped in water becomes a pearl", that is, take a bit of the heated medicated oil and drip it in water, where the oil drop will disperse and gather again.

Adding Minium and Preparing Plasters

Remove the pot with the oil from fire and place it in a steady position, add slowly the yellow lead by even speading and continual stirring in a certain direction to avoid precipitation of minium in the bottom of the pot. At this time the oil temperature is likely to remain at about 320℃ and a lot of irritative fume may be given off. When the white fume disappears and the oil turns from brown to black, take out a bit of the plaster and place it in cold water, and pull with a hand the plaster out of the water a few seconds later. Provided that the plaster is not stuck to the hand and is in an adequate thickness, the plaster is considered to be the finished one. This method is the common one which is called fire—leaving—and—minium—adding method. Another one is on—fire—minium—adding method, meaning that after the oil is slightly heated, the minium is added gradually while the oil is being heated. All of minium having been placed in the oil, heating is continued until the content becomes plaster. As far as the dosage of yellow lead goes, it should be 150−210g when 1 kg of oil is used, and it may be less in winter and greater in summer. The lead should be parched dry before it is used.

Removing "fire—evil"

Pour the resulting plaster slowly into cold water, stir continuously with a wooden rod in order to make it in the form of a band, which facilitates cooling. The cold water should be frequently replaced. After being condensed the plaster is taken out of the water and made into a mass by repeated pressing. The mass is left in cold water for 24 hours to a few days(the water has to be replaced every day)so as to remove all the five—evil. Otherwise the plaster when applied to the skin would cause local stimulation, marked by red rash and itch, even vesiculation or ulcer.

Coating

Put the plaster mass in a suitable vessel and place the vessel on water bath to melt the mass. Add to it ground materials, such as the powders of *She Xiang* (Moschus)and *Bing Pian* (Borneolum Syntheticum)and stir the content evenly. Take a certain quantity of the medicinal plaster with a bamboo stick and coat it on a piece of paper or cloth, which is the final step for preparing the plaster.

When one administrates the ready plaster, he may either warm it on fire or heat the cloth cover with a cup full of boiling water in order to make the plaster soft and sticky. As a result, it can stick to the skin. It should be pointed out that before the application the local skin must be cleaned.

Conventional plasters contain many, often up to several dozens of drugs, including such rare and precious ones as *She Xiang* (Moschus)and *Hu Gu* (Os Tigris). Therefore the plaster is not easy for the individual to prepare and it is more convenient to buy the ready—made plaster in a Chinese drugstore. Some simple ones will be introduced here and you may make them yourself with the methods described above.

1. Yang Xin Gao

Source

The book *Li Yue Pian Wen*

Ingredients

Dang Shen (Radix Codonopsis)
Bai Zhu (Rhizoma Atractylodis Macrocephalae)
Yun Ling (Poria)
Gan Cao (Radix Glycyrrhizae)
Sheng Di (Radix Rehmanniae)
Bai Shao (Radix Paeoniae Alba)
Dang Gui (Radix Angelicae Sinensis)
Chuan Xiong (Rhizoma Chuanxiong)
Huang Lian (Rhizoma Coptidis)
Gua Lou (Fructus Trichosanthis)
Ban Xia (Rhizoma Pinelliae)
Chen Xiang (Lignum Aquilariae Resinatum)
Zhu Sha (Cinnabaris)
Zhi Zi (Fructus Gardeniae)

Preparation

Boil the above ingredients in sesame oil and condense the medicated oil with yellow lead.

Administration

To be applied to the point Danzhong(RN17).

Effect

Tranquilizing the mind, promoting blood circulation, eliminating phlegm, clearing away heat.

Indications

Deficiency of the heart with phlegm-fire.

It is good for chest pain(i. e. coronary heart disease)caused by blood stasis, which results from deficiency of *Qi* and heat accumulation due to retention of phlegm.

2. *Xin Shen Shuang Bu Gao*

Source

The book *Li Yue Pian Wen*

Ingredients

Tu Si Zi (Semen Cuscutae)	90 g
Niu Xi (Radix Achyranthis Bidentatae)	30 g
Shu Di (Rhizoma Rehmanniae Praeparata)	30 g
Rou Cong Rong (Herba Cistanchis)	30 g
Fu Zi (Radix Aconiti Lateralis Preparata)	30 g
Lu Long (Cornu Cervi Pantotrichum)	30 g
Dang Shen (Radix Codonopsis)	30 g
Yuan Zhi (Radix Polygalae)	30 g
Fu Shen (Poria Cum Ligno Hospite)	30 g
Huang Qi (Radix Astragali)	30 g
Shan Yao (Rhizoma Dioscoreae)	30 g
Dang Gui (Radix Angelicae Sinensis)	30 g
Long Gu (Os Draconis)	30 g
Wu Wei Zi (Fructus Schisandrae)	30 g

Preparation

Boil all the above ingredients in sesame oil and condense the medicated oil with yellow lead into plaster. Mix the plaster with 30g of *Zhu Sha* (Cinnabaris) and stir the mixture thoroughly.

Administration

This plaster is applied to the areas of the stomach and elixir field.

Effect

Warming mainly and invigorating *Yang* of the heart and

kidney.

Indications

Overstrain of the heart and kidney, deficiency complicated by cold pathogen.

Those who are suffering the syndrome due to deficiency of the heart—*Qi* and the kidney—*Yang* may use this kind of plaster to supplement *Qi* and build up health.

3. *Zhuan Yi Yuan Qi Gao*

Source

The book *Li Yue Pian Wen*

Ingredients

Niu Du (ox tripe)	one
Ma You (Oleum Sesami)	
Huang Qi (Radix Astragali)	240 g
Dang Shen (Radix Codonopsis)	180 g
Sheng Bai Zhu (Rhizoma Atractylodis Macrocephalae)	180 g
Dang Gui (Radix Angelicae Sinensis)	180 g
Shu Di (Rhizoma Rehmanniae Praeparata)	120 g
Ban Xia (Rhizoma Pinelliae)	120 g
Xiang Fu (Rhizoma Cyperi)	120 g
Mai Dong (Radix Ophiopogonis)	120 g
Wu wei Zi (Fructus Schisandrae)	30 g
Fu Ling (Poria)	30 g
Bai Shao (Radix Paeoniae Alba)	30 g
Yi Zhi Ren (Fructus Alpiniae Oxyphyllae)	30 g
Bu Gu Zhi (Fructus Psoraleae)	30 g
Hu Tao Rou (Semen Juglandis)	30 g
Chen Pi (Pericarpium Citri Reticulatae)	30 g

Rou Gui (Cortex Cinnamomi)	30 g
Gan Cao (Radix Glycyrrhizae)	30 g
Sha Ren (Fructus Amomi)	21 g
Mu Xiang (Radix Aucklandiae)	21 g
Gan Jiang (Rhizoma Zingiberis)	15 g
Da Zao (Fructus Jujubae)	10 dates

Preparation

Boil *Niu Du* in sesame oil to get the oil and remove the boiled *Niu Du*. Mix the processed oil with all the other ingredients into a mixture. Decoct the mixture to get the medicated oil. Condense the medicated oil with yellow lead into plaster.

Administration

To be applied to the point Danzhong(RN17)or the region below the umbilicus.

Effect

Invigorating the kidney, supporting *Yang*, strengthening the spleen and stomach, nourishing vital essence and blood, promoting functioning of the five—Zang organs.

Indications

Syndrome due to deficiency of primordial *Qi*, marked by mental decline and weakness of the five—*Zang* organs.

Notes

The primordial *Qi* is the source of motive force for life activities. It has been produced by congenital essence and is maintained by taking in nutrients.

4. *Yong Quan Gao*

Number One

Source

The book *Li Yue Pian Wen*

Ingredients

Hai Long (Syngnathus)	1 pair
Fu Zi (Radix Aconiti Lateralis Preparata)	30 g
Ling Ling Xiang (Lysimachia foenum-graecum)	9 g
Chuan Shan Jia (Squama Manitis)	9 g
Suo Yang (Herba Cynomorii)	9 g

Yang Qi Shi (Actinolitum)
Dong Chong Xia Cao (Cordyceps)
Gao Li Shen (Korean Radix Ginseng)
Chuan Jiao (Pericarpium Zanthoxyli)
Ding Xiang (Flos Caryophylli)

Preparation

Boil the first five ingredients in sesame oil. Condense the medicated oil with yellow lead. While condensing, stir the content with *Huai Zhi* (Ramulus Sophorae). Then put the powder of all the other ingredients into the content and stir the final mixture evenly into the plaster.

Administration

To be applied to the centre of the sole.

Number 2

Source

The book *Li Yue Pian Wen*

Ingredients

Hai Ma (Hippocampus)
Lu Rong (Cornu Cervi Pantotrichum)
Ren Shen (Radix Ginseng)
Da Hui Xiang (Fructus Illicii Veri)
Rou Cong Rong (Herba Cistanchis)
Shu Di (Rhizoma Rehmanniae Praeparata)

Di Long (Lumbricus)
Chen Xiang (Lignum Aquilariae Resinatum)
Rou Gui (Cortex Cinnamomi)

Preparation

Boil the first seven ingredients in sesame oil to get medicated oil and condense the medicated oil with yellow lead into plaster. Put the fine powder of the last two ingredients into the plaster and stir it evenly.

Administration

To be applied to the centre of the sole.

Effect

The two plasters have the action of warming the kidney, supplementing body fire and expelling *Yin*—cold, because most of their ingredients are drugs with the action of supporting *Yang* and warming the interior.

Indications

Syndrome due to deficiency of the kidney—*Yang* and decline of the fire from the gate of life, marked by soreness and weakness of the loins and knees, chills, cold limbs, impotence, night emission, tinnitus, deafness, loss of hair, loose teeth, edema of the face and feet, and frequent urination at night.

Notes

Hai Long in Number 1 may be replaced with *Hai Ma*.

The centre of the sole is where the acupoint Yongquan(KI1)is located. This point is the *Jing*xue of the Kidney Meridian of Foot—Shaoyin. Applying this plaster to this point will strengthen its action of increasing body fire and supplementing *Yang*.

Teenagers who are in good health and have no the syndrome

of *Yang*—deficiency should not use this plater. If they do, it will have the ministerial fire become hyperactive, causing dizziness, dysphoria with feverish sensation in the chest, palms and soles, as well as night emission and premature ejaculation, all due to the hyperactivity of *Yang*.

Those drugs with no dosage indicated may be used in adequate amounts according to the needs.

5. Si Yin Bai Bing Gao

Source

The book *Li Yue Pian Wen*

Ingredients

Chuan Wu (Radix Aconiti)	30 g
Cao Wu (Radix Aconiti Kusnezoffii)	30 g
Qiang Huo (Rhizoma seu Radix Notopterygii)	30 g
Du Huo (Radix Angelicae Pubescentis)	30 g
Nan Xing (Rhizoma Arisaematis)	30 g
Ban Xia (Rhizoma Pinelliae)	30 g
Ma Huang (Herba Ephedrae)	30 g
Gui Zhi (Ramulus Cinnamomi)	30 g
Cang Zhu (Rhizoma Atractylodis)	30 g
Da Huang (Radix et Rhizoma Rhei)	30 g
Xi Xin (Herba Asari)	30 g
Dang Gui (Radix Angelicae Sinensis)	30 g
Bai Zhi (Radix Angelicae Dahuricae)	30 g
Xi Xian Cao (Herba Siegesbeckiae)	30 g
Hai Feng Teng (Caulis Piperis Kadsurae)	30 g
Jiang (Rhizoma Zingiberis)	500 g
Cong (Allium Fistulosi)	500 g
Suan (Bulbus Allii)	500 g

Huai Zhi (Ramulus Sophorae)	500 g
Song Xiang (Colophonium)	60 g
Mu Xiang (Radix Aucklandiae)	15 g
Ru Xiang (Resina Olibani)	15 g
Mo Yao (Myrrha)	15 g
Qing Fen (Calomelas)	15 g
Chuan Jiao (Pericarpium Zanthoxyli)	15 g

Preparation

Boil the first nineteen ingredients in sesame oil. Remove the dregs and get medicated oil. Condense the medicated oil with yellow lead into plaster. Grind the last six ingredients into fine powder and add the powder to the plaster.

Administration

To be applied to the acupoint Shenshu(BL23).

Effect

Applied to the point Shenshu, this kind of plaster will exert the action of reinforcing the kidney, supplementing primordial *Qi*, building up constitution, keeping exogenous evils out, preventing diseases and maintaining health.

Indications

All the diseases due to wind, cold and summer-dampness.

Notes

Most of the drugs contained in this plaster have the action of eliminating the pathogens of wind, dampness and cold, and promoting the flow of blood to remove stasis.

6. *Bao Yuan Gu Ben Gao*

Source

The book *Ci Xi Guang Xu Yi Fang Xuan Yi*

Ingredients

Dang Shen (Radix Codonopsis)	45 g
Chao Bai Zhu (Rhizoma Atractylodis Macrocephalae parched)	45 g
Lu Jiao (Cornu Cervi)	45 g
Dang Gui (Radix Angelicae Sinensis)	45 g
Xiang Fu (Rhizoma Cyperi)	45 g
Chuan Xiong (Rhizoma Chuanxiong)	30 g
Zhi Fu Zi (Radix Aconiti Lateralis Preparata)	30 g
Du Huo (Radix Angelicae Pubescentis)	30 g
Gan Jiang (Rhizoma Zingiberis)	30 g
Chuan Jiao (Pericarpium Zanthoxyli)	30 g
Du Zhong (Cortex Eucommiae)	30 g
Bie Jia (Carapax Trionycis)	30 g
Bi Bo (Fructus Piperis Longi)	30 g
Cao Guo Ren (Fructus Tsaoko)	30 g
Bai Shao (Radix Paeoniae Alba)	30 g
Sheng Huang Qi (Radix Astragali)	45 g
Rou Gui (Cortex Cinnamomi)	9 g
Chen Xiang (Lignum Aquilariae Resinatum)	9 g
Ding Xiang (Flos Caryophylli)	9 g

Preparation

Boil the first sixteen ingredients in 1500g of sesame oil until they turn brown. Get rid of the residue and continue to heat the medicated oil up to the point that if a drop of the oil drips into water, it will be in the form of a pearl. Put 560g of refined yellow-lead into the oil. When the content has cooled, add the fine powder of the last three ingredients. Stir the final content evenly and make it into masses, each weighing 120—150g. Only three days later when the fire—evil has gone away, can the masses be spread on pieces of cloth or paper.

Administration

To be applied to the umbilicus.

Effect

This kind of plaster can strengthen body resistance to diseases and reinforce the primordial *Qi*, because the drugs it contains have the action of strengthening the spleen, invigorating the kidney, supporting *Yang*, nourishing *Yin*, replenishing *Qi*, enriching blood, expelling cold and promoting blood circulation.

Indications

Dysfunction of the intestines and stomach due to deficiency of the spleen and kidney.

Notes

This plaster may be used for health care of middle-aged and old people who are debilitated.

The plaster was first made by several imperial physicians to treat Empress Dowager Ci Xi on May 21 of the 7th year after Emperor Guang Xu ascended the throne.

7. *Yu Lin Gu Ben Gao*

Source

The book *Qing Tai Yi Yuan Pei Fang* and the book *Ci Xi Guang Xu Yi Fang Xuan Yi*

Ingredients

Du Zhong (Cortex Eucommiae)	120 g
Shu Di (Rhizoma Rehmanniae Praeparata)	120 g
Fu Zi (Radix Aconiti Lateralis Preparata)	120 g
Cong Rong (Herba Cistanchis)	120 g
Niu Xi (Radix Achyranthis Bidentatae)	120 g
Bu Gu Zhi (Fructus Psoraleae)	120 g

Xu Duan (Radix Dipsaci)	120 g
Guan Gui (Cortex Cinnamomi)	120 g
Gan Cao (Radix Glycyrrhizae)	120 g
Sheng Di (Radix Rehmanniae)	45 g
Da Hui Xiang (Fructus Illicii Veri)	45 g
Xiao Hui Xiang (Fructus Foeniculi)	45 g
Tu Si Zi (Semen Cuscutae)	45 g
She Chuang Zi (Fructus Cnidii)	45 g
Tian Ma Zi (Fructus Gastrodiae)	45 g
Zi Shao Hua (Spongilla fragilla fragillis)	45 g
Lu Jiao (Cornu Cervi)	45 g
Yang Yao Zi (sheep kidney)	a pair
Chi Shi Zhi (Halloysitum Rubrum)	30 g
Long Gu (Os Draconis)	30 g
Xiong Huang (Realgar)	30 g
Ding Xiang (Flos Caryophylli)	30 g
Chen Xiang (Lignum Aquilariae Resinatum)	30 g
Mu Xiang (Radix Aucklandiae)	30 g
Ru Xiang (Resina Olibani)	30 g
Mo Yao (Myrrha)	30 g
She Xiang (Moschus)	0.9 g
Yang Qi Shi (Actinolitum)	1.5 g

Preparation

Boil the first twenty ingredients in 4000g of sesame oil until they turn brown. Remove the residue to get the medicated oil. Condense the medicated oil with 1500g of yellow-lead into plaster. Grind the last eight ingredients into fine powder and mix the powder with the plaster into a mixture. Spread the mixture on pieces of cloth or paper to obtain the finished plasters for application.

Administration

For a female 1 piece of the plaster is applied to the area above the umbilicus; for a male 2 pieces are placed over both the left and right Shenshu(BL23)points and 1piece over Dantian(the elixir field three *Cun* below the umbilicus). The applied plasters are fixed with sweat towels and replaced with fresh ones every two weeks.

Effect

The book *Qing Tai Yi Yuan Pei Fang* describes the effect of this plaster as follows: reinforcing the kidney, stopping emission, promoting the flow of *Qi* and blood, strengthening the ability of reproducing semen and marrow, protecting the kidney—*Yang*, consolidating body resistance, enhancing *Yang*, increasing strength, thus maintaining health; or activating the liver, warming the uterus to induce fertilization, thus promoting pregnancy; or enriching *Qi* and blood, brightening complexion, preventing diseases, blackening hair, thus slowing down the process of ageing. Still, the book says: "If one applies this plaster for all his life, he will keep himself as fit as a youth, even at the age of 80 or so; he will be likely to be healthy enough, having good vision and not feeling tired after walking. ··· Having applied this plaster for a hundred days, an ageing person will enjoy its remarkable effect." Probably, the above words are exaggerated to some extent. But for those who are weak or ageing, this plaster is indeed worth testing as a simple and convenient medication for maintaining their own health.

The book *Ci Xi Guang Xu Yi Fang Xuan Yi* classifies this plaster as the semen—cultivating one suitable for Emperor Guang

Xu. Emperor Guang Xu suffered from emission for a long time and had no offspring. He had applied this plaster in order to have his kidney supplemented and the symptom of emission stopped, expecting himself to have the ability of causing his wives to become pregnant.

Indications

According to the book *Qing Tai Yi Yuan Pei Fang*, the indications of this plaster in the male are as follows: deficiency and coldness of the kidney—*Yang*, all kinds of disorders and impairments due to deficiencies and other factors, impotence, or weak erection of the penis, long infertility, turbid urine, hernia, emission, night sweating, numbness of the limbs, hemiplegia, simple abdominal distention, and pain of the loins and legs, while in the female: deficiency and weakness of the spleen and stomach, irregular menstruation, reddish leucorrhea, insufficiency of *Qi* and blood, long infertility, emaciation due to chronic blood stasis, frequent abortion, and metrorrhagia and metrostaxis with blood clots.

8. Yi Shou Bi Tian Gao

Source

The book *Qing Tai Yi Yuan Pei Fang*

Ingredients

Niu Xi (Radix Achyranthis Bidentatae)	30 g
Du Zhong (Cortex Eucommiae)	30 g
Zhi Hu Gu (prepared Os Tigris)	30 g
Mu Bie Zi (Semen Momordicae)	30 g
She Chuang Zi (Fructus Cnidii)	30 g
Rou Dou Kou (Semen Myristicae)	30 g
Tu Si Zi (Semen Cuscutae)	30 g

Zi Shao Hua (Spongilla fragilla fragillis)	30 g
Xu Duan (Radix Dipsaci)	30 g
Chuan Shan Jia (Squama Mantis)	30 g
Yuan Zhi (Radix Polygalae)	30 g
Tian Ma Zi (Rhizoma Gastrodiae)	30 g
Lu Rong (Cornu Cervi Pantotrichum)	30 g
Cong Rong (Herba Cistanchis)	30 g
Sheng Di (Radix Rehmanniae)	30 g
Shu Di (Rhizoma Rehmanniae Praeparata)	30 g
Guan Gui (Cortex Cinnamomi)	30 g
Chuan Lian Zi (Fructus Toosendan)	30 g
Shan Yu Rou (Fructus Corni)	30 g
Ba Ji Tian (Radix Morindae Officinalis)	30 g
Bu Gu Zhi (Fructus Psoraleae)	30 g
Hai Qu (little Hippocampus Kelloggi)	15 g
Gan Cao (Radix Glycyrrhizae)	60 g
Sang Zhi (Ramulus Mori)	22 cm
Huai Zhi (Ramulus Sophorae)	22 cm
Xiong Huang (Realgar)	6 g
Long Gu (Os Draconis)	6 g
Chi Shi Zhi (Halloysitum Rubrum)	6 g
Mu Ding Xiang (Fructus Caryophylli)	12 g
Chen Xiang (Lignum Aquilariae Resinatum)	12 g
Mu Xiang (Radix Aucklandiae)	12 g
Ru Xiang (Olibanum)	12 g
Mo Yao (Myrrha)	12 g
Yang Qi Shi (Actinolitum)	12 g
She Xiang (Moschus)	12 g
Huang La (Cera Flava)	15 g

Preparation

Steep the first twenty-five ingredients in 3000g of sesame oil for one night and heat the content over gentle fire until the colour of the ingredients becomes black. Get rid of the residue. Put yellow-lead into the medicated oil, every 195 g of yellow-lead being put into every 500g of the oil. While doing so, keep stirring the content by hand with a willow rod. And then add the fine powder of the last eleven ingredients and another 6g of yellow-lead. Finally spread the content on pieces of cloth or paper.

Administration

Two pieces of the plaster are separately applied to the two acupoints Yaoyan(EX-B7), or one piece to the umbilicus instead. The applied pieces of plaster are replaced with new ones every two weeks.

Effect

Supplementing essence and marrow, consolidating the kidney to keep kidney-essence, being good at enhancing the kidney-*Yang*, smoothing the skin, strengthening the tendons and bones, regulating the waist and knees, removing stasis in the 24 blood vessels, thus building up and rejuvenating the body.

Indications

Deficiency and coldness of the kidney-*Yang*, all kinds of impairments, hemiplegia, or weakness of the legs, soreness and numbness of the feet and knees, impotence, dream with emission, as well as reddish leukorrhea, stranguria from urolithiasis, metrorrhagia, etc.

Notes

In the palace of the Qing Dynasty, a number of plasters of this kind were administrated externally for health-preserving and life-prolonging. Among them were *Yi Shou Gao* made up of the two prescriptions mentioned above and *Pei Yuan Yi Shou Gao*, which were once used to treat Emperor's Mother Ci Xi.

This kind of plasters contain a great number of drugs and are very similar in preparation and administration, so only a few of them are introduced here for reference. A few rare or precious drugs used in them may be omitted or replaced with their substitutes.

2.10 Medicated Pillows for Health Care

Medicated pillows are those that are filled with suitable traditional Chinese medicines and used as the ordinary ones. They have the action of treating and preventing diseases or building up health. This has been one of conventionally external treatments in traditional Chinese medicine, and has been attached importance to since ancient times. Among the relics unearthed from Mawangdui No 1 Tomb of the Han Dynasty in the suburb of Changsha, Hunan province, there is an embroidered silk pillow filled with the drug *Pei Lan* (Herba Eupatorii). A pillow coated with gold, set with jade and filled with the medicinal herb *Hua Jiao* (Pericarpium Zanthoxyli)has also been unearthed from the tomb of Duke Liu Sheng of the Han Dynasty, which is situated in Lingshan Mountain, Mancheng county of Hebei province. Thus it has been established that medicated pillows were used 2,100years ago. Later, various kinds of medicated pillows were in succession recorded in medical books such as the book *Sheng Ji Zong Lu* (General Collection for Holy Relief)and the book *Bao Sheng Yao Lu* (Essentials for Life-saving)of the Song Dynasty, the book *Yu Yao Yuan Fang* (Prescriptions of Imperial Drug Institution)of the Yuan Dynasty, the book *Shen Shi Yao Han* (A Valuable Manual of Ophthalmology) and the book *Ben Cao Gang Mu* (Compendium of Materia Medica)of the Ming Dynasty, the book *Li Yue Pian Wen* (Rhymed Discourses on External Therapy)of the Qing Dynasty, etc. In recent years researchers in all parts of China have developed one after another kind of medicated pillows favourably received at home, many of which have been exported to foreign markets, making a contribution to the health of the poeple both in and outside China.

Medicated pillows have unique characteristics in maintaining health and treating diseases. A medicated pillow is simple and easy to use. It gives off its effect on the user while he, she is sleeping. The user is treated in such a way that he needn't decoct any drugs nor take any decoction, thus avoiding a lot trouble. Drugs with which to fill a pillow weigh less than one kilo and will retain their effectiveness for several months. So the average amount of the drugs consumed in a pillow is a few grams per day, which is much lower that that in the corresponding decoction. In addition, medicated pillows are especially suitable for the prevention and treatment of chronic diseases and for the protection of health, for it is the most easy thing for one to use a pillow for a long time.

Plenty of clinical observations have demonstrated that medicated pillows have reliable and lasting effects. The observations made by the author himself and his colleagues on specially–developed medicated pillows for health care have shown that these pillows exert remarkable effects on hypertension in one–month, two–month and six–month periods. It has also been discovered that medicated pillows may give excellent regulative action. For example, when the above–mentioned antihypertensive pillows are used by those with normal blood pressure, their normal blood pressure is actually maintained rather than being lowered.

Medicated pillows have found extensive purposes. Not only can they be used to treat hypertension, cervical spondylopathy, headache of nervous origin, neurosism, coronary heart disease and diseases of the respiratory system, but also to prevent common cold, etc. There are different kinds of medicated pillows. Some are for health care and suitable for children; others are effective for middle—aged and old people in eliminating illnesses and keeping good health or in antiageing and prolonging life. Medicated pillows also have another advantage that they are easier to make. That's the reason middle—aged and old people like to use them for the purpose of self—maintain ence of health.

The composition of drugs in medicated pillows is strictly based on the principle of differentiation, and a compatible application of the drugs is needed. Most drugs used in a pillow are of fragrant nature, they contain various sorts of volatile oil, and for this reason a medicated pollow is also called a "fragrant pillow". Since the effect of a pillow depends to some extent on the volatile oil, when drugs with which to fill a pillow are selected, what should be taken into consideration is not only their nature, taste, channel tropism and effects but also the volatile oil they contain and its pharmacological action. The number of the drugs in different pillows varies greatly. For example, there are pillows filled with one drug, such as *Ju Hua Zhen* and *Jue Ming Zhen*, and pillows filled with several dozens of drugs, such as *Shen Zhen* containing 32 drugs recorded in the book *Sheng Ji Zong Lu*. At present, each of the commonly used medicated pillows usually contains about 10 drugs.

When you make a medicated pillow yourself, you should first process in a suitable way the drugs which are required according to the prescription, and the process is usually to crush the drugs into rough powder. If the drugs are not crushed, their effects will be difficult to exert. If they are crushed too finely, their effects will exert too rapidly, shortening the pillow's effective period. Furthermore, if the powder is too fine, it tends to leak out from the pillow. Before being crushed, the drugs must be freed from impurities and dust. Drugs which have been contaminated or deteriorated must not be used. The pillowcase is better made of pure—cotton cloth. The bag filled with processed drugs is used as a pillow bag which is covered with a pillowcase easy to wash. Usually a pillow bag is 35—45cm long and 20—30cm wide, depending on the amount of the drugs and the user's habit. Pillows for children are smaller. The total amount of the drugs used in a pillow is in general 500—1000grams.

When used, a medicated pillow should be placed on an ordinary one whose height is to be regulated in order to make the total height of the two's moderate and comfortable, and the drugs inside the medicated pillow should be kept even and smooth and rearranged after the pillow is used for a few days. The pillowcase and the towel used to cover it should be frequently washed. Furthermore, a medicated pillow should be kept from wetness, mildewing and being moth—eaten. It should remain dry but must not be overheated in the sun. The drugs inside a pillow are necessarily replaced with fresh ones after the pillow is used for six to twelve months. To ensure the curative effects from a medicated pillow one must use it 6 hours per day for a long period of time.

One should choose a medicated pillow according to his disease condition, his contitution and age, and other relevant factors. Before doing so, one shohld ask a physician for advice. Generally, critical and acute conditions should not be treated with a mere medicated pillow, and for serious diseases, it seems to be a subsidiary therapy or to be used in their convalescence.

According to the theory of traditional Chinese medicine, the medicated—pillow therapy is a "treatment by smelling fragrance", i. e. odour therapy, or one of fragrance therapies. From the point of view of modern knowledge, the drugs inside a pillow can send out various kinds of volatile oil or other biologically active substances that form a small climate with mild medicinal fragrance round the pillow. The fragrance absorbed through mucous membrane of the respiratory tract or the skin may act locally, in the body fluids, or reflectively, producing better regulative actions on the functions of the heart and brain blood bessels and on other functions of the body. These actions are either against diseases and ageing, or for prolonging life. As for the actual mechanism of these actions, it still needs further investigating.

Here are some kinds of medicated pillows for reference for those who will buy or make them themselves, The dosage of the drugs used in the pillows of ancient times was calculated in an old measuring system and it is converted into the metric system which is convenient for those who make their own to adopt.

1. *Qi Huang Pai Gao Xiao Bao Jian Yao Zhen*

Source

This pillow is developed by Shandong College of Traditional Chinese Medicine, Jinan City, Shandong Province, China.

Main Ingredients

Ju Hua (Flos Chrysanthemi)

Bo He (Herba Menthae)
Chuan Xiong (Rhizoma Chuanxiong)
Xi Xin (Herba Asari)
Bai Zi Ren (Semen Platycladi)
Gao Ben (Rhizoma Ligustici)
Bai Zhi (Radix Angelicae Dahuricae)

Manufacturer

Experimental Pharmaceutical Factory Affiliated to Shandong College of Traditional Chinese Medicine

Effect

Calming the liver, suppressing *Yang*, clearing away heat, cooling blood, nourishing the heart, tranquilizing the mind, restoring consciousness, removing obstacles from the channels, promoting blood circulation, expelling wind, relieving numbness, stopping pain.

Indications

Hypertension, cerebral arteriosclerosis, cervical spondylopathy, coronary heart disease, hyperlipemia, neurosism, nervous headache, etc.

This kind of pillow has the effects of preventing and treating the above diseases. Middle-aged and old people can use it to maintain their health.

Clinical Observations

It has been proved that this pillow is markedly effective in relieving headache, dizziness, rigidity and pain in the neck, tinnitus, insomnia, etc. It tends to lower greatly the blood pressure of the hypertensive who use it, and after one month or two months of application, their systolic pressure has been found to decrease by 14.86% to 12.92%, and their diastolic pressure by 16.11% to

11.88%. If non—hypertensives use the pillow, their blood pressure will not change considerably. It has also been noted that following one—month—and—a—half use of this pillow, the rising time of rheoencephalogram will be significantly shortened, indicating the improvement of the elasticity of the blood vessels in the skull, or the reduction of vasotonia, the decrease of peripheral resistance, and the increase of free passages of inflow, all of which mean the improvement of blood circulation in the brain to a certain extent. The differential impedance cardiogram has indicated that after the use of the medicated pillow for one month and a half the function of the left side of the heart seems to be improved and the peripheral resistance to the blood vessels in the patients with hypertension decreases. The improvement of the objective indexes plays an important role in keeping good health of the middle—aged and the aged, thus meaning the positive effects of medicated pillows.

Notes

Shandong College of TCM developed this pillow by referring to the following prescriptions in the classics: the prescription *Shen Zhen Fang* in the book *Sheng Ji Zong Lu* (General Collection for Holy Relief)and the prescription *Yao Zhen Fang* in the book *Bao Sheng Yao Lu* (Essentials for Life—saving)of the Song Dynasty, the prescription *Shen Zhen Fang* in the book *Yu Yao Yao Fang* (Prescriptions of Imperial Drug Institution)of the Yuan Dynasty, the prescription *Yao Zhen Fang* in the book *Shen Shi Yao Han* (A Valuable Manual of Ophthalmology)of the Ming Dynasty, and the prescription *Ding Gong Xian Zhen* in the book *Li Yue Pian Wen* (Rhymed Discourses on External Therapy)of the Qing Dynasty. In addition, the college also studied many prescriptions for making modern medicated pillows, analyzed the feature of the drugs in these prescriptions, investigated their chemical compositions, pharmacologic actions and clinical effects and finally developed this kind of pillow of the choice drugs.

2. *Shen Zhen Fang*

Source

The book *Sheng Ji Zong Lu*

Ingredients

Dang Gui (Radix Angelicae Sinensis)	18.65 g
Chuan Xiong (Rhizoma Chuanxiong)	18.65 g
Bai Zhi (Radix Angelicae Dahuricae)	18.65 g
Xin Yi (Flos Magnoliae)	18.65 g
Du Zhong (Cortex Eucommiae)	18.65 g
Gao Ben (Rhizoma Ligustici)	18.65 g
Rou Cong Rong (Herba Cistanchis)	18.65 g
Bai Zi Ren (Semen Platycladi)	18.65 g
Mi Wu (shoot of Ligusticum wallichii Franch)	18.65 g
Ren Shen (Radix Ginseng)	18.65 g
Yi Yi Ren (Semen Coicis)	18.65 g
Qin Jiao (Radix Gentianae Macrophyllae)	18.65 g
Mu Lan Pi (Cortex Magnoliae)	18.65 g
Shu Jiao (Pericarpium Zanthoxyli)	18.65 g
Rou Gui (Cortex Cinnamomi)	18.65 g
Gan Jiang (Rhizoma Zingiberis)	18.65 g
Fei Lian (Herba seu Radix Cardui Crispi)	18.65 g
Fang Feng (Radix Saposhinkoviae)	18.65 g
Kuan Dong Hua (Flos Farfarae)	18.65 g
Jie Geng (Radix Platycodi)	18.65 g
Bai Wei (Radix Cynanchi Atrati)	18.65 g

Man Jing Zi (Fructus Viticis)	18.65 g
Bai Zhu (Rhizoma Atractylodis Macrcephalae)	18.65 g
Bai Xian Pi (Cortex Dictamni)	18.65 g
Wu Tou (Radix Aconiti)	18.65 g
Fu Zi (Radix Aconiti Lateralis Preparata)	18.65 g
Li Lu (Rhizoma et Radix Veratri)	18.65 g
Zao Jia (Gledistsia sinensis)	18.65 g
Mang Cao (Shikimmi)	18.65 g
Ban Xia (Rhizoma Pinelliae)	18.65 g
Fan Shi (Alumen)	18.65 g
Xi Xin (Herba Asari)	18.65 g

Preparation

Remove the rough bark of *Du Zhong*, the soil carried by *Gao Ben*, the broken and solid particles of *Qin Jiao* and *Chuan Jiao*, the fork of *Fang Feng*, the bark of *Wu Tou*, the tip and bark of *Fu Zi*, the head of *Li Lu*, and the shoot leaves of *Xi Xin*.

Pound the ingredients soft and make them into rough powder, and place them into a pillow, with those having poison being lower and those smelling fragrant being upper.

Administration

Contain all the drugs in a pillow made of cypress, on which 120 holes have been drilled. Wrap the pillow in three layers of deep-red cloth. One hundred days later, remove the first layer; two hundred days later, the second layer; three hundred days later, the third layer. Replace the drugs with fresh ones yearly. This is for your reference when you use this kind of pillow.

Notes

In the book *Sheng Ji Zong Lu*, there is a description of the effects of the pillow: If the aged used the pillow for 100 days, their muscles and bones would be stronger and their skins and faces would look lustrous, and then one of the three layers was removed; if they used it for 200 days, their blood and Qi were to increase, and all illnesses would be cured, and another layer of cloth was taken off; up to 300 days, the last layer was removed. The pillow was yearly replaced with a new one. After 3 years of using this kind of medicated pillow, the teeth and hair of them would be more healthy and their complexions would seem to be like those of children.

A legend goes that in the Western Han Dynasty, there lived an old man at the foot of *Taishan* mountain. When 85 years old, he had had grey hair and no teeth. One day he met with a Taoist priest by chance and he was taught to eat fruit instead of grain, drink water and adopt the medicated pillow. After doing so, the old man's grey hair turned black and his new teeth grew and he was even able to walk 300 *Li* a day. When the old man was 180 years old he gave the formula for the pillow to Han Wu Emperor, who had gone to *Taishan* mountain for hunting. The efficacy of the pillow, though exaggerated in the legend, merits some importance. It does have the effect of keeping fit and prolonging life. If the pillow is used, the formula may be modified in accordance with particular requirements.

3. Bao Sheng Yao Lu Yao Zhen Fang

Source

The book *Bao Sheng Yao Lu*

Ingredients

Man Jing Zi (Fructus Viticis)	3 g
Gan Ju Hua (Flos Chrysanthemi)	3 g
Xi Xin (Herba Asari)	2.2 g

Xian Bai Zhi (Radix Angelicae Dahuricae)	2.2 g
Bai Zhu (Rhizoma Atractylodis Macrocephalae)	1.5 g
Xiong Qiong (Rhizoma Chuanxiong)	2.2 g
Tong Cao (Medulla Tetrapanacis)	3 g
Fang Feng (Radix Saposhinkoviae)	3 g
Gao Ben (Rhizoma Ligustici)	3 g
Ling Yang Jiao (Cornu Antelopis)	3 g
Xi Jiao (Cornu Rhinoceri)	3 g
Shi Shang Chang Pu (Rhizoma Acori Tatarinowii)	3 g
Hei Dou (Glycine Max)	0.33 litre

Preparation

Rub the ingredients and separate them from the fine powder. Mix them evenly and put them in a silk bag where they remain for their smell to give off. Then place them in another silk bag and sew the bag as a pillow in which the drugs are compacted as tightly as possible. Put the pillow in a pillow-shaped box whose upper lips are 1.5 inches lower than the upper surface of the pillow. Close the box with a special cover.

Administration

Take off the cover and sleep with the head on the pillow in the box. Put the cover on the box after getting up to retain the fragrance. The pillow will lower as time passes by. As this occurs, add more of the same herbs to the pillow until it is as tight as before, returning the pillow to its original height. The fragrance of the herbs will be exhausted in 3 or 5 months. By then new herbs will have to be used to replace the old ones.

Effect and Indications

The book *Bao Sheng Yao Lu* points out that one who uses this kind of medicated pillow regularly will enjoy its curative effects of treating long-standing intermittent headache, dizziness, heavy head, cold pain, poor vision, stuffy nose, as well as warding off pathogens. In the light of the herbs, the effect and indications of the pillow must be true. The introduced methods of preparing and using this pillow are worth mimicking.

Notes

The drugs *Ling Yang Jiao* and *Xi Jiao* are rare and precious. They might be replaced with something like a magnet, or their dosage might be reduced according to the condition of illness.

4. Ding Gong Xian Zhen

Source

The book *Li Yue Pian Wen*

Ingredients

Chuan Jiao (Pericarpium Zanthoxyli)	37.3 g
Jie Geng (Radix Platycodi)	37.3 g
Man Jing Zi (Fructus Veticis)	37.3 g
Bai Zi Ren (Semen Biotae)	37.3 g
Jiang Huang (Rhizoma Curcumae Longae)	37.3 g
Wu Yu (Fructus Euodiae)	37.3 g
Bai Zhu (Rhizoma Atractylodis Macrocephalae)	37.3 g
Bo He (Herba Menthae)	37.3 g
Rou Gui (Cortex Cinnamomi)	37.3 g
Chuan Xiong (Rhizoma Chuanxiong)	37.3 g
Yi Zhi Ren (Fructus Alpiniae Oxyphyllae)	37.3 g
Zhi Shi (Fructus Aurantii Immaturus)	37.3 g
Dang Gui (Radix Angelicae Sinensis)	37.3 g
Chuan Wu (Radix Aconiti)	37.3 g
Qian Nian Jian (Rhizoma Homalomenae)	37.3 g
Wu Jia Pi (Cortex Acanthopanacis)	37.3 g

Li Lu (Rhizoma et Radix Veratri)	37.3 g
Qiang Huo (Rhizoma seu Radix Notopterygii)	37.3 g
Fang Feng (Radix Saposhinkoviae)	37.3 g
Xin Yi (Flos Magnoliae)	37.3 g
Bai Zhi (Radix Angelicae Dahuricae)	37.3 g
Fu Zi (Radix Aconiti Lateralis Preparata)	37.3 g
Bai Shao (Radix Paeoniae Alba)	37.3 g
Gao Ben (Rhizoma Ligustici)	37.3 g
Cong Rong (Herba Cistanchis)	37.3 g
Xi Xin (Herba Asari)	37.3 g
Ya Zao (Spina Gleditsiae)	37.3 g
Wu Yi (Ulmus macrocarpa)	37.3 g
Gan Cao (Radix Glycyrrhizae)	37.3 g
Jing Jie (Herba Schizonepetae)	37.3 g
Ju Hua (Flos Chrysanthemi)	37.3 g
Du Zhong (Cortex Eucommiae)	37.3 g
Wu Yao (Radix Linderae)	37.3 g
Ban Xia (Rhizoma Pinelliae)	37.3 g

Preparation

Break all the drugs into small pieces and grind the pieces into powder. Put the powder into a spun—silk bag and place the bag into a pillow.

Effect

Treating all diseases, prolonging life, strengthening the reproductive organs.

Notes

This prescription has different ingredients from the prescription of *Shen Zhen Fang*. It may be a reference for developing modern medicated pillows.

5. *Gao Xue Ya Bing Yao Zhen*

Source

The book *Zhong Cao Yao Wai Zhi Yan Fang Xuan*

Ingredients

Tu Ju Hua (Flos Chrysanthemi)	500 g
Wan Can Sha (Excrementum Bombycis)	500 g
Guo Huai Hua (Flos Sophorae)	500 g
Zheng Chuan Xiong (Rhizoma Chuanxiong)	200 g
Xiang Bai Zhi (Radix Angelicae Dahuricae)	300 g

Preparation

Grind the last two ingredients into powder and mix the powder with the other three thoroughly into a mixture. Put the mixture into a small bag made of gunny cloth. Sheathe the small bag in a fine linen pillowcase to form a medicated pillow.

Administration

Use this medicated pillow in the same way as an ordinary one.

Effect

Calming the liver, cooling blood, expelling wind, promoting blood circulation, relieving pain.

Indications

Hypertension.

6. *Bao Jian Yao Zhen*

Source

This pillow was developed by Dr. Jin Yacheng and reported in Zhejiang Journal of Traditional Chinese Medicine in 1986.

Ingredients

Ye Ju Hua (Flos Chrysanthemi Indici)	500 g
Ai Rong (mugwort floss)	200 g

Ye Jiao Teng (Caulis Polygoni Multiflori)	100 g
Mu Dan Pi (Cortex Moutan)	20 g
Gou Qi Zi (Fructus Lycii)	20 g
Shan Hai Luo (Codonopsis lanceolata)	20 g
Hu Zhang (Rhizoma Polygoni Cuspidati)	20 g
Bai Zhi (Radix Angelicae Dahuricae)	20 g
Zhang Nao (Camphora)	5 g
Xiang Jing (essence)	small amount
Ruo Ke Si (indocalamus bark)	500 g

Preparation

Cut *Ruo Ke* into slivers. Grind *Ye Jiao Teng* into rough powder. Put the slivers and the rough powder into a gauze pillow together with *Ye Ju Hua* and *Ai Rong*, with the slivers beneath the other three. Grind the remaining drugs into fine powder and mix it evenly with *Xiang Jing* into a mixture. Put the mixture into five small tightly woven cotton cloth bags of the same size, and sew them tightly. Place one in each corner of the pillow and one in the centre. Sheathe the pillow in a pillowcase made of bluish cotton cloth.

The pillow made of gauze tends to release the medicinal fragrance. The pillowcase made of bluish cotton cloth is for calming emotion and dispelling fatigue.

Effect and Indications

This pillow has proved to be effective for chronic bronchitis, hyperlipemia and neurosism of the aged, the clinically effective rate being 73—87%, and it is also good for antiageing, leading to marked decreasing of ageing symptoms. Those with the above illnesses or the middle—aged may consider using this pillow.

7. Jian Kang Chang Shou Yao Zhen

Source

The basic prescription was established by Wang Jiansheng and reported in No. 1 issue of Journal of Zhejiang College of Traditional Chinese Medicine published in 1986.

Ingredients

Hang Ju Hua (Flos Chysanthemi)	500 g
Dong Sang Ye (Winter Folium Mori)	500 g
Ye Ju Hua (Flos Chrysanthemi Indici)	500 g
Xin Yi (Flos Magnoliae)	500 g
Bo He (Herba Menthae)	200 g
Hong Hua (Flos Carthami)	100 g
Bing Pian (Borneolum)	50 g

Preparation

Grind all the drugs except *Bing Pian* into small pieces. Mix the pieces with *Bing Pian* into a mixture. Put the mixture into a cloth bag.

Administration

Use the bag as an ordinary pillow.

Effect

Calming the liver, suppressing *Yang*, dispersing wind, expelling heat, relieving swelling, detoxifying, promoting blood circulation, inducing menstruation to alleviating pain.

Indications

Hypertension, arterosclerosis, concussion of brain, discomfort in the head and headache or hemicrania due to sequela from cerebral thrombosis, dizziness, neurosism, alopecia areata, conjunctivitis with pain, acute and chronic rhinitis, laryngopharyngitis and folliculitis on the back of the neck.

8. Jing Zhui Bing Yao Zhen

Source

This prescription was introduced by Yao Changhua in No. 1 issue of Chinese Journal of Rehabilitation Medicine published in 1986.

Ingredients

Tong Cao (Medulla Tetrapanacis)	300 g
Ju Hua (Flos Chrysanthemi)	200 g
Bai Zhi (Radix Angelicae Dahuricae)	100 g
Hong Hua (Flos Carthami)	100 g
Pei Lan (Herba Eupatorii)	100 g
Chuan Xiong (Rhizoma Chuanxiong)	100 g
Hou Po (Cortex Magnoliae Officinalis)	100 g
Shi Chang Pu (Rhizoma Acori Tatarinowii)	80 g
Gui Zhi (Ramulus Cinnamomi)	60 g

Preparation

Process all the drugs and put them in a bag, which is made adequately soft.

Administration

Use the bag as an ordinary pillow.

Modification

In case of soreness and discomfort in the neck, add 60g of *Cang Zhu* (Rhizoma Atractylodis) and 100g of *Xi Xian Cao* (Herba Siegesbeckiae) to the pillow; in case of dizziness and stuffy nose, add 60g of Ge Gen (Radix Puerariae) and 60g of *Xin Yi Hua* (Flos Magnoliae); in case of numbness of the limbs, add 50 g of *Ma Huang* (Herba Ephedrae), 100 g of *Sang Zhi* (Ramulus Mori), 100 g of *Fang Feng* (Radix Saposhinkoviae) and 100 g of *Qiang Huo* (Rhizoma seu Radix Notopterygii).

Effect

Inducing resuscitation by means of its aromatics, clearing the head, expelling wind, promoting blood circulation, regulating *Qi*, relieving stagnation of *Qi* and blood.

Indications

Cervical spondylosis.

9.　*Xiao Er Bi Yuan Yao Zhen*

Source

These prescriptions were introduced by Zhao Xiaoming in No. 6 issue of Jiangsu Journal of Traditional Chinese Medicine published in 1985.

Ingredients

Prescription One

Su Ye (Folium Perillae)	60 g
Bai Zhi (Radix Angelicae Dahuricae)	60 g
Jing Jie (Herba Schizonepetae)	60 g
Fang Feng (Radix Saposhinkoviae)	60 g
Chen Pi (Pericarpium Citri Reticulatae)	60 g
Huo Xiang (Herba Agastachis)	60 g
Gui Zhi (Ramulus Cinnamomi)	30 g
Chuan Jiao (Pericarpium Zanthoxyli)	30 g
Chuan Xiong (Rhizoma Chuanxiong)	30 g
Ju Hua (Flos Chrysanthemi)	30 g
Tan Xiang (Lignum Santali)	20 g
Xi Xin (Herba Asari)	15 g

Prescription Two

Huo Xiang (Herba Agastachis)	100 g
Ju Hua (Flos Chrysanthemi)	60 g
Bo He (Herba Menthae)	60 g

Jing Jie (Herba Schizonepetae)	60 g
Fang Feng (Radix Ledebouriellae)	60 g
Bai Zhi (Radix Angelicae Dahuricae)	60 g
Chuan Xiong (Rhizoma Chuanxiong)	30 g
Chen Pi (Pericarpium Citri Reticulatae)	30 g
Xin Yi Hua (Flos Magnoliae)	20 g
Tan Xiang (Lignum Santali)	20 g
Xi Xin (Herba Asari)	15 g

Indications

Rhinorrhea with turbid discharge in children due to exogenous wind—cold, wind—heat or heat derived from wind—cold.

Notes

Rhinorrhea with turbid discharge is considered to be a serious case of sinusitis in TCM. It is mainly manifested as stuffy nose, frequent purulent nasal discharge with foul smell, which may be accompanied by headache, dizziness and blurred vision. And it is similar to parasinusitis. The adults with the same disorder may also use this pillow.

10. *Li Shizhen Yao Zhen*

Source

This pillow was introduced by Ge Huopu in No. 12 issue of Journal of Traditional Chinese Medicine published in 1984.

Ingredients

Bo He (Herba Menthae)
Ye Ju Hua (Flos Chrysanthemi Indici)
Qing Mu Xiang (Radix Aristolochiae)
Dan Zhu Ye (Herba Lophatheri)
Sheng Shi Gao (Gypsum Fibrosum)

Bai Shao (Radix Paeoniae Alba)
Chuan Xiong (Rhizoma Chuanxiong)
Dong Sang Ye (Folium Mori)
Man Jing Zi (Fructus Viticis)
Ci Shi (Magnetitum)
Wan Can Sha (Excrementa Bombycum)

Effect and Indications

When the pillow is used to treat hypertension, remarkable effect of reducing blood pressure will be achieved with significant relief of the relevant symptoms, the effective rate being 88.5%.

Manufacturer

Shangrao City Hospital of Traditional Chinese Medicine and Shangrao City Healthy Product Service Corporation

11. *Shen Nong Pai Bao Jian Yao Zhen*

Kinds

1. Healthy pillows for the aged to prolong their lives,
2. Healthy pillows for the middle-aged and young to divert themselves,
3. Healthy pillows for children to keep themselves fit and to improve their intelligence.

Special Indications

Headache, vertigo, dizziness, insomnia and neurosism.

Manufacturer

Xindu County Health Product Plant in Chengdu City of Sichuan Province

12. *Yi Shou Yao Zhen*

Ingredients

Hang Ju (Flos Chrysanthemi)
Zhu Ru (Caulis Bambusae in Taeniam)

Xia Ku Cao (Spica Prunellae)
Deng Xin (Medulla Junci)
and other nearly thirty ones

Effect

Nourishing *Yin,* calming fire, improving eye—sight, clearing away heart—fire, tranquilizing and refreshing the mind, detoxifying, preventing heatstroke, expelling pathogenic factors.

Indications

Hypertension, neurosism, neurosis, Meniere's syndrome, etc. The aged with the symptoms of headache, dizziness, tinnitus and insomnia will enjoy its sure curative effects if they use this pillow.

Manufacturer

Pucheng County Plant for Making Life—prolonging Medicated Pillows in Shanxi Province

3 Health Care Independent of Medicines

3.1 Acupuncture and Moxibustion for Health Care

Acupuncture and moxibustion, as a medical and health-care method unique to the Chinese nation, has made great contributions to our Chinese people. More than 1,400 years ago, its introduction to Korea and Japan began; more than 4 centuries ago, to Europe, serving the people there. Now it has been well accepted and highly appreciated throughout the world.

Acupuncturology involves two therapies: acupuncture and moxibustion, which were formed and developed gradually in the struggle of human beings against diseases. As early as in the Stone Age 10 000years ago, the Chinese already knew the fact that puncturing some parts of the body with chipped stone instruments could alleviate the sufferings due to disorders. This was the beginning of acupuncture. Up to the New Stone Age, they had used polished stone needles as a special medical instrument, which was then called as *Bian Shi*. Later on, with the development of social productive forces and science and technology, they kept improving acupuncture instruments until the following kinds of needles came into being one after another: bamboo needles, bone needles.

Bronze needles, iron needles, gold needles, silver needles and stainless steel needles. Combustion therapy appeared also about in the Old Stone Age. After fire came into use, it was found out that the sufferings due to disease could be relieved when some parts of the body were, by chance, smoked, roasted or burned. This was the budding of combustion therapy, which was later developed into moxibustion and other kinds of combustion therapies. The ancient Chinese people summarized their rich practical experiences in preventing and treating diseases with the therapy of acupuncture and moxibustion into a whole series of integrated scientific theroies. In recent years, modern scientific research in acupuncture and moxibustion has been carried out both theroretically and clinically, resulting in more rapid development.

Both acupuncture and moxibustion can be used to protect health and prevent diseases. Moxibustion, by comparison, is more suitable for self-protecting health. In this case, it is called as moxibustion for health care.

3.1.1 The Effects of Acupuncture and Moxibustion in Health Care

When one is healthy, in his body, *Yin* and *Yang* coordinate, *Qi* and blood exuberate, *Zang* and *Fu* function well, channels and collaterals are smooth, and *Ying* and *Wei* harmonize. Under these conditions, he will not be ill, nor will be become senile early. But when he is unhealthy, the conditions in his body are just the opposite. And he will be susceptible to all diseases, and become senile early, shortening his life span. Acupuncture and moxibustion acts on acupoints, channels and collaterals to clear the channels and collaterals which are closely related to *Zang* and *Fu* organs so as to promote the flow of *Qi* and blood, coordinate *Yin* and *Yang*, regulate *Zang* and *Fu*, harmonize *Ying* and *Wei*, eliminate diseases and expel pathogenic factors. These regulating effects of acupuncture and moxibustion can, of course, ensure perfect health, thus preventing early ageing and prolonging life.

Moxibustion for health care is convenient and highly effective. In China, it has been appreciated since ancient times. Its effects of preserving health and prolonging life are summarized as follows:

1. Warming and Clearing Channels and Collaterals to Remove *Yin*-cold

Moxibustion is a kind of warm stimulation plus moxa's action of warm-dispersing cold pathogens. Thus it can be used to warm and clear the channels, collaterals and blood vessels, expel wind-dampness and *Yin*-pathogens of wind-cold type, prevent invasion of wind, cold and dampness pathogens, prevent and treat arthralgia-syndrome and promote recovery.

2. Supplementing Fire and Strengthening *Yang* to Retard Senility

The fire from the gate of life and *Yang-Qi* of the aged and middle-aged will decline day by day with senile symptoms and signs appearing one after another. Moxibustion aciting on the acupoints Shenque(RN8), Guanyuan(RN4), Qihai (RN6), Mingmen(DU4)and Shenshu (BL23)can enhance their life vitality and slow down the process of their ageing, for the heat given off by the moxa burning over the acupoints, combining with the warm nature and fragrant taste of the moxa, exerts the effects of strengthening the fire from the gate of life and warming and reinforcing *Yang-Qi*.

3. Supporting Vital-*Qi* to Prevent Diseases

It is very hard for the weak or the old to guard themselves

against the invasion of exogenous evils because they have deficient vital-*Qi*, weakened *Zang* and *Fu*, and loose striae of the skin. Therefore, the six evils may take the opportunity to break through their body's defenses, causing them to be ill or even die. Moxibustion for health care can be used, in this case, to support vital-*Qi*, supplement primordial-*Qi*, close the striae of the skin properly, and improve the functions of *Zang* and *Fu* organs, thus strengthening their ability to prevent exogenous evils and diseases. People who are susceptible to diseases due to poor health, especially those over middle age, should keep treated with moxibustion for the purpose of warding off diseases and prolonging life.

4. Invigorating the Spleen and Stomach to Strengthen the Acquired *Qi* after Birth

Regular application of moxibustion over the acupoints Zusanli(ST36), Zhongwan(RN12), etc. will have spleen-Yang warmed, stomach-*Qi* replenished and digestion promoted. The spleen and stomach are the material basis of the acquired constitution. If they function normally in receiving, transporting and digesting food, they will provide the body with enough essential substances including essence and blood and build up health. Just as the book *Jing Yue Quan Shu* says, "After birth, one depends on nothing but his acquired constitution. This acquired constitution may not be strong enough. But if he will only keep his spleen and stomach regularly strengthened, he can certainly live a long life."

5. Promoting the Flow of *Qi* and Blood to Resolving Masses and Relieve Swelling

In the healthy body, *Qi* and blood move freely. Any

stagnation of them will obstruct the channels and collaterals, resulting in blood stasis and phlegm retention, which in turn leads to mass in the abdomen, swelling, apoplexy an all kinds of pain, If moxibustion is regularly applied, *Qi* and blood will be kept flowing and the channels and collaterals will remain clear and smooth, which will prevent the above mentioned syndromes. In case these syndromes occur, regular moxibustion can be applied as an accessory treatment to promote recovery.

3.1.2 Mechanism of Acupuncture and Moxibustion for Health Care

Plenty of clinical experimental research carried out with modern scientific methods have shown that acupuncture and moxibustion can regulate the functions of the whole body so as to build up health and slow down the process of ageing.

1. Improving Immunologic Function

Acupuncture and moxibustion can enhance cellular immune function and adjust humoral immune function. For example, they can regulate the count and the activity and its relevant indices of lymphocytes in peripheral blood, adjust the total of leucocytes and their phagocytosis in peripheral blood flow, strengthen the function of the reticuloendothelial system, control the content of immunoglobulin in blood sera, and increase the content of complements in blood sera and the content of some specific complements. Thus acupuncture and moxibustion can produce the effects of preventing diseases, preserving health and slowing down the process of ageing.

2. Adusting Cardiovascular Function to Improve Microcirculation

Acupuncture and moxibustion have good regulative effects on the functions of the heart and blood vessels. For instance, they can cause vasoconstriction, adjust blood pressure, improve the function of the heart, coronary circulation and microcirculation so as to protect cardiac muscles without enough blood supply, and prevent and treat experimental myocardiac infarction. For this reason acupuncture and moxibustion may be used to prevent cardiovascular diseases and promote the recovery of the patients who have been ill with those diseases.

3. Improving the Function of Digestion and Absorption

Application of acupunction and moxibustion to the acupoints for health care such as Zusanli(ST36), etc. may Attain the effect of regulating gastrointestinal peristalsis to promote the digestion of food and the absorption of nutrients, thus harmonizing the whole digestive system so as to build up constitution and strengthen the resistance to diseases.

4. Improving the Functions of Many Other Systems

Application of acupuncture and moxibustion can regulate the function of the nervous system, the functions of endocrine glands such as the pituitaria and the adrenal gland, and the functions in respiration, urination and reproduction, all for the good of health care.

3.1.3 Commonly Selected Acupoints in Health Care

The theoretical basis of acupuncture and moxibustion is the therory of channels and collaterals. Channels and collaterals are the passages through which *Qi* and blood of the body flow. They are everywhere in the body, throughout the *Zang—Fu* organs in the interior and all over the organism in the exterior, uniting all the tissues and organs into an organic whole. The channel system includes twelve regular channels, Eight Extra-channels, etc.

Acupoints, usually called points for short, are specific locations on (or over) which acupuncture or moxibustion is applied. When they are stimulated, they will play a part in promoting the flow of *Qi* and blood, reacting on disease, and strengthening the body resistance to eliminate pathogenic factors. Application of acupuncture and moxibustion on (or over) acupoints will cause stimulation which results in the effect of regulating the body through the channel system, thus preventing and treating diseases to preserve health. The acupoints include 361 ones from the fourteen channels (the twelve channels plus *Du* channel and *Ren* channel), extra-points and *Ashi* points. Locating or selecting the acupoints accurately or not is closely related to the curative effects. So how to locate points is most important in acumoxibustion. There are three methods in the following

1. *Gu Du Fen Cun Ce Liang Fa*

Measure different parts of the body and convert the measurements into *Cun*. For example the measurement of the length from the centre of the navel up to the juncture between pectus major and xiphoid process is converted into 8 *Cun*; down to the upper border of the symphysis pubis, 5 *Cun*. Use the length of this *Cun* to locate points.

2. *Shou Zhi Tong Shen Cun Fa*

In this method, the lengths of patients' fingers are regarded as *Cun*. There are three kinds of this Cun.

(1) *Zhong Zhi Tong Shen Cun*

The length between the two tips of the two striae appeared at the first and second knuckles and in the inner lateral side of the middle finger when it is bent is regarded as one *Cun*.

(2) *Mu Zhi Tong Shen Cun*

The width of the knuckle of the thumb of a patient himself is regarded as one *Cun*.

(3) *Heng Zhi Tong Shen Cun*

Ask a patient to stretch out naturally his forefinger, middle finger, ring finger and small finger. The width of the four fingers measured through the tranverse striae at the second knuckle of the middle finger is regarded as three *Cun*.

3. *Ti Biao Biao Zhi Fa*

Anatomic marks of the body, fixed or appeared when the body is in a certain posture, are regarded as the basis of point—selecting.

In the following we attach importance to the description of the points selected in health care. As to the details of all the other points and the channels and collaterals, please consult the relevant works on acumoxibustion.

1. Zusanli(ST36)

Location

3 *Cun* directly below Dubi(ST35), one finger—breadth from the anterior crest of the tibia, or in the anterior tibia muscle.

Method

Puncture perpendicularly 0.5—1.2 *Cun*. Moxibustion is applicable.

Effect

Regular application of acupuncture and moxibustion on this point will strengthen the function of the spleen and stomach, build up the body and enhance the immunity to disease.

Indications

Disorders of the spleen, stomach, kidney, liver, heart, lung and brain, especially those of the digestive system such as stomachache, vomiting, hiccup, abdominal distension, bowel sound, diarrhea, dysentery, constipation, acute appendicitis and indigestion, as well as apoplexy, paralysis, dizziness, insomnia, mania, cough, dyspnea, edema, acute mastitis, beriberi, soreness of the knees and calves, emaciation due to consumption, infantile malnutrition.

Notes

This is an essential point commonly chosen for health care.

Legend has it that there was an old man who had moxibustion done on the point Zusanli once daily in the first eight days of each month. He ensured a life span of more than 174 years.

2. **Shenque** (RN8)

Location

At the centre of the umbilicus.

Method

Puncture is prohibited. Moxibustion is applicable.

Effect

Application of moxibustion on this point will reinforce *Yang*, supplement *Qi*, warm the kidney and strengthen the function of the spleen.

Indications

Abdominal pain, bowel sound, flaccid type of apoplexy, prolapse of the rectum.

Notes

For health care, moxibustion is regularly applied on this point.

It is recorded in medical literature that there was an old man who had moxibustion done on the point Shenque every year and still kept fit at the age of over 100 years old.

3. **Zhongji (RN3)**

Location

4 *Cun* below the centre of the umbilicus.

Method

Puncture perpendicularly 0.5—1.0 *Cun*. Moxibustion is applicable.

Indications

Impotence, enuresis, nocturnal emission, frequent urination, retention of urine, metrorrhagia and metrostaxis, irregular menstruation, dysmenorrhea, morbid leukorrhea, pruritus vulvae, prolapse of uterus, pain in the lower abdomen, hernia.

4. **Guanyuan (RN4)**

Location

3 *Cun* below the centre of the umbilicus.

Method

Puncture perpendicularly 0.8—1.2 *Cun*. Moxibustion is applicable.

Indications

Impotence, enuresis, nocturnal emission, frequent urination, retention of urine, uterine bleeding, irregular menstruation, dysmenorrhea, morbid leukorrhea, postpartum hemorrhage, lower abdominal pain, hernia, indigestion, diarrhea, prolapse of the rectum, flaccid type of apoplexy.

Notes

This is an essential point for building up health.

5. **Qihai(RN6)**

Location

1.5 *Cun* below the centre of the umbilicus.

Method

Puncture perpendicularly 0.8—1.2 *Cun*. Moxibustion is applicable.

Effect

Supplementing the kidney, supporting *Yang*, replenishing *Qi*, controlling nocturnal emission.

Indications

Impotence, enuresis, nocturnal emission, uterine bleeding, irregular menstruation, dysmenorrhea, amenorrhea, morbid leukorrhea, postpartum hemorrhage, abdominal pain, hernia, diarrhea, dysentery, constipation, edema, flaccid type of apoplexy, dyspnea.

Notes

This is an essential point for strengthening the body and preserving health.

6. Shenshu (BL 23)

Location

On the low back, below the spinous process of the 2nd lumbar vertebra and 1.5 *Cun* lateral to the posterior midline.

Method

Puncture perpendicularly 0.8—1.2 *Cun*. Moxibustion is applicable.

Effect

Tonifying the kidney, strengthening *Yang*, replenishing vital essence.

Indications

Impotence, nocturnal emission, enuresis, irregular

menstruation, morbid leukorrhea, lumbar pain, weakness of the loins and knees, dizziness, tinnitus, deafness, edema, dyspnea, diarrhea.

7. Mingmen (DU 4)

Location

On the low back, on the posterior midline, and in the depression below the spinous process of the 2nd lumbar vertebra.

Method

Puncture perpendicularly 0.5—1.0 *Cun*. Moxibustion is applicable.

Effect

Tonifying the kidney, strengthening *Yang*, reinforcing the stomach.

Indications

Stiffness of the back, lumbago, impotence, nocturnal emission, irregular menstruation, morbid leukorrhea, diarrhea, indigestion, edema, dizziness, tinnitus.

8. Sanyinjiao (SP 6)

Location

Posterior to the medial border of the tibia, 3 *Cun* above the tip of the medial malleolus.

Method

Puncture perpendicularly 0.5—1.0 *Cun*. Moxibustion is applicable. Acupuncture on this point is contraindicated in pregnant women.

Indications

Impotence, nocturnal emission, enuresis, dysuria, uterine bleeding, irregular menstruation, dysmenorrhea, morbid leukorrhea, abdominal pain, borborygmus, abdominal distension, diarrhea, edema, hernia, pain in the external genitalia, paralysis and pain of the lower extremities, headache, dizziness, insomnia.

Regular application of moxibustion on the above six points will have the effects of invigorating and supporting the kidney—*Yang*, reinforcing the kidney and spleen, replenishing vital essence and *Qi*, supplementing bone marrow, strengthening tendons and bones, nourishing the blood, consolidating the teeth and blackening hair, which greatly benefits the middle—aged and the aged. The book *Bian Que Xin Shu* says, " If one apply moxibustion regularly on the points Guanyuan, Qihai Mingmen and Zhongwan, he will enjoy a long life of more than 100 years.

9. Zhongwan (RN 12)

Location

4 *Cun* or 3 *Cun* below the xiphoid process (on the midline of the abdomen, 4 *Cun* above the umbilicus).

Method

Puncture perpendicularly 0.5—1.2 *Cun*. Moxibustion is applicable.

Indications

Stomachache, acid regurgitation, regurgitation of food from the stomach, vomiting, indigestion, borborygmus, diarrhea, dysentery, jaundice, insomnia.

Notes

Regular application of moxibustion on this point and Zusanli may strengthen the spleen and stomach, and build up the acquired constitution.

10. Tianshu (ST 25)

Location

In the depression 2 *Cun* lateral to the centre of the umbilicus.

Method

Puncture perpendicularly 1.0—1.5 *Cun*. Moxibustion is applicable.

Indications

All diseases of the digestive system such as abdominal pain and distension, borborygmus, pain around the umbilicus, diarrhea, dysentery and constipation, as well as irregular menstruation and edema.

11. Quchi (LI 11)

Location

On the lateral end of the cubital crease and at the midpoint of the line connecting Chize (LU5) and the external humeral epicondyle, when the elbow is flexed. (When the elbow is flexed, it is in the depression at the lateral end of the transverse cubital crease.).

Method

Puncture perpendicularly 1.0—1.5 *Cun*. Moxibustion is applicable.

Indications

Sore throat, toothache, redness and pain of the eye, scrofula, urticaria, motor impairment of the upper extremities, abdominal pain, vomiting, diarrhea, febrile disease.

Notes

Regular application of moxibustion on this point and Zusanli may regulate blood pressure, prevent apoplexy and enhance resistance to disease.

12. Neiguan (PC6)

Location

On the palmar side of the forearm, on the line connecting Quze (PC3) and Daling (PC7), 2 *Cun* above the crease of the wrist, between the tendons of the long palmar muscle and radial flexor muscle of the wrist. (2 *Cun* above the transverse crease of the wrist, between the tendons of m. palmaris longus and m. flexor radialis.)

Method

Puncture perpendicularly 0.5—0.8 *Cun*. Moxibustion is applicable.

Effect

Regulating effectively the cardiovascular system, preserving health.

Indications

Cardiac pain, palpitation, stuffy chest, mania, epilepsy, insomnia, pain in the hypochondriac region, stomachache, nausea, vomiting, hiccup, febrile disease, irritability, malaria, contracture and pain of the elbow and arm.

13. Shenmen (HI 7)

Location

At the ulnar end of the crease of the wrist, and in the depression on the radial side of the tendon of the ulnar flexor muscle of the wrist.

Method

Puncture perpendicularly 0.3—0.5 *Cun*. Moxibustion is applicable.

Indications

Cardiac pain, irritability, palpitation, hysteria, amnesia, insomnia, mania, epilepsy, dementia, pain in the hypochondriac region, yellowish sclera.

14. Dazhui (GB 14)

Location

Below the spinous process of the 7th cervical vertebra, approximately at the level of the shoulders.

Method

Puncture obliquely upward 0.5–1.0 *Cun*. Moxibustion is applicable.

Effect

This is a main point for regulating all the *Yang* channels. Acupuncture and moxibustion on this point may support *Yang*, regulate the *Qi* in the channels and collaterals.

Indications

Neck pain and rigidity, malaria, febrile disease, epilepsy, afternoon fever, cough, dyspnea, common cold, back stiffness.

15. Feishu (BL 13)

Location

On the back, below the spinous process of the 3rd thoracic vertebra, and 1.5 *Cun* lateral to the posterior midline.

Method

Puncture obliquely 0.5–0.7 *Cun*. Moxibustion is applicable.

Indications

Cough, dyspnea, fullness in the chest, chest pain, spitting of blood, afternoon fever, night sweating.

Notes

Regular moxibustion on the above two points may replenish *Qi*, support *Yang*, reinforce the lung, consolidate the superficial resistance, and enhance resistance to exogenous evils, which is especially beneficial to those who are susceptible to common cold owing to their weak constitutions.

16. Xinshu (BL 15)

Location

On the back, below the spinous process of the 5th thoracic vertebra, and 1.5 *Cun* lateral to the posterior midline.

Method

Puncture obliquely 0.5–0.7 *Cun*. Moxibustion is applicable.

Indications

Cardiac pain, amnesia, palpitation, irritability, mania, epilepsy, cough, spitting of blood, nocturnal emission, night sweating.

Notes

Acupuncture and moxibustion on this point benefits the heart and lung.

17. Ganshu (BL 18)

Location

On the back, below the spinous process of the 9th thoracic vertebra, and 1.5 *Cun* lateral to the posterior midline.

Method

Puncture obliquely 0.5–0.7 *Cun*. Moxibustion is applicable.

Indications

Pain in the hypochondriac region, jaundice, redness of the eye, blurring of vision, night blindness, mania, epilepsy, backache, spitting of blood, epistaxis.

Notes

Acupuncture and moxibustion on this point benefits the liver and gallbladder.

18. Pishu (BL 20)

Location

On the back, below the spinous process of the 11th thoracic

vertebra, and 1.5 *Cun* lateral to the posterior midline.

Method

Puncture obliquely 0.5—0.7 *Cun*. Moxibustion is applicable.

Indications

Epigastric pain, abdominal distension, anorexia, vomiting, diarrhea, dysentery, bloody stools, jaundice, profuse menstruation, edema, backache.

19. Weishu (BL 21)

Location

On the back, below the spinous process of the 12th thoracic vertebra, and 1.5 *Cun* lateral to the posterior midline.

Method

Puncture obliquely 0.5—0.7 *Cun*. Moxibustion is applicable.

Indications

Epigastric pain, anorexia, abdominal distension, regurgitation, of food from the stomach, vomiting, borborygmus, diarrhea, pain in the hypochondriac region.

Notes

Acupuncture and moxibustion on the above two points benefits the spleen and stomach.

20. Huantiao (GB 30)

Location

When the patient lies on his side with the hip flexed, Huantiao is located on the lateral side of the thigh, at the middle third and lateral third of the line connecting the prominence of the great trochanter and the sacral hiatus when the patient lies on his side with the thigh flexed.

Method

Puncture perpendicularly 1.5—2.5 *Cun*. Moxibustion is applicable.

Indications

Pain of the lumbar region and thigh, muscular atrophy of the lower limbs, hemiplegia.

21. Yongquan (KI 1)

Location

On the sole in the depression appearing on the anterior part of the sole when the foot is in plantar flexion, approximately at the junction of the anterior third and the posterior two thirds of the line connection the base of the 2nd and 3rd toes and the heel.

Method

Puncture perpendicularly 0.3—0.5 *Cun*. Moxibustion is applicable.

Indications

Headache, dizziness, blurring of vision, sore throat, dryness of the tongue, loss of voice, constipation, dysuria, infantile convulsions, loss of consciousness, feverish sensation in the sole.

Notes

Regular moxibustion on this point may reinforce the kidney—*Yang*, and strengthen the body.

22. Baihui (DU 20)

Location

4.5 *Cun* directly above the midpoint of the anterior hairline.

Method

Puncture subcutaneously 0.3—0.5 *Cun*. Moxibustion is applicable.

Indications

Headache, vertigo, tinnitus, nasal obstruction, coma, aphasia by apoplexy, mania, prolapse of the rectum and the uterus.

23. Danzhong (RN 17)

Location

On the anterior midline, on the level of the 4th intercostal space and at the midpoint of a line connecting both nipples.

Method

Puncture subcutaneously 0.3−0.5 *Cun*. Moxibustion is applicable.

Indications

Pain and fullness in the chest, cardiac pain, palpitation, dyspnea, hiccup, difficulty in swallowing, insufficient lactation.

3.1.4 Acupuncture and Moxibustion for Health Care

1. Acupuncture for Health Care

(1) Filiform Needle Puncturing

Needles with loose handles or hooked tips are not to be used, and they should be straight, smooth, tough and elastic. Before application, a suitable posture should be chosen for a patient; the needles and the located points should be strictly disinfected. In application, different acupuncture manipulations are used according to the locations of the points and the length of the needles. There is a variety of acupuncture manipulations, among which are *Zhiqie* Insertion, *Pianzhi* Insertion, *Shuzhang* Insertion, *Jiachi* Insertion, etc. While a needle is being inserted, its angle and depth should be properly controlled. After the insertion, a certain kind of needle transmission is needed to a certain degree so that the stimulation induced in this way may be felt by the patient. When the patient has a sense of numbness, distention and compression, the acupuncturist must also have in his finger a sense of sinking and tension. This is called *Deqi,* a state in which the therapeutic efficacy has been achieved. Only when this state appears can a satisfactory curative effect be obtained. After *Deqi,* the needle is generally retained for 15—20 minutes or a little longer, during which the needle may be manipulated intermittently, keeping or enhancing the stimulation. When withdrawing the needle, press the skin around the point with the thumb and forefinger of the left hand and twist the needle slowly first to the subcutaneous layer and then out with the right hand. Then, press with disinfected cotton ball the point slightly to prevent bleeding. There are different acupuncture manipulations such as reinforcing and reducing. When filiform needle puncturing is used in health care, the points Zusanli (ST 36), Sanyinjiao(SP 6) and Quchi(LI 11) rather than others are usually chosen, and the reinforcing method is often used. As far as reinforcing method is concerned, it means inserting the needle quickly and with a little more strength to certain depth, twisting the handle slowly and within a narrow range and withdrawing it slightly and slowly.

(2) Cutaneous Needle Puncturing

Plum—blossom needles and seven—star needles are both called cutaneous needles. They are used to tap on the skin the points and the superficial meridians so as to promote flowing of *Qi* and blood through the meridians and regulate the functions of *Zang* and *Fu* organs. This is practical in health care.

A Seven—star needle has a handle 17—20 centimeters long and with a tiny plate in the shape of a seedpod of the lotus at one end on which are set 7 short pins made of stainless steel.

A plum—blossom needle has a handle about 33 centimeters long and with 5—7 stainless steel pins bound tightly together at one end. It may be home-made with a chopstick and several small-sized sewing needles.

The tips of these two kinds of needles must be neither too sharp nor hooked.

In the course of acupuncture, the acupuncturist should disinfect strictly the needle and the skin around the located points, hold the back end of the handle and jerk the wrist quickly to let the other end of the needle quickly tap vertically down and up on the skin. Tap either slightly until the skin becomes congested or heavily until bleeding is about to appear. Finally disinfect the skin.

The location which cutaneous needles are used to tap is usually the route along which the relevant meridian goes and the related points are distributed, or the affected place of a disorder. For building up constitution, the midline of the back and waist (The *Du* Channel) and the 4 channels(The Urinary Bladder Channel of Foot-Taiyang), 2 at the either side with one 1.5 *Cun* and the other 3 *Cun* away from the midline, are often chosen for tapping.

Cutaneous needle puncturing is also administered to prevent and treat headache, dizziness, insomnia, gastrointestinal diseases, women's diseases, cutaneous diseases, faccidity and arthralgia syndromes, or in the convalescence for promoting recovery.

(3) In tradermal Needle Puncturing

Intradermal needles, usually made of 30-32 sizes of stainless steel wire, are short and in two shapes: thumbtack-shaped and wheatgrain-shaped. The former is about 0.3 cm long and used mainly on the auricles and the latter, 1 cm, used on acupoints or pressure pain points all over the body. In application, the needles are buried under the skin and this kind of puncturing is also called needle—embedding therapy. Because the needles buried under the skin are always retained for a certain time, continuous stimulation is then achieved, which meets the purpose of health care and the treatment of various chronic and ache—causing diseases among which are headache, stomachache, insomnia, asthma, enuresis, dysmenorrhea and some menstrual disturbances.

The method of operation is as follows: Disinfect thoroughly the needle and the local skin. Insert the needle with a pair of sterilized tweezers into the skin with its handle remaining outside and fixed with a piece of adhesive plaster. In summer, the needle is not to be retained for more than two days lest infection occur but in winter or autumn, longer if necessary. In the course of retaining the needle, bath is avoided lest infection occur. Needle—embedding near the joints and on the purulent skin is not allowed.

2. Moxibustion for Health Care

There are a few of combustion methods. Here is mainly introduced moxibustion commonly used in health care. Moxibustion consists of the following three kinds: moxa cone moxibustion, moxa roll moxibustion and needle warming through moxibustion. As its name indicates, needle warming though moxibustion is a treatment in which needling and moxibustion are used in combination. It is not introduced here in detail. Leaves of moxa, belonging to those of the composite family, are warm in nature, fragrant and acrid in flavor. They have the action of supporting *Yang—Qi*, warming the meridians, expelling cold, dredging the meridian passages to regulate *Qi* and blood. Chinese mugwort leaves are pounded into mugwort floss which is easily lit. When burning, it produces moderate heat which tends to penetrate the skin and enter the muscles. That's why Chinese mugwort leaves are usually used as the material for moxibustion. Moxa cones are made in the following ways. A small amount of mugwort floss is put over a flat surface and moulded into circular cones with the thumb, forefinger and middle finger. The small ones, as big as wheat grains or half date cores, are used in direct moxibustion. The larger ones, as big as thumbs, each about 1 cm high and with a base whose diameter is 0.8 cm, are used in indirect moxibustion. Moxa rolls are made by putting mugwort floss on pieces of mulberry paper and rolling up the pieces into rolls of cigarette shape, each 20 cm long and with a base whose diameter is 1.5 cm. These rolls are easy to use in moxa roll moxibustion.

(1) Moxa Cone Moxibustion

There are two ways of moxa cone moxibustion: direct and indirect. To burn one cone up is termed as one *Zhuang*.

A. Direct Moxibustion

A moxa cone is put directly on the point chosen and then lit. This method was popular in ancient times. There are also two ways of direct moxibustion: nonscarring moxibustion and scarring moxibustion. In the application of the former, the cone is burned to one half or two-thirds of the total length, the remaining part being replaced with a new one. In so doing, the skin will be neither blistered nor festered later. In the application of the latter, on the other hand, some scallion or garlic juice is first applied to the point and the moxa cone is put on it and lit. After the cone has burnt out, place another one. Use 5-10 *Zhuang* for each administration. In addition to burning and blistering the skin, festering is to be expected following this kind of moxibustion. Though both the methods are used in curing chronic and deficient—cold diseases as well as in preserving health, scarring moxibustion is less commonly used because of the pain it causes and the damage it does to the skin.

B. Indirect Moxibustion

Indirect moxibustion is also called indirect contact moxibustion. It is applied by placing adequate medicines between the skin and moxa cone, preventing the skin from being directly burned and bringing the medicines effects into play. Indirect moxibustion varies with the different medicines used. For example, there is ginger moxibustion, garlic moxibustion, moxibustion with salt and moxibustion with *Fu Zi Bing,* etc. Ginger moxibustion is applied to treat the syndrome due to *Yang*—deficiency, such as weakness of the spleen and stomach, diarrhea, abdominal pain and stagnation of *Qi;* garlic moxibustion, to treat insect—bites, skin and external diseases in the early stage, impairment of the lung caused by overstrain and scrofula; moxibustion with *Fu Zi Bing,* to treat impotence, premature ejaculation due to deficiency of the kidney—*Yang* and obstinate syndromes due to *Yin*—cold or deficiency; moxibustion with salt applied on the acupoint Shenjue (RN 8), having the effect of recuperating depleted *Yang,* to treat collapse as well as abdominal pain, hernia, diarrhea and long—standing dysentery. It was recorded in the classics that one who was treated with 300—500 *Zhuang* of moxibustion with salt would have his disease cured and his life prolonged. *Peng Zu Gu Yang Gu Di Chang Sheng Yan Shou Dan* introduced by Li Yan, a physician in the Ming Dynasty, in his book *Yi Xue Ru Men* under the title of *Lian Qi Fa* is also used for navel moxibustion. Its ingredients are as follows:

Ren Shen (Radix Ginseng)	21 g
Fu Zi (Radix Aconiti Praeparata)	21 g
Hu Jiao (Piper Nigrum)	21 g
She Xiang (Moschus)	15 g
Ye Ming Sha (Faeces Vespertilions)	15 g
Mo Yao (Resina Commiphorae Myrrhae)	15 g
Hu Gu (Os Tigris)	15 g
She Gu (Os Serpentis)	15 g
Long Gu (Os Draconis)	15 g
Zhu Sha (Cinabaris)	15 g
Bai Fu Zi (Rhizoma Typhonii)	15 g
Wu Ling Zhi (Faeces Trogopterorum)	15 g
Qing Yan (Halite)	12 g
Xiao Hui Xiang (Fructus Foeniculi)	12 g
Ding Xiang (Flos Syzygii Aromatici)	9 g
Ru Xiang (Resina Boswelliae Carterii)	6 g
Mu Xiang (Radix Aucklandiae)	6 g
Xiong Huang (Realgar)	3 g

Grind the above drugs into powder. Surround the navel with a strip made of wheat flour paste. Put into the navel 1.5 g of the powder of *She Xiang*. Put one-third of the above powder onto the surrounded navel, press the powder and then make in it several holes and finally cover the powder with a piece of pagoda tree bark. Put a moxa cone near to the bark and light it. Change the burnt-up cone regularly in order to keep the navel hot enough. In the course of treatment, the patient must be sure to refrain from wind-cold and not to eat food either greasy, raw or cold. If women are to be treated in this way, replace *She Xiang* with 3 g of *Shao Nao* (Camphora). It is stated in Li's book, "To use this method once each season may guarantee sufficient primordial *Qi*, prevent all diseases and prolong life. This method is also effective for chronic cough and dyspnea, emission and impotence, whitish and turbid urine, deficiency of the kidney—*Yang*, mental disorder, accumulation of phlegm, leukorrhea with reddish discharge, women's sterility and uterine—cold." The ingredients in the prescription may vary depending on different cases. For instance, *Zheng Qi Zhi Bing Fa* recorded in the book *Zhen Jiu Da Cheng* involves the following ingredients instead:

Wu Ling Zhi (Faeces Trogopterorum)
Qing Yan (Halite)
Ru Xing (Resina Boswelliae Carterii)
Mo Yao (Resina Commiphorae Myrrhae)
Ye Ming Sha (Faeces Vespertilions)
Di Shu Fen (Faeces Ochotona Thibetana)
Cong Tou (Allium Fistulosum)
Mu Tong (Caulis Akebiae)
She Xiang (Moschus)

In *Jiu Qi Gu Ji Fa* recorded in the book *Ming Yi Xuan Yao Ji Shi Qi Fang*, the prescription is modified as follows:

Ye Ming Sha (Faeces Vespertilions)	30 g
Wu Ling Zhi (Faeces Trogopterorum)	30 g
Ku Fan (Alunite)	60 g
She Xiang (Moschus)	6 g

which is for 4 times's dosage, once each season.

(2) Moxa Roll Moxibustion

Moxa roll moxibustion is commonly used in modern times, particularly in health care. In application, special points are chosen to be heated with a lit moxa roll. This method consists of mild moxibustion and bird-pecking moxibustion.

A. Mild Moxibustion

Smoke and heat the points chosen with the lit end of a moxa roll at a certain distance from the skin until the skin feels hot and becomes reddish. The duration is generally from 5-10 minutes.

B. Bird-pecking Moxibustion

Move the lit end of a moxa roll up and down above the point as if a bird were pecking grains, or move it evenly from the right to the left, or stir it horizontally over the point.

The application of any kind of moxibustion must be adequate in its amount. Therefore, be sure to decide properly how big the moxa cone should be and how long the moxa roll moxibustion should last according to the constitution, the disease condition and the age of a patient, and the the location of the points. Over-moxibustion is avoided in case blisters occur, except for scarring moxibustion. Let blisters, if any, be absorbed and scarred naturally, never repture them and be sure to keep them clean. Prick bigger blisters with a clean filiform needle after disinfecting the skin, let the watery fluid go out, and then cover them with sterilized dressing. If the point becomes festered after the administration of scarring moxibustion, disinfect it and then cover it with clean dressing so as to ensure a smooth recovery.

3. Selection and Compatibility of Points in Acupuncture and Moxibustion for Health Care

(1) Points Selected for the Purpose of Strengthening Health and Prolonging Life

Zusanli (ST 36)   Shenque (RN 8)
Guanyuan (RN 4)   Qihai (RN 6)

Dazhui (GB 14)　　　Yongquan (KI 1)

(2) Points Selected for the Purpose of Invigorating the Kidney—*Yang* to Stop Nocturnal Emission

Mingmen (DU 4)　　Shenshu (BL 23)
Zhongji (RN 3)　　Guanyuan (RN 4)
Qihai (RN 6)　　　Sanyinjiao (SP 6)
Yongquan (KI 1)

(3) Points Selected for the Purpose of replenishing *Qi* of the Spleen and Stomach to Strengthen the Digestive System

Zusanli (ST 36)　　Zhongwan (RN 12)
Tianshu (ST 25)　　Pishu (BL 20)
Weishu (BL 21)　　Shenque (RN 8)

(4) Points Selected to Keep the Circulatory System Healthy

Xinshu (BL 15)　　Neiguan (PC 6)
Danzhong (RN 17)　Shenmen (HT 7)

(5) Points Selected to Keep the Respiratory System Healthy

Feishu (BL 13)　　Dazhui (GB 14)
Xinshu (BL 15)　　Danzhong (RN 17)

(6) Points Selected to Keep the Urinary and Reproductive Systems Healthy

Shenshu (BL 23)　　Mingmen (DU 4)
Sanyinjiao (SP 6)　　Zhongji (RN 3)
Guanyuan (RN 4)　　Qihai (RN 6)

(7) Points Selected for Regulating the Mind

Shenmen (HT 7)　　Neiguan (PC 6)
Xinshu (BL 15)　　Sanyinjiao (SP 6)

(8) Points Selected for the Prevention and Recovery of Apoplexy

Zusanli (ST 36)　　Quchi (LI 11)

Baihui (DU 20)   Huantiao (GB 30)

(9) Points Selected for the Prevention and Recovery of Gallbladder Diseases

Ganshu (BL 18)   Pishu (BL 20)

Zusanli (ST 36)

(10) Points Selected for the Prevention of Cold

Dazhui (GB 14)   Feishu (BL 13)

Zusanli (ST 36)

(11) Points Selected for the Auxiliary Treatment and Recovery of Collapse

Shenque (RN 8)   Guanyuan (RN 4)

Zhongji (RN 3)

(12) Points Selected for the Prevention and Recovery of Head Diseases

Baihui (DU 20)   Yongquan (KI 1)

(13) Points Selected for the Prevention and Recovery of Waist and Leg Disorders

Shenshu (BL 23)   Mingmen (DU 4)

Huantiao (GB 30)   Sanyinjiao (SP 6)

(14) Points Selected for the Prevention and Recovery of Insanity, Mania and Epilepsy

Neiguan (PC 6)   Shenmen (HT 7)

Dazhui (GB 14)   Xinshu (BL 15)

Ganshu (BL 18)   Baihui (DU 20)

It is not necessary to use all the points listed above every time in clinical treatment. 1-3 points are enough in each practical treatment, 1-2 of which are usually the ones for long term use, and 1-2 additional ones may be considerably added each time.

4. Cautions in Acupuncture and Moxibustion for Health

Care

(1) Moxibustion is more frequently used than acupuncture in health care, especially for the weak and old. Puncturing must be avoided and moxibustion must be carefully conducted whenever the subject is too weak or over-hungry, exhausted, and drunk, or has over-eaten.

(2) Comfortable and durable postures are to be chosen for a subject; supine and sitting postures being the common ones.

(3) Points in the lower abdominal and lumbosacral areas are not to be chosen for pregnant women. Special care should be taken to avoid hurting the important internal organs when points on the chest, abdomen of back are being punctured, and to keep off blood vessels, inflammation areas, ulcers and wounds. Disinfection of puncturing instruments and the skin is always indispensable.

(4) Be careful not to hurt the skin when applying moxibustion. If infection occurs after scarring moxibustion is applied, measures should be taken to prevent it from diffusing. Moxibustion is not allowed for patients who are suffering from asthenia-syndrome, heat-syndrome or fever due to *Yin*-deficiency. The elderly or those who have difficulty getting about should be careful not to burn clothes or things or even cause fire when they themselves conduct moxibution. Moxibustion should not be done in a pregnant woman's abdominal and lumbosacral areas. Scarring moxibustion is not allowed on the face or where major blood vessels are located.

(5) Nursing after application of acupunture and moxibustion is considered essential in the classics. After the application of moxibustion, the subject shouldn't have tea or food

immediately. He should lie on bed in his bed-room, not meeting anybody and not to be bothered by anything. Overanger, overstrain, overhunger, overeating, exposure to heat and cold, raw and cold fruit, overdrinking, and excessive sexual intercourse are all to be avoided. Diggestible and tasty food nourishing the stomach is recommended.

(6) Regular application of acupuncture and moxibustion for health care is exceptionally important. One course of treatment consists of ten times of application. An interval of several days is needed between two courses. The application may be given every day or every other day. Curative effects will be seen after several courses. In the classics there is record that moxibustion may be given at a certain time, daily, seasonally or yearly. But this needs further verification.

3.1.5 Magnetotherapy for Health Care

According to some clinical observations and experimental research, magnetotherapy can serve to promote and regulate the flow of *Qi* and blood so as to prevent and cure diseases as well as to prolong life-span. In health care, an appropriate permanent magnetic body is fixed on a certain point for health care, which is called Point Magnetotherapy for Health Care. Among Point Magnetotherapies the commonly used one is *Sanlici*, which is carried out by fixing a permanent magnetic body on the point Zusanli. It was reported that about 90% of those, sick or healthy, treated with *Sanlici* gained to different extent in appetite, sleep, muscular strength and blood pressure. In application, however, the magnetic induction intensity and the administration duration should be carefully controlled. As to the diameter of the magnet to be used, 1 centimeter is considered adequate. This magnet should have proper magnetic induction intensity. While applying, sew the magnet in one layer of a band of cloth. Tie the band around the leg with the magnet right on the point Zusanli. For those who are not severely sick, the magnetic induction intensity should remain 0.01—0.03 T for 2—4 hours daily. For those who suffer from hypotension or leukopenia not accompanied by any other diseases, the magnetic induction intensity should be reduced to 0.005—0.02 T. 0.04—0.1 T is suggested with a prolonged administration duration for patients who suffer from stomach and intestine troubles, hypertension and arthritis, and for them regular *Sanlici* is even recommended. From this method, the healthy effects of a permanent magnet with proper mangetic induction intensity on other important points for health care may be studied and observed, which should be with small magnetic induction intensity at the beginning.

3.2 *Qigong* Exercises for Health Care

Qigong is a traditional exercise created by the labouring people of China for the purpose of keeping fit. It is good for people of all ages, especially for the elderly and the middle-aged. *Qigong*, the present-day popular term, was also referred to in ancient China as *Daoyin* (inducement of *Qi* by the mind), *Tuna* (breathing out and in), *Zuochan* (sitting in meditation), *Anqiao* (self-massage at certain acupoints plus *Daoyin* through special posture), *Jing Zuo* (sitting still, similar to *Zuochan*), etc. Based on a series of TCM theories (the theories of *Yin* and *Yang*, Five Elements, *Zang* and *Fu*, Channels and Collaterals, *Qi* and Blood, etc.), with *Qi* functioning as the power, *Qigong* can help an exerciser achieve self-control, self-adjustment, self-repair and self-building-up, and enable him or her to prevent and combat diseases, preserve good health and procur longevity as long as the exerciser can regulate his posture, his mental activities and his respiration (doing the Three Regulations of *Qigong*) and enter the state of *Rujing* and relaxation when he or she is doing *Qigong* exercise.

Qigong exercises date from the time of Tang Yao. The basic patterns were formed during the periods of the Spring-Autumn and Warring States and have continuously been developed ever since. Many schools have been formed because of different views in theory and different ways of exercising. There are, for example, dynamic *Qigong* and static *Qigong* in regard to the form of exercises, health-preserving *Qigong* and hard *Qigong* in regard to the method of exercising (gentle or intense), pneumatic *Neigong* and vocal *Qigong* in regard to breathing type, *Qigong* for building up health and *Qigong* for treating diseases in regard to *Qigong*'s functions, and internal *Qigong* and out-going-*Qi Qigong* in regard to *Qigong*'s properties. The ways of exercising of a particular school may differ from those of other schools; they, however, correlate to each other in fundamentals.

All schools emphasize the way of exercising endogenously for ever-improving "*Jing* (essence), *Qi* (vital energy) and *Shen* (vitality)" and the way of exercising exogenously for ever-toughening "*Jin* (muscles and tendons), *Gu* (bones) and *Pi* (skin)". In doing *Qigong* exercises, two points must always be kept in mind, that is, putting stress on self-training and paying full attention to the correlation between the mind and the body as an integral. By practising *Qigong* exercises, the exerciser can maintain a sound mind, regulate *Qi* and blood, establish good balance between *Yin* and *Yang*, activate blood circulation to remove blood stasis, which will make it possible for him / her to prevent and combat diseases and ensure a long life.

Included in this section is but a brief introduction to ways of exercising and schools of *Qigong* exercises. For detailed information, please refer to related treatises on *Qigong*.

3.2.1 Ways of Exercising

Ways of exercising refer to ways in doing *Qigong* exercises. They are too many to enumerate. On the basis of selecting the most essential and most prominent, we can summarize them into the following: Regulation(regulation of *Yin* and *Yang*, of *Qi* and blood, and of *Ying* and *Wei*), "Practising"(in posture, aiming at mildness, relaxedness and stillness; in breath, aiming at delicateness, deepness and prolonged duration; in training of the mind, aiming at concentration of the mind on the lower *Dantian* and lastly "Mastery" of the skills in performing the exercises. In a word, to do *Qigong* exercises means to train oneself both mentally and physically by giving full play to one's subjective initiative to reach the goal of preserving good health and overcoming diseases.

Qigong exercises, whatever school they may pertain to, include Three Regulations that associate, influence and promote each other, namely, the regulation of posture, the regulation of mental activities and the regulation of respiration .Of the three, the latter two are the key ones though they are performed simultaneously.

1. **Regulation of Posture**

Regulation of posture means to choose a specific posture when doing exercises. There are normally four basic postures to take: standing, sitting, lying and walking. As a rule, sitting is the most frequently selected posture in practice. And which is the best? It depends upon individual conditions as well as upon when and where you do the exercises.

(1) Standing Posture

This is usually taken by healthy exercisers for the purpose of building up a strong constitution. It can further be classified into three modes, i.e., standing with three "circles", natural standing, and standing at will, of which the first is the most commonly selected. The pricinples of its performance are as follows:

A. Stand with the feet separated from each other at shoulder-width, the knee joints flexing a little and the toes slightly directed inwards.

B. Withdraw the chest properly.

C. Raise the arms first to the level of the shoulders and then let them down slowly with the hands about 30cm apart from each other and both at the height of the nipples.

D. Keep this posture as if there were a ball in the arms "held" by the fingers.

E. Narrow the eyes and mouth with a smile in the face.

(2) Sitting Posture

This can be taken by both healthy exercisers and patients in convalescence for rehabilitation. The commonly selected modes include sitting upright on a stool, sitting cross-legged freely on a board bed, and sitting on a board bed with one sole upward.

A. Sitting Upright

In taking this posture, the exerciser is required to sit upright on a stool with the feet on the ground, the legs apart from each other. A right angle must be formed between the body trunk and the legs and between the thighs and the calves. The hands should be put on the knees or placed before the lower abdomen in fist—making manner. The chin is drawn back, the shoulders relaxed and the chest withdrawn. The eyes as well as the mouth are narrowed while the tongue tip sustains the hard palate, and a smile is on the face.

B. Sitting Cross—legged Freely

This posture requires the exerciser to sit upright cross—legged (knees outward and soles inward) on a hard board. However, he / she should do this as naturally as possible. The other principles are the same as those in the above mentioned mode.

C. Sitting Cross—legged with One Sole Upward

This mode also requires the exerciser to sit upright cross—legged on a bed of hard board, but he / she needs to do this with the knees outward and either of the soles upward crossing the calf of the other leg. The rest of the requirements are the same as those in the first mode.

(3) Lying Posture

This is the usual posture preferred by patients who are weak due to prolonged illness or by patients who suffer from insufficiency of *Yang—Qi* or from chronic diseases. This posture has two modes.

A. Lying in Dorsal Position

This mode requires the exerciser to lie dorsally on a bed of hard board, but the upper part of the body should be raised to an oblique position. The legs are stretched straight with the hands on either side of the body. Narrowed eyes and mouth, and a smile are also required.

B. Lying in Lateral Recumbent Position

This mode requires the exerciser to lie on one side on a bed of hard board with the head resting on a pillow or the like and kept at the same level as the body. The upper part of the body should be kept straight with one leg flexed and riding on the other (which is extended). The upper hand is placed against the hip while the lower hand on the pillow with the palm upward. The requirements for narrowed eyes and mouth and a smile are the same as in the posture of sitting upright. It makes no difference as to lie on the right or left side. However, patients with heart trouble are advised to lie on the right side.

(4) Walking Manner

This posture is used in both *Qigong* exercises and *Wushu* (martial art). Activities vary with schools. The requirements of the performance for the usual mode are as follows:

A. Stand still for 2–3 minutes before "walking".

B. Step a pace forward with the left foot (but be sure that the heel touches the ground first) while the upper part of the body and the hands swing to the right, inhale through the nose and exhale through the mouth.

C. Take the second step with the right foot and repeat the other movements in B except that the swinging is towards the left.

D. Repeat the steps in B and C alternately until it is time to finish the exercises (that is, for about 20–30 minutes).

2. Regulation of Mental Activities

Regulation of mental activities is also spoken of as "training of the mind" or "concentration of the mind on certain part of the body". It is a method by which the exerciser can regulate his / her physiological functions through training of the mind. In doing *Qigong* exercises, to regulate mental activities to reach the state of *Rujing* is most essential as well as most important. The level of *Rujing* attained determines the result the exerciser can achieve. The better the state is, the greater the result will be. The meaning of *Rujing* here is a stable state of stillness of the exerciser resulting from his / her concentration of the mind on a single part of the body, for instance, on *Dantian,* or on breathing itself, without any distracting thought. When the exerciser is in this state, he / she is practically insensitive to external stimulations such as sound and light, sometimes even entirely unconscious of the existance of position and weight, i.e., the cerebral cortex has entered a protective depressive state. Usually, there are five methods to reach the state of *Rujing*.

(1) Method of Concentration

This method requires the exerciser to concentrate the mind highly on a certain point of the body. The frequently selected point is Dantian or Qihai (RN 6). When concentrating the mind on the selected point, the exerciser should expel all distracting thoughts. However, he / she need not get nervous about this. The best way to perform concentration is to do it naturally as well as relaxedly.

(2) Method of Attention to Respiration

In practising this method, what the exerciser must do is just to concentrate the mind on breathing, paying attention to process of inhaling and exhaling of abdominal respiration. But he / she must in no case try to control it at will. To reach the state *Rujing,* a harmonious relationship between mind concentration and natural process of breathing should be established.

(3) Method of Counting Breathing Times

The process of inhaling followed by exhaling is counted as one breathing. By counting in mind the times of breathing from 1–10 and from 10–100 and from 100–as many as necessary where the exerciser perceives no sound, no sight, and no disturbance, the state of *Rujing* will naturally be reached.

(4) Method of Recitation in Mind

Some simple and positive words or expressions, short and easy to recite, are selected in advance. When doing *Qigong* exercises, the exerciser, concentrates his / her attention to nothing else but reciting in mind these simple words again and again. In doing so the exerciser has already expelled all distracting thoughts from the mind, which will help him / her reach the state of *Rujing*.

(5) Method of Listening to Breathing

In following this method, the exerciser should try to listen to his / her own breathing. If he / she finds it hardly possible to hear the breathing, so much the better, and even so he / she should continue to listen, for this will help reach the state of *Rujing*.

For beginners, it is recommended to choose the Method of Concentration at first. They can gradually practise the other methods after a period of transition from one method to another. An exerciser can also persist in the method that he / she likes best.

3. Regulation of Respiration

Regulation of respiration is also known as deep respiration or training of breathing. It is one of the most important steps in doing *Qigong* exercises. Regulation means here to change the usual thoracic respiration to abdominal respiration, that is, to change shallow breathing into deep breathing through exercises;

and to establish spontaneous Dantian respiration finally so as to expand vital capacity and promote air metabolism and blood circulation. The new-type respiration will also give "massage" to the internal organs and help digestion and absorption. All this will contribute to preservation of health and prevention of diseases. There are eight commonly employed methods of breathing.

(1) Natural Breathing

This is what physiological respiration means. In doing this breathing, the exerciser respires naturally without any interference by the mind. The process of breathing is even and mild though not deep and prolonged enough.

(2) *Shun* Breathing (breathing with diaphragm-down inhaling)

In this breathing, the diaphragm moves down and the abdomen expands when the exerciser inhales, and when he/she exhales, the diaphragm moves up and the belly contracts in. This type of breathing enables the diaphragm to move up and down to a larger extent as the diaphragm muscles are doing greater amount of work in forward and backward directions. Abdominal respiration can be formed gradually on the basis of this type of breathing.

(3) *Ni* Breathing (breathing with diaphragm-up inhaling)

This type of breathing may be regarded as the counter-type of *Shun* Breathing. The diaphragm moves up when the exerciser inhales and down when he/she exhales. Correspondingly, breathing in makes the abdomen contract and breathing out makes it expand. This type of breathing requires greater amount of exercise and more strength than *Shun* Breathing.

(4) *Tingbi* Breathing (breathing with prolonged inhalation

or exhalation)

This method needs prolonged inhalation or exhalation for a respiration.

(5) Breathing with Nasal Inhalation and Oral Exhalation

This type of breathing is particularly applicable for patients ill with diseases of the respiratory tract which has narrowed the air passage, causing unsmooth respiration.

(6) Breathing with *Qi* Travelling through the *Ren* and *Du* Channels

This type of breathing begins with *Ni* Breathing. The exerciser breathes in air by the nose and imagines that it is led by the mind down to *Dantian* and further down to the perineum; when the exerciser exhales, it is conducted to travel from the perineum through the spine to the point Baihui (DU20) and then is breathed out though the nose. As the "air" has circulated vertically once within the body, this method is also termed as *Xiao Zhoutian* Breathing (small circle of the evolution).

(7) *Qian* Breathing (sub—breathing)

This is a type of breathing naturally formed after having exercised *Shun* Breathing or *Ni* Breathing for a period of time. It is characterized by extremely mild and considerably prolonged inhalation and faint exhalation. The breathing is extremely even. It is called sub—breathing because you can hardly perceive the air current even if you put a finger directly under the nose to test it.

(8) Essential Breathing (very mild abdominal breathing)

This is a state of breathing as expressed in "when visible ordinary breathing ceases, internal essential breathing will naturally begin", a conclusion drawn through experience by some ancient Chinese *Qigong* exercisers. Instead of stopping breathing by force, what "ordinary breathing ceases" actually means here is a state of extreme stillness and extraordinary concentration of the mind in which all activities of the body have become unperceivable: superficially, the breathing seems to have ceased, but it has in fact transformed into navel breathing, a very gentle abdominal breathing form, also known as "fetal breathing". This is the breathing which only those who have reached the high stage in *Qigong* exercises can do.

Training of respiration must be combined with protection of respiration. No matter what type of breathing is selected for *Qigong* exercises, it has to be changed into natural breathing when it has been practised for 10—20 minutes; the respiratory muscles will be exhausted otherwise. It is an elemental principle to do training of respiration in a mild and natural manner. Only by patient practising can the exerciser gradually learn to make breathing deep, long, gentle, even and slow. No hasty attempt can be successful.

3.2.2 Types of *Qigong* Exercises

There are many types of *Qigong* exercises. Such types as *Songjing Gong* (exercises for relaxation and stillness), *Neiyang Gong* (exercises for internal adjustment), and *Qiangzhuang Gong* (exercises for building up a strong constitution) are commonly used to preserve good health, prevent diseases and procure longevity.

1. *Songjing Gong*

This type of exercises puts stress on training to get relaxed.
Preparations
The place for doing the exercises should be as quiet as possi-

ble, with fresh air. If it happens to be in a room or the like, it must be of good ventilation, but the exerciser should keep him—/her—self from direct wind to avoid catching cold. In order to make every part of the body comfortable and assure smooth blood circulation, he/she should wear loose clothing and unfasten such things as the necktie, belt, brassiere, etc. A rest for about 20 minutes before doing the exercises is necessary to get calm and delighted.

Posture

The exerciser can take any of the postures described in "Regulation of Posture." Whichever posture is preferred, the exerciser has to perform it correctly and properly without feeling a shade of discomfort, for this will help him/her reach the state of *Rujing*. Apart from keeping correct posture, the exerciser needs to narrow the eyes as well, gazing at the tip of the nose. The mouth should be slightly open with the tongue touching the hard palate.

The Way to Get Relaxed

In any of the four postures, the exerciser can get relaxed, but the proper procedure is to relax the body from the head down to the feet. The head is slightly bowed so as to let the neck get as relaxed as possible, the shoulders naturally dropping and elbows hanging down. There should be no chest—out and the abdomen should contract in while the waist extends straight. There must not be any strain in any part of the body, nor in the mind, but there must be a smile on the face.

Breathing

Songjing Gong exercises require *Shun* Breathing, the exerciser saying "still" when inhaling and "relaxed" when exhaling. The more relaxed, the sooner the exerciser will reach the state of *RuJ-*

ing. The breathing should be natural and mild that it makes the exerciser comfortable and delighted and the "air" should be led by the mind to go down to *Dantian*. Breathing is one of the key aspects in doing *Qigong* exercises, so it must be practised step by step. It is recommended to do breathing training 20—30 minutes at a time

Sitting Still

This exercise follows breathing training. Sitting Still requires concentration of the mind on the navel or Qihai (RN 6) without any interference of distracting thoughts. However, "stillness" is a relative concept, and the state of *Rujing* varies with individuals. For a beginner, hasty attempt to reach the "real" state of *Rujing* with great effort will never help. When necessary, the exerciser can rid him—/her—self of all distracting thoughts by concentrating the mind on one positive idea. This method has proved quite effective.

Concluding a Time of Exercising

On completion of the exercises, the exerciser should do the following before standing up: press the navel with one palm and ride on it with the other; then, move both hands, with the navel as the center, first to the left to form larger and larger whirlings slowly for 30 circles; then, after a pause, to the right to form 30 smaller and smaller whirlings and stop circling at the navel. This can be followed by moderate free activities. Other supplementary exercises such as *Taiji* boxing, *Baduanjin* exercises, slow running, etc. will help obtain better results.

Songjing Gong is applicable for people of normal health as well as for the elderly and middle aged, the less able—bodied, and individuals with chronic cardiovascular, respiratory or digestive diseases.

2. *Neiyang Gong*

This type of exercise puts stress on regulation of respiration. The requirements for preparations, posture and the way to get relaxed are the same as those in *Songjing Gong*.

Breathing

In doing *Neiyang Gong* exercise, the exerciser has to practise *Tingbi* Breathing, whether he / she may choose the breathing way of inhaling—pause—exhaling—inhaling or the way of inhaling—exhaling—pause—inhaling, prolonging inhalation or exhalation. The breathing must be deep and long, soft and gentle, even and smooth. A conditional reflex should be established that he / she breathes completely through the nose and conducts through the mind the "air" down to *Dantian* whenever the exerciser does the breathing. If he / she can really lead the "air" down to the lower abdomen (Qihai Point), there will be an apparent expansion of that part. Nevertheless, it must be noted that he / she is by no means advised to expand the lower abdomen by intentional effort. It is entirely wrong to think that greater expansion of the abdomen would produce better result, because the level of expansion is a matter of individual difference; it, too, varies at different stages in the course of doing *Qigong* exercises.

In practising Sitting Still in *Neiyang Gong,* the exerciser can use one or two methods to regulate respiration. The other requirements for Sitting Still and Concluding Exercises are the same as those in *Songjing Gong*.

Neiyang Gong is particularly preferable for the elderly, the less able—bodied and patients with chronic diseases of the digestive system.

3. *Qiangzhuang Gong*

Qiangzhuang Gong puts stress on training to reach the state of *Rujing*. As a rule, to do this type of exercise on the basis of *Songjing Gong* will be successful. The key to achieve success lies in correct posture, good regulation of respiration and high concentration of the mind on *Rujing* state. The requirements for preparations, posture and the way to get relaxed are the same as those in *Songjing Gong*.

Breathing

Generally, *Shun* Breathing is more suitable for males whereas *Ni* Breathing, for females though it should be born in upon the exerciser that those who are used to *Shun* Breathing should change to *Ni* Abdominal Breathing and those who are used to *Ni* Breathing should change to *Shun* Abdominal Breathing. Breathing practice can last 10—20 minutes before normal respiration is restored. Regulation of respiration in *Qiangzhuang Gong* requires attention to be paid to mild natural exhalation rather than to inhalation.

Sitting Still

As this type of exercises aims at training to reach the state of *Rujing*, the exerciser may as well do Sitting Still directly without performing its breathing exercise. In order to reach the state of *Rujing*, exercisers can employ any of the ways in Regulation of Mental Activities described in an earlier part of the text (see: 2 in 3.2.1.) that will help them get into a state between sleeping and awakening, oblivious of themselves. Sitting Still exercise can take 30—40 minutes.

To conclude the exercises, related performances described in *Songjing Gong* can be made with slight modification: instead of 30 circles, 24 will be sufficient.

Qiangzhuang Gong is a unique type of exercise effective in building up a strong constitution, maintaining health, preventing and combatting diseases and ensuring longevity. Its curative effects have proved satisfactory in the treatment of such nervous disorders as neurasthenia, neurosis, vegetative functional disturbance, etc.

3.2.3 Principles in Doing *Qigong* Exercises

Exercisers must have a good command of the principles in doing *Qigong* exercises before they can expect desirable results.

1. They must confident, resolute and persistent in doing the exercises, firmly believing that the exercises are effective in prevention and treatment of diseases, in keeping fit and ensuring longevity.

2. They should live a regular life and try to avoid interference from any of the pathogenic "Seven Emotions" so that they can keep themselves in good humour. They are also advised to give up smoking and drinking.

3. Before doing the exercises, they must be free from any bands or restraints from the clothing. They also need to relax themselves completely, expel any distracting thought from the mind, settle down for the exercises, and defecate or urinate if necessary.

4. They should choose the postures that are most appropriate for them and do the exercises for 30—60 minutes a time, 1—2 times a day. The place for them to do the exercises must be quiet and ventilated with fresh air.

5. The exercises must be preceded by preparatory activities

and followed by concluding exercises. During the course of practising the exercises, stillness, relaxedness and naturalness can never be over—emphasized and no attempt to hasten success is acceptable.

6. They should not pay too much attention to (not to say strongly desire) spontaneous dynamic activities during the course of doing exercises. If any such activities are to be expected, they must be under the tutor's supervision: there should be both lithe and vigorous, both slow and quick activities because constant variability accounts. Only by forming regular patterns can deviant activities be reduced remarkably.

3.3 TCM Massage for Health Care

TCM massage is the English translation of the term *Tuina* in traditional Chinese medicine which is similar to, but different from, massage in Western medicine. It is an effective therapy to preserve health created by ancestors of the Chinese people through long-term practice. TCM massotherapy refers to a method used to treat diseases or to keep good health by application of continuous skillful actions of the hands or fingers of a practitioner to the skin or the muscular tissues of him—/ her--self or others. As it is a treatment economical, safe, effective, easy and convenient to perform with no need of drugs or medical apparatus. TCM massage is particularly applicable for old people ill with certain chronic diseases. It is also a good practice fot the aged to keep good health and for the healthy to build up the body.

TCM massage has a long history. It was already in wide medical use in China more than 2,000 years ago and has kept developing ever since. Today a complete theoretical system has been formed along with a set of practical and effective manipulative maneuvers.

TCM massage is used as a therapy to treat diseases or as a method to preserve health because it can cause local or general responses of the body so as to regulate the body functions and overcome pathogenic factors. In modern medicine, it is concluded that massage manipulation can produce a physiological stimulation on the affected area where subsequent biophysical and biochemical changes and physiological actions of the local tissues will occur; these actions can then be reinforced through regulation of nerve reflexes and body fluids circulation; furthermore, they will result in secondary systemic responses of the body which in turn will change the pathological and physiological courses that contribute to combatting diseases and keeping good health. According to TCM theory, massage manipulation applied to human body may have such effects as balancing *Yin* and *Yang*, regulating functions, re-adjusting the actions of the meridians, strengthening the body resistance, eliminating pathogenic factors, promoting blood circulation to remove blood stasis, invigorating the bones and muscles, and calming and relieving pains.

The general principle of TCM massotherapy is based on the conception of "searching for the primary cause of diseases in treatment". Choice and performance of manipulative maneuvers depend upon such factors as the patient's age and constitution, the nature and course of the disease, the time, etc.

TCM massage is too broad a text to discuss in this section. We will but concentrate on a brief introduction to self-preservation of health by application of TCM massage. For detailed information, please refer to treatises on *Tuina*.

3.3.1 Classification and Manipulation

TCM massage can be classified as Active Massage and Passive Massage.

If one performs massage manipulative maneuvers on one's own body to keep oneself in good health, this is termed as Active Massage, which is primarily employed to preserve health.

If a doctor performs massage manipulative maneuvers on a patient as a treatment, this is termed as Passive Massage, which is primarily employed to treat diseases.

Difference in performing manipulative maneuvers exists between schools of different views. There are, therefore, various manipulative maneuvers in practising TCM massage. In general, the following maneuvers can be found in clinical practice: pushing (*Tui*), symmetric pinching (*Na*), pressing (*An*), palm-rubbing(*Mo*), rotatory kneading(*Rou*), mobile finger-pinching(*Nie*), rolling(*Gun*), rubbing(*Ca*), acupoint finger-pushing(*Yun*), foulaging(*Cuo*), holding-and-twisting(*Yao*), rotating(*Nian*), scraping(*Gua*), clapping(*Pai*), piling(*Die*), fingertip-pressing(*Dian*), pulse pressing(*Ya*), moderate pulling(*Chen*), finger-flicking(*Tan*), separating(*Fen*) and uniting(*He*); though only the first eight of them are commonly used and a few of them are frequently selected for self-massage, for instance, clapping, finger-pressing and pulse pressing.

1. Pushing Maneuver

The massagist presses with a finger (usually the thumb) / palm / elbow on a definite part of the patient's body and moves it straight and unidirectionally along a certain line for a desired distance. The exertion of strength should be steady and slow, and the finger / palm / elbow must be kept touching closely the part being massaged. This maneuver can be applied to any part of the body and increase the excitability of the muscles and promote blood circulation. In TCM terms, this is expressed as relieving the rigidity of the muscles and activating the channels and collaterals.

2. Symmetric Pinching Maneuver

The massagist holds between the fingers (the forefinger plus middle finger or all of the four) and the thumb a certain part or point of the patient's body and pinches tightly and loosely alternately. The performance should be in a moderate and continual way, any interruption being avoided, and the exertion should be made with gradual increase of strength. Sudden violent action must be avoided. As a maneuver with considerably strong stimulation, it is frequently accompanied with other maneuvers and applied to the points in the neck, shoulders and limbs. Symmetric pinching can produce such effects as expelling wind and clearing away cold, causing resuscitation and relieving pain, and remitting spasm of the muscles and tendons.

3. Pressing Maneuver

The massagist presses a certain part / acupoint of the patient's body with the fingers (or the thumb only) or the palm-base and gradually exerts strength downward while rotating, and keeps the hand there for as long as necessary. This maneuver has the following modes: thumb pressing, palm-base pressing, four-finger pressing and two-finger pressing. The pressing can provide a relatively strong stimulation and it is frequently combined with rotatory kneading, forming a compound maneuver "pressing-rotatory-kneading". Thumb pressing can be applied to any part of the body; palm-base pressing to the back, waist and the lower limbs; four-finger pressing to the neck or the costal part, and thumb-and -forefinger pressing to the fingers or the parts with slim and soft muscles. This maneuver can produce such effects as alleviating pain through inducement, relieving syndromes of stroke and easing constipation or dysuria, relaxing the muscles, and correcting spinal deformity.

4. Palm-rubbing Maneuver

The massagist puts the palm or the palmar surface of the forefinger, middle finger and ring finger on a certain part of the patient's body and does rhythmic circular rubbing. The palm is tracted by movement of the wrist joint and the forearm. The massagist has to make sure that the elbow joint flexes slightly, that the wrist is relaxed and that the fingers stretch straight naturally. The rubbing palm or finger surface should move in a circulor way under traction of the wrist and forearm. Natural exertion of strength is needed and the rubbing must be mild and harmonious at a rate of about 120 circles per minute. Palm rubbing provides mild stimulation and is frequently applied to the thoracico-abdominal part and hypochondriac region. This maneuver can produce such effects as normalizing the function of the stomach-*Qi*, promoting digestion and removing stagnated food, and regulating peristalsis of the intestines.

5. Rotatory Kneading Maneuver

The massagist kneads rotatorily a certain part or a acupoint of the patient's body with the thenar and palm-base or the palmar surface of the fingers. The performance should be gentle and soft. When the palmar part rotates at 120—160 circles a minute under the drive of the wrist joint and forearm, the wrist must be in a relaxed state and its range of movement can be increased gradually. The pressure applied should be gentle and mild. As this maneuver provides just a mild stimulation, it can be applied to any part of the body. The main effects of this maneuver includes relieving stuffiness of the chest and regulating the flow of Qi, promoting digestion and removing stagnated food, activating blood flow and eliminating blood stasis, subduing swelling and alleviating pain.

6. Mobile Finger-pinching Maneuver

The massagist holds between the finger(s) and the thumb a muscle or tendon of the patient's body, pinches or squeezes tightly and loosely alternatively while moving the pinching fingers along the muscle or tendon, and repeats this as many times as necessary. The performance can be made with the thumb and the forefinger or the thumb and forefinger plus the middle finger or the thumb and all the four fingers according to how strong a stimulation is needed. Mobile finger-pinching is usually applied to the thigh, calf, shoulders or back. It can produce such effects as relieving rigidity of the muscles and dredging the channels and collaterals, promoting the flow of Qi and activating blood circulation.

7. Rolling Maneuver

The massagist lays on a certain part of the patient's body the dorsal side of a hand adjacent to the small finger or to the knuckles of the middle finger, ring finger and small finger, and rolls the hand to and fro continually under the drive of the wrist joint, twisting in-and-out-ward to let the strength evenly act on the treated area. During the performance, it is required to keep the wrist joint relaxed and to flex the elbow joint slightly (forming an angle of about 120 degrees) with the arm and shoulders mobilized but not too much strained. The rolling part (hypothenar) should closely adhere to the patient's body. Beating or rubbing with the hand-back is not permissible. The pressure applied should be even and the manipulation must be harmonious and rhythmic at 120-160 rolls a minute. As this maneuver exerts relatively great pressure and makes quite broad contact surface, it can be applied to such parts with rich muscles as the shoulders and the back, the waist and buttocks or the limbs. Rolling maneuver can produce such effects as relieving rigidity of the muscles and joints, activating the flow of blood, alleviating spasms, promoting the circulation of blood and helping to recover from exhaustion.

8. Rubbing Maneuver

The massagist puts on a certain part of the patient's body the palmar surface and the thenar or the hypothenar of a hand and rubs to and fro along a certain line. The moving should be straight rather than crooked, and the rubbing distance sufficiently long. Though excessive pressure is not suitable in case the skin of the patient get injured, the palm or thenar should be closely on the patient's body. Steady exertion of strength is significant and even and continual rubbing at 100-120 times a minute is most important. This maneuver is characterized by mild and warm stimulation with such effects as promoting the flow of Qi by warming the channels and collaterals, subduing swelling and alleviating pain, strengthening the spleen and stomach, lifting local temperature of the body, and promoting the circulation of blood and lymph. Palmar rubbing is mostly applied to the thoracico-hypo-chondriac part and the abdomen and hypothenar rubbing to the shoulders, back, waist, clunis and lower limbs and thenar rubbing to the thoracico-abdominal part, waist, back and limbs. During the performance, the treated part should be exposed and some lubrication or unguent is needed.

9. Clapping Maneuver

The massagist claps the body surface of the patient with the palm which is shaped like an upside-down cup, that is, the fingers clench close naturally with slight bending of the metacarpophalangeal joints. The clapping should be steadly and rhythmic. This maneuver can be applied to the shoulders, back, clunis and the lower limbs and it can produce such effects as relieving rigidity of the muscles and tendons, activating the collaterals, promoting the flow of *Qi* and blood, alleviating spasms and helping to recover from exhaustion.

10. Fingertip Pressing Maneuver

The massagist presses the areas about a certain part of the patient's body with one or two finger tips (the tips of the thumb and forefinger). This maneuver can provide very strong stimulation. As it is performed with one or two fingers, this maneuver is usually applied to bone raphae where there are fewer or thinner muscles, producing such effects as relieving syndromes of stroke and easing constipation or dysuria, activating the flow of blood and alleviating pain, and regulating the function of *Zang* and *Fu* organs.

11. Pulse Pressing Maneuver

The massagist presses the part of the patient's body to be treated in a way like pulsebeat with the finger(s) or palm. Finger pressing can be performed with the middle finger or other fingers, applicable to the face or other parts of the head; palm pressing can be performed with one or two palms, applicable to any part of the body trunk. This maneuver can produce such effects as relaxing the muscles, activating the circulation of blood, and relieving pain.

3.3.2 Self-massage for Health Care

Self-massage is one of the commonly used methods for preservation of health. It includes local self-massage and general self-massage. The former refers to giving massage to small areas of the body by the practitioner him-/her-self for the treatment of local disorders while the latter means to provide self-massage to greater areas, such as the head, trunk and limbs, for the prevention of diseases or preservation of good health. General self-massage is among those ideal methods for people to keep fit. It is particularly applicable for the aged with less able-body.

1. Indication of Self-massage

Local self-massage is usually prescribed to treat local disorders such as pain, numbness, atrophy and hypofunction of the muscles due to invasion of the evils of wind-cold. It can also be applied to treat indigestion, local neuralgia, etc.

General self-massage is mainly employed to prevent diseases or to preserve health, to build up constitutions and to obtain longevity though it can also be applied to treat diseases.

2. Method of Practising Self-massage

What is discussed here is a method to keep strong and healthy and to prevent diseases by means of practice of general self-massage. This method is particularly applicable for the aged and less able-bodied. The performance includes 20 actions in series:

(1) Tapping of the Teeth

Shut the mouth softly and do tapping of the teeth rhythmically for 30—40 times.

(2) Cleaning of the Mouth

Shut the mouth softly and wash the surface of the teeth and the teeth ridges with the tongue from the right to the left and vice versa, each 30 times.

(3) Rubbing of the Palms

Rub the palmar surfaces energetically and gradually increase the frequency until both palms are warmed up (about 30—40 times).

(4) Wiping the Face

Wipe the face with the warmed palms. Be sure that the fingers cling together with the knuckles flexing slightly and the palms move from the forehead to the chin 20—30 times.

(5) "Combing" the Hair

"Comb" the hair with the ten finger tips of the hands from the forehead backward to the occiput and then from the temples up to the vetex, each 20—30 times.

(6) Kneading the Temples

Knead the temples with the tips of the middle fingers rotatorily, clockwise and counterclockwise, each direction 7—8 circles.

(7) Kneading the Eyes

Knead the eyes around the orbits rotatorily with the knuckles of the forefingers, middle fingers and ring fingers counterclockwise and then clockwise for 7—8 rounds.

(8) Pressing the Jingming (UI 1) Points

Press the Jingming points with the forefinger tips and then release the tips for a pause. Do this 15—30 times.

(9) Pressing the Temples Rotatorily

Press the temples rotatorily with the forefinger tips, clockwise and then counterclockwise, each direction 10—15 circles.

(10) *Ming Tiangu* (Auricular Drilling)

Press tightly the ears with the palms while beating the occiput 15 times with the forefingers, middle fingers and ring fingers and then release the palms a little but press the fingers tightly on the occiput for a while and suddenly remove them. Do this 15 times. Finally, insert the tips of the middle fingers or the forefingers into the ears, make three turns and suddenly withdraw the tips. Repeat this 3—5 times.

(11) Kneading the Breast

Put the palms on the breast parts (above the nipples and to the outer sides) and knead rotatorily, clockwise and then counterclockwise, each direction 10 circles. Be sure to press the breast firmly and not to let the palms make slides.

(12) Pinching the Shoulder Muscles

Hold the left shoulder muscle about the point Jianjing with the thumb and the forefinger and the middle finger of the right hand and pinch. Change sides and do the same, that is, pinch the right shoulder muscle with the left hand. Do the above modes alternately, 10—15 times on each side. Be sure that the pinching is sufficiently energetic.

(13) Broadening the Chest

Place the hands on either side of the sternum with the fingers slightly apart from each other and move the tips of the fingers along the intercostal spaces from the breastbone to the sides. Do this 10—15 times.

(14) Kneading the Abdomen

Knead the abdomen with one hand (fingers apart from each other and finger tips downwars) from the stomach part down the left side of the navel to the lower abdomen, then rightward, upward, leftward and downward, the round route corresponding to the trend of the large intestine. Do this 10—15 times.

(15) Rubbing the Lumbar Region

Press the lumbar region tightly with the palms that have been warmed by rubbing each other beforehand and move one of the palms down to the caudal end. When this hand rubs up back, the other rubs down simultaneously. Keep the hands rubbing the loins up and down each after the other 30 times.

(16) Pressing the Huantiao (GB 30) Points

Lie down on the right lateral position with the right leg stretching straight and the left leg flexing and press the left Huantiao point with the left thumb tip. Change the Lying side and press the corresponding right point with the right thumb tip. Do these alternately, 10 times on either side.

(17) Rubbing the Thigh

Hold a thigh tightly between the hands and rub it energetically from the hip to the knee and vice versa for 20 times. Be sure that the strength is evenly exerted; excessive or insufficient strength is in no case acceptable.

(18) Kneading the Calf

Hold a calf tightly between the palms and knead it energetically in a rotatory way 20—30 rounds. Change to the other calf and do the same as above.

(19) Rubbing the Yongquan (KL 1) Points

Rub the palms to warm them up and then rub the left Yongquan point quickly and energetically with the palms until the sole is warmed up, too. Do the same as above to the other Yongquan point.

(20) Breathing

Stand straight with the feet apart from each other at shoulder-width and breathe in while raising the head, stretching the waist and lifting the hands from the belly to the throat, then breathe out uttering "*Ha, Ho, Xi, Xu*" while lowering the head, stooping down, and letting the hands down from the throat back to the abdomen. Do this three times.

Practise the above exercises in the order they are presented here. Those who are less able-bodied can choose some of the exercises at first and gradually cover them all.

3. Precautions in Practising Self-massage

(1) Never do self-massage after overeating or in great hunger.

(2) Be sure that the place for performing self-massage is ventilated with fresh air.

(3) As a rule, do self-massage twice a day: once in the morning and again in the evening, about 20 minutes a time; one can prolong or shorten the time according to his own condition.

(4) The amount of massage performance varies with individuals. That which feels most comfortable, pleasurable and brightening is the best to be recommended.

(5) Concentrate the mind, calm the feelings and get relaxed when doing self-massage.

(6) Eat enough nutritive food, avoid exhaustion and control sexual life.

(7) Keep the skin clean. Wash hands before self-massage. Nails must be cut short and rounded. Talcum powder can be used on the skin of the limbs or other parts with much hair to prevent injure to the skin.

(8) Direct skin-contact is significant. Massage outside the clothing is barely effective.

3.3.3 Indications and Contraindications

1. Indications

Massotherapy can be utilized in internal medicine, surgery, pediatrics, traumatology, health protection, etc. It can also be used as an auxiliary treatment. In dealing with internal diseases, especially chronic or functional diseases, massotherapy is one of the best choices. Self-massage is quite effective in treatment of certain diseases during their acute stage such as protrusion of intervertebral disc, acute sprain, acute mastitis, infantile fever, indigestion or diarrhea of children, etc. This therapy has proved a good method in prevention of diseases, preservation of good health and making longevity.

2. Contraindications

Among the contraindications of massotherapy are acute infectious diseases, local lesion of malignant tumours, ulcerative dermatoses, burns, scalds, all contagious and suppurative diseases, tubercular arthritis, serious heart disease, hepatic diseases, serious psychoses, gastric or duodenal perforation, hemorrhagic or other fatal diseases. In addition, females during menstrual period or in pregnancy are cautioned not to massage the abdomen or the lumbosacaral portion.

9
自 我 保 健

序

《英汉实用中医药大全》即将问世，吾为之高兴。

歧黄之道，历经沧桑，永盛不衰。吾中华民族之强盛，由之。世界医学之丰富和发展，亦由之。然而，世界民族之差异，国别之不同，语言之障碍，使中医中药的传播和交流受到了严重束缚。当前，世界各国人民学习、研究、运用中医药的热潮方兴未艾。为使吾中华民族优秀文化遗产之一的歧黄之道走向世界，光大其业，为世界人民造福，徐象才君集省内外精英于一堂，主持编译了《英汉实用中医药大全》。是书之问世将使海内外同道欢呼雀跃。

世界医学发展之日，当是歧黄之道光大之时。

吾欣然序之。

中华人民共和国卫生部副部长
兼国家中医药管理局局长
世界针灸学会联合会主席
中国科学技术协会委员
中华全国中医学会副会长
中国针灸学会会长

胡熙明
1989年12月

序

　　中华民族有同疾病长期作斗争的光辉历程，故而有自己的传统医学——中国医药学。中国医药学有一套完整的从理论到实践的独特科学体系。几千年来，它不但被完好地保存下来，而且得到了发扬光大。它具有疗效显著、副作用小等优点，是人们防病治病，强身健体的有效工具。

　　任何一个国家在医学进步中所取得的成就，都是人类共同的财富，是没有国界的。医学成果的交流比任何其他科学成果的交流都应进行得更及时，更准确。我从事中医工作30多年来，一直盼望着有朝一日中国医药学能全面走向世界，为全人类解除病痛疾苦做出其应有的贡献。但由于用外语表达中医难度较大，中国医药学对外传播的速度一直不能令人满意。

　　山东中医学院的徐象才老师发起并主持了大型系列丛书《英汉实用中医药大全》的编译工作。这个工作是一项巨大工程，是一种大型科研活动，是一个大胆的尝试，是一件新事物。对徐象才老师及与其合作的全体编译者夜以继日地长期工作所付出的艰苦劳动，克服重重困难所表现出的坚韧不拔的毅力，以及因此而取得的重大成绩，我甚为敬佩。作为一个中医界的领导者，对他们的工作给予全力支持是我应尽的责任。

　　我相信《英汉实用中医药大全》无疑会在中国医学史和世界科学技术史上找到它应有的位置。

中华全国中医学会常务理事
山东省卫生厅副厅长
张奇文
1990年3月

出版前言

中国医药学是我中华民族优秀文化遗产之一，建国以来由于党和国家对待中医药采取了正确的政策，使中医药理论宝库不断得到了发掘整理，取得了巨大的成绩。当前，世界各国人民对中国医药学的学习和研究热潮日益高涨，为促进这一热潮更加蓬勃的发展，为使中国医药学能更好地为全人类解除病痛服务，就必须促进中医中药在世界范围内的传播和交流，而要使这一传播和交流进行得更及时、更准确，就必须首先排除语言障碍。因此，编译一套英汉对照的中医药基本知识的书籍，供国内外学习、研究中医药时使用，已成为国内外医药学界和医药学教育界许多人士的迫切需要。

多年来，在卫生部门的号召下，在"中医英语表达研究"方面，已经作出了一些可喜的成绩。本书《英汉实用中医药大全》的编辑出版就是在调查上述研究工作的历史和现状的基础上，继续对中医药英语表达作较系统、较全面的研究，以适应中国医药学对外传播交流的需要。

这部"大全"的版本为英汉对照，共有21个分册，一个分册介绍论述中国医药学的一个分科。在编著上注意了中医药汉文稿的编写特色，在内容上注意了科学性、实用性、全面性和简明易读。汉文稿的执笔撰写者主要是有20年以上实践经验的教授、副教授、主任医师和副主任医师。各分册汉文稿撰写成后，均经各学科专家逐一审订。各分册英文主译、主审主要是国内既懂中医又懂英语的权威人士，还有许多中医院校的英语教师及医药卫生部门的专业翻译人员。英译稿脱稿后，经过了复审、终审，有些译稿还召开全国22所院校和单位人员参加的英译稿统稿定稿研讨会,对英译稿进行细致的研讨和推敲,对如何较全面、较系统、较准确地用英语表达中国医药学进行了探讨,从而推动整个译文达到较高水平,因此,这部"大全"可供中医院校高年级学生作为泛读教材使用。

这部"大全"的编纂得到了国家教育委员会、国家中医药管理局、山东省教育委员会、山东省卫生厅等各部门有关领导的支持。在国家教委高等教育司的指导下,成立了《英汉实用中医药大全》编译领导委员会。还得到了全国许多中医院校和中药生产厂家领导的支持。

希望这部"大全"的出版,对中医院校加强中医英语教学,对国内卫生界培养外向型中医药人才,以及在推动世界各国人民对中医药的学习和研究方面,都将产生良好的影响。

高等教育出版社
1990年3月

前 言

《英汉实用中医药大全》是一部以中医基本理论为基础,以中医临床为重点,较为全面系统、简明扼要、易读实用的中级英汉学术性著作。它的主要读者是:中医药院校高年级学生和中青年教师,中医院的中青年医生和中医药科研单位的科研人员,从事中医对外函授工作的人员和出国讲学或行医的中医人员,西学中人员,来华学习中医的外国留学生和各类进修人员。

由于中国医药学为我中华民族之独有,因此,英译便成了本《大全》编译工作的重点。为确保译文能准确表达中医的确切含义,我们邀集熟悉中医的英语人员、医学专业翻译人员、懂英语的中医药人员乃至医古文人员于一堂,共同翻译、共同对译文进行研讨推敲的集体翻译法,这样,就把众人之长融进了译文质量之中。然而,即使这样,也难确保译文都能尽如人意。汉文稿虽反映了中国医药学的精髓和概貌,但也难能十全十美。我衷心地盼望读者能提出批评和建议,以便《大全》再版时修改。

参加本《大全》编、译、审工作的人员达200余名,他们来自全国28个单位,其中有山东、北京、上海、天津、南京、浙江、安徽、河南、湖北、广西、贵阳、甘肃、成都、山西、长春等15所中医学院,还有中国中医研究院,山东省中医药研究所等中医药科研单位。

山东省教育委员会把本《大全》的编译列入了科研计划并拨发了科研经费,山东省卫生厅和一些中药生产厂家也给了很大支持,济南中药厂的资助为编译工作的开端提供了条件。

本《大全》的编译成功是全体编译审者集体劳动的结晶,是各有关单位主管领导支持的结果。在《大全》各分册即将陆续出版之际，我诚挚地感谢全体编译审者的真诚合作，感谢许多专家、教授、各级领导和生产厂家的热情支持。

愿本《大全》的出版能在培养通晓英语的中医人才和使中医早日全面走向世界方面起到我所期望的作用。

主编　徐象才

于山东中医学院

1990年3月

目　录

说明 451
1 中医保健原则 453
  1.1　精神保健 453
    1.1.1　豁达乐观 454
    1.1.2　清心寡欲 456
    1.1.3　喜怒有节 457
    1.1.4　省思少虑 459
    1.1.5　忌忧伤悲 459
    1.1.6　避免惊恐 460
  1.2　饮食保健 461
    1.2.1　食宜清淡 461
    1.2.2　谨和五味 463
    1.2.3　按时节量 464
    1.2.4　调适寒热 466
    1.2.5　清洁卫生 467
    1.2.6　饮食宜忌 468
  1.3　起居保健 474
    1.3.1　起居有常 474
    1.3.2　安卧有方 475
    1.3.3　衣适寒温 478
    1.3.4　讲究卫生 479
  1.4　劳逸保健 481
    1.4.1　勿劳伤形体 481
    1.4.2　勿劳伤心神 483
    1.4.3　勿房劳过度 483
    1.4.4　勿过度安逸 486

1.5 运动保健 ····· 487
1.5.1 坚持参加劳动 ····· 488
1.5.2 参加体育锻炼 ····· 489
1.5.3 常用运动方法简介 ····· 489
1.6 顺应自然保健 ····· 490
1.6.1 顺应四时 ····· 491
1.6.2 调适环境 ····· 494
2. 实用保健方药 ····· 498
2.1 常用保健中药 ····· 498
2.1.1 补气药 ····· 498

1. 人参
2. 西洋参
3. 太子参
4. 刺五加
5. 党参
6. 黄芪
7. 白术
8. 甘草
9. 山药
10. 黄精
11. 大枣
12. 饴糖
13. 蜂蜜

2.1.2 养血药 ····· 503

1. 阿胶
2. 当归
3. 熟地黄
4. 何首乌
5. 白芍
6. 龙眼肉
7. 桑椹

2.1.3 助阳药 ····· 505

1. 鹿茸
2. 蛤蚧
3. 巴戟天
4. 杜仲
5. 冬虫夏草
6. 紫河车
7. 菟丝子
8. 胡桃仁
9. 阳起石
10. 补骨脂
11. 淫羊藿

2.1.4 滋阴药 ··· 509

1. 沙参
2. 天冬
3. 石斛
4. 麦冬
5. 玉竹
6. 百合
7. 枸杞子
8. 女贞子
9. 黑芝麻
10. 鳖
11. 银耳

2.1.5 其他保健中药 ································· 513

1. 酸枣仁
2. 山楂
3. 莲子
4. 灵芝
5. 茯苓
6. 薏苡仁
7. 芡实
8. 香菇
9. 木耳
10. 菊花
11. 丹参
12. 三七
13. 天麻
14. 花粉

2.2 常用保健中成药 ····································· 518

2.2.1 补气成药 ··· 518

1. 补中益气丸
2. 参苓白术丸
3. 四君子丸
4. 十全大补丸
5. 两参精
6. 人参蜂王浆
7. 北京蜂王精
8. 延年益寿精
9. 五加参冲剂
10. 大力士补液
11. 人参 VitC 滋补片
12. 青春宝
13. 万年青滋补浆

2.2.2 养血成药 ··· 521

1. 八珍丸
2. 复方阿胶浆
3. 康宝
4. 参芪王浆养血精
5. 人参首乌精
6. 阿胶滋补精
7. 两仪冲剂
8. 益寿滋补浆

· 445 ·

9. 补血宁神片　　10. 参归枣汁

2.2.3 助阳成药 ... 523
1. 金匮肾气丸　　2. 海龙蛤蚧精
3. 男宝　　　　　4. 参茸鞭丸
5. 阳春药　　　　6. 益肾糖浆
7. 参茸大补丸　　8. 雏凤精
9. 海马补肾丸　　10. 梅花鹿茸血
11. 海参丸

2.2.4 滋阴成药 ... 525
1. 六味地黄丸　　2. 人参固本丸
3. 健脑冲剂　　　4. 参杞蜂皇浆
5. 滋阴百补丸　　6. 康复丸
7. 清宫寿桃丸

2.2.5 其他保健成药 ... 527
1. 灵芝片　　　　2. 益脑复健丸
3. 脑灵素　　　　4. 优康平
5. 安神补心丸　　6. 益春宝口服液
7. 灵芝强体片　　8. 丹七片
9. 女宝　　　　　10. 更年安

2.3 保健药酒 ... 529

2.3.1 药酒的保健作用 ... 530
1. 协调阴阳　　　2. 补益气血
3. 滋补五脏　　　4. 祛病驱邪
5. 延年益寿

2.3.2 药酒保健的机理 ... 531

2.3.3 药酒保健的特点 ... 532
1. 酒助药势，提高药效 ... 532
2. 作用广泛，应用灵活 ... 533
3. 药性稳定，服用方便 ... 533

  2.3.4 保健药酒的适用范围 ························· 533
   1. 补气药酒   2. 养血药酒
   3. 滋阴药酒   4. 助阳药酒
   5. 补五脏药酒 6. 延年益寿药酒
   7. 防治疾病的保健药酒
  2.3.5 药酒的制作方法 ····························· 534
  2.3.6 服用药酒注意事项 ·························· 536
  2.3.7 常用保健药酒 ································ 538
   1. 补气药酒 ··································· 538
    人参酒 参芪益气酒 三圣酒 黄芪生脉酒 长生固本酒
   2. 养血药酒 ··································· 539
    阿胶酒 龙眼桑椹酒 归圆酒 圆肉补血酒 胶艾酒
   3. 滋阴药酒 ··································· 541
    女贞子酒 二冬酒 银耳香菇酒 枸杞药酒 洋参固本酒 春寿酒 固精酒
   4. 助阳药酒 ··································· 542
    仙灵脾酒 蛤蚧酒 鹿茸酒 复方鹿茸虫草酒 羊肾二仙酒 三鞭补酒 东北三宝酒 琼浆
   5. 气血双补药酒 ······························· 544
    芪归双补酒 八珍酒 十全大补酒
   6. 阴阳双补药酒 ······························· 545
    虫草酒 二仙酒 滋阴百补药酒
   7. 补益五脏药酒 ······························· 546
    茯苓酒 神仙药酒丸 养心安神酒 参蛤虫草酒 复方海马酒 首乌杞菊酒 补血顺气药酒
   8. 延年益寿药酒 ······························· 548
    百岁酒 延寿九仙酒 疗百疾延寿酒 精神药酒
   9. 防治疾病保健药酒 ··························· 549

菊楂益心酒　健心灵酒　屠苏酒　独活寄生酒　参茸酒

2.4 保健膏滋 ······ 551
2.4.1 补气膏滋 ······ 553
1. 人参膏　2. 代参膏　3. 益气开胃膏
2.4.2 养血膏滋 ······ 554
1. 桑椹膏　2. 杞圆膏　3. 首乌补血膏　4. 当归补血膏
2.4.3 滋阴膏滋 ······ 555
1. 二冬膏　2. 二至膏　3. 养阴膏
2.4.4 助阳膏滋 ······ 556
1. 锁阳膏　2. 苁蓉二仙膏　3. 蛤蚧党参膏
2.4.5 气血双补膏滋 ······ 556
1. 两仪膏　2. 十全大补膏　3. 洋参双补膏
2.4.6 补益五脏膏滋 ······ 557
1. 枸杞膏　2. 苍术膏　3. 茯苓膏　4. 润肺膏
2.4.7 其他补益延寿膏滋 ······ 558
1. 琼玉膏　2. 益寿养真膏　3. 河车膏　4. 龟鹿二仙膏
5. 红玉膏　6. 加减扶元和中膏　7. 加减扶元益阴膏
2.4.8 防治疾病保健膏滋 ······ 561
1. 菊花延龄膏　2. 明目延龄膏　3. 加竹沥梨膏　4. 利咽膏
5. 首乌菊楂膏　6. 益气活血膏　7. 老鹳草膏

2.5 保健药茶 ······ 562
2.5.1 补气、养血药茶 ······ 564
1. 参芪代茶饮　2. 五宝茶汤　3. 观音面茶　4. 五香奶茶
5. 术冬代茶汤　6. 桑龙代茶饮　7. 益气生津代茶饮
8. 补血和胃代茶饮
2.5.2 滋阴、助阳药茶 ······ 566
1. 玉石代茶饮　2. 二参二冬代茶饮　3. 参苓代茶饮　4. 仙灵脾茶
5. 复方杜仲茶　6. 新二仙代茶饮　7. 复方枸杞茶
2.5.3 调理脾胃、消食化积药茶 ······ 567

1. 和胃代茶饮　2. 二神代茶饮　3. 五仙代茶饮　4. 甘露茶

2.5.4　安神药茶 ·· 568

1. 安神代茶饮　2. 圆肉二仁茶　3. 清心代茶饮

2.5.5　防治常见病症的药茶 ································ 568

1. 菊楂代茶饮　2. 首乌决明茶　3. 复方玉米须茶　4. 减肥代茶饮　5. 消肥健身茶　6. 复方罗布麻茶　7. 黄玉石代茶饮　8. 荷佩防暑茶　9. 温中茶　10. 健胃茶　11. 清解茶

2.6　保健药粥 ·· 570

1. 人参粥　2. 补虚正气粥　3. 大枣粥　4. 参苓粥　5. 山药粥　6. 白扁豆粥　7. 黄芪粥　8. 落花生粥　9. 珠玉二宝粥　10. 糯米阿胶粥　11. 龙眼肉粥　12. 仙人粥　13. 乳粥　14. 海参粥　15. 桑仁粥　16. 鸡汁粥　17. 菟丝子粥　18. 苁蓉羊肉粥　19. 胡桃粥　20. 荔枝粥　21. 栗子粥　22. 雀儿药粥　23. 鹿角胶粥　24. 枸杞羊肾粥　25. 山萸肉粥　26. 玉竹粥　27. 天门冬粥　28. 沙参粥　29. 百合粉粥　30. 莲子粉粥　31. 酸枣仁粥　32. 山楂粥　33. 薏苡仁粥

2.7　保健药糕 ·· 580

1. 阳春白雪糕　2. 秘传二仙糕　3. 九仙王道糕　4. 八仙白云糕　5. 八仙早朝糕　6. 八珍糕　7. 健脾养心糕　8. 和中消食糕

2.8　保健药饼 ·· 583

1. 天门冬饼子　2. 黄精饼　3. 壮阳暖下药饼　4. 期颐饼　5. 益脾饼　6. 益寿饼　7. 九仙保健饼

2.9　外用保健膏药 ·· 586

1. 养心膏　2. 心肾双补膏　3. 专益元气膏　4. 涌泉膏　5. 四淫百病膏　6. 保元固本膏　7. 毓麟固本膏　8. 益寿比天膏

2.10　保健药枕 ·· 591

1. 歧黄牌高效保健药枕　2. 神枕方　3. 《保生要录》药枕方　4. 丁公仙枕　5. 高血压病药枕　6. 保健药枕　7. 健康长寿药枕　8. 颈椎病药枕　9. 小儿鼻渊药枕

· 449 ·

10. 李时珍药枕　　11. 神农牌保健药枕　　12. 益寿药枕

3　非药物保健方法 ································· 599
3.1　针灸保健 ··································· 599
3.1.1　针灸的保健作用 ·························· 599
3.1.2　针灸保健的机理 ·························· 601
3.1.3　常用保健穴位 ···························· 602

　　1. 足三里　　2. 神阙　　3. 中极　　4. 关元　　5. 气海　　6. 肾俞

　　7. 命门　　8. 三阴交　　9. 中脘　　10. 天枢　　11. 曲池

　　12. 内关　　13. 神门　　14. 大椎　　15. 肺俞　　16. 心俞

　　17. 肝俞　　18. 脾俞　　19. 胃俞　　20. 环跳　　21. 涌泉

　　22. 百会　　23. 膻中

3.1.4　针灸保健方法 ···························· 606

　　1. 针刺保健法　　2. 保健灸法　　3. 针灸保健的穴位选配　　4. 针灸保健注意事项

3.1.5　穴位磁疗保健 ···························· 612

3.2　气功保健 ··································· 613
3.2.1　气功的功法 ······························ 613

　　1. 调身　　2. 调心　　3. 调息

3.2.2　气功的功种 ······························ 617

　　1. 松静功　　2. 内养功　　3. 强壮功

3.2.3　气功锻炼的要领 ·························· 619

3.3　推拿保健 ··································· 619
3.3.1　推拿的种类与常用手法 ···················· 620
3.3.2　自我推拿保健方法 ························ 623
3.3.3　推拿的适应症和禁忌症 ···················· 626

英汉实用中医药大全（书目） ······················· 628

说　　明

　　《自我保健》是《英汉实用中医药大全》的第9分册。

　　本分册共有"中医保健原则","实用保健方药","非药物保健"等3章,介绍了适合自我实施或运用的精神保健,饮食保健,起居保健,劳逸结合保健,运动保健以及顺应自然保健的方法;还介绍了56种常用保健中药,51种常用保健中成药,47种常用保健药酒,34种保健膏滋,33种保健药茶,33种保健药粥,8种保健药糕,7种保健药饼,8种外用保健膏药,12种保健药枕,以及针灸保健,气功保健,推拿保健。

　　本分册中文稿著者参考大量医著的有关资料并结合他们自己的经验和学识著成,由著名专家陈可冀教授审定。由来自全国若干院校的包括冯秀萍、姜文英、黄庆娴女士等在内的若干译者译成英文初稿。为了统一全书英文稿,又邀请刘强、曹会来、约翰·布莱克等另外7名译者和审校者,共同连续不断地工作了一年,重新整理和翻译了部分文稿,经过对全书的审校、修改,形成了现在的译稿。亓秀恒、王正忠等教授曾帮助审校过英文初稿。

　　在本分册英文稿中,中药名称一律用汉语拼音和拉丁语表示。为方便海外读者,汉语拼音一律采用单音节词和斜体字。拉丁语单词首字母大写以便同英语单词区别。大部分中药拉丁语名称来自1990年出版的《中华人民共和国药典》,针灸穴位和标号来自1990年发布的《中华人民共和国国家标准——经穴部位》。

编　者

1 中医保健原则

中医保健的原则是古人在长期的养生保健实践中逐渐形成并日趋完善的,《内经》曾将古人的养生长寿之道高度概括为:"法于阴阳,和于术数,食饮有节,起居有常,不妄作劳","虚邪贼风,避之有时;恬淡虚无,真气从之,精神内守,病安从来",受到历代养生家的推崇,成为人们养生保健所必须遵循的准则与宗旨。许多养生保健的内容与方法就是在上述原则的指导下产生并不断完善的。

1.1 精神保健

中医历来十分重视精神情志活动对人体健康的密切关系,提出"形神合一"学说,认为精神与形体是一个有机的整体,养神必须养形,而养形必须调神,强调调节精神在养生保健中占有主导地位。认为"精、气、神"为人身之三宝,是祛病延年的内在因素,提出"养精、爱气、惜神",精力充沛,五脏六腑就能各司其功能,人体才能健康无病。而精神失调,则可导致机体真气的耗散而百病滋生,乃至夭折短寿,即所谓:"一切犯邪者,皆是神失守之故也"。"得守者生,失守者死;得神者昌,失神者亡"。因此,必须保全精神,使精神内守,以祛病延年。人有七情六欲,而喜怒忧思悲惊恐七情的偏激常常可以导致脏腑功能的失调,使气血逆乱而产生相应的病理变化,给人体健康带来极大的危害,如《内经》所言:"余知百病皆生于气也。怒则气上,喜则气缓,悲则气消,恐则气下,……惊则气乱,……思则气结。"并指出"怒伤肝","喜伤心","思伤脾","悲伤肺,""恐伤肾"。足见精神情志的失调对健康的影响。

精神保健作为养生益寿的主要方法，历来受到人们的重视和运用。通过人为的调节，避免过激的情志刺激，保持良好的心境与心态平衡，以达到却病强身、延年益寿的目的。历代中医养生文献和医书中记载了丰富多彩的有关精神调养的论述和许多行之有效的精神调养方法，对于作好精神保健具有现实的指导意义。

1.1.1 豁达乐观

谚云"乐以忘忧"，乐观稳定的情绪，良好的心理平衡可以安定神气，促进气血周流，增进人体健康。《管子》说："凡人之生也，必以其欢。忧则失纪，怒则失端。忧悲喜怒，道乃无处。爱欲静之，遇乱正之。勿引勿催，福将自归。"《内经》指出"无患嗔之心……内无思想之患，以恬愉为务。"说明不要有愤怒的心情，思想不要有所负担，一切以安静乐观为目的，使情志舒畅，才能做到"形体不敝，精神不散，亦可以百数"，即形体不易衰老，精神不易耗散，可以活至百岁。《淮南子》主张"和愉"，认为人"性有一乐也"，《遵生八笺》提出"安神宜悦乐"，这些论述说明了乐观宁静的心态是人体健康的正常需要与基本保证，而要保持乐观的情绪，就必须具备高尚的情操与远大的理想，做到目光宏远，性格开朗活泼，心胸开阔，襟怀坦荡，为人处事，不斤斤计较，不以一己之得失而忧患无穷，做到如《稽中散集》中所说的："修性以保神，安心以保身，爱憎不栖于情，忧喜不留于意，泊然无恙。"能做到这一点，就会减少许多无谓的烦恼，使身心保持宁静与健康。

保持乐观情绪，要做到遇事泰然处之，即如《寿世青编》所说："未事不可先迎，遇事不可过忧，既事不可留住，听其自来，应以自然，任其自去，忿憶恐惧，好乐忧患，皆得其正，此养生之法也。"

知足常乐，"知足"既是修身养性的重要内容，也是保持乐观情绪的主要因素，《道德经》记载："祸莫大于不知足；咎莫大于欲得。故知足之足，常足矣"，《遵生八笺》则认为"知足不辱，知止不殆"，都说明只有知足才能常乐。在现实生活中，一切烦恼忧愁多数来自名誉地位、物质享受等方面的不知足与贪心不止，对待待遇和享受，应当经常想想"不如我者何限"，不作非分追求与争夺，做到随遇而安，豁达开朗，这样才能消除烦忧，使内心恬静，使精神处于乐观、稳定、自守的良好状态。

加强道德情操的自我修养也是保持乐观的一个重要内容。古人十分重视养性养德，提出"仁者寿"，"仁者"就是有道德的人。道德修养有十分丰富的内涵，古人论及的"寡欲"、"知足"、"忍让"、"性善"、"仁礼"等等，都是养性修身的重要内容，古人认为"大德必得其寿"，道德高尚的人之所以能够长寿，主要也是在于他们"善养浩然之气"，胸怀博大，意志坚定，有远大的理想与抱负，同时敬人人敬，知足常乐，忍让减忧等，都有益于情绪稳定和精神乐观。

培养广泛的爱好与兴趣，不断充实生活内容也是保持乐观情绪的有力保证。如读书、会友、漫游、垂钓、奕棋、书画、吟诗、歌唱、弹琴、浇花种竹等。古人多有论述，认为这些爱好与活动可以畅心悦性，怡养情志。《怡情小录》云："冬日之阳，夏日之阴，良辰养景，负杖蹑履，逍遥自乐，临池观鱼，披林听鸟，浊酒一杯，弹琴一曲，求数刻之乐"，这段文字说明应当放松精神，根据自己的实际情况，选择与培养爱好，不断增加生活情趣，使情感畅怡，精神稳定，情绪乐观，以利寿康。

总之，豁达乐观是精神调养与保健的重要内容，正如《内经》所言："是以圣人为无为之事，乐恬澹之能，从欲快志于虚无之守，故寿命无穷，与天地终，此圣人之治身也"，指出了善于养生的人不做勉强的事情，不胡思乱想，有乐观愉快的情绪，有丰富多彩的情趣，过平静安定的生活，常使心旷神怡，豁达乐观、就能长寿命，尽享天年。

1.1.2 清心寡欲

我国历代养生家十分重视清心寡欲,认为这是调摄精神,益寿延年的重要环节。《理论要纪》云:"养生莫若寡欲。"

私心、嗜欲出于心,私心太重,嗜欲不止,则会扰动神气,破坏精神的清静。故老子特别强调养生要清心寡欲,主张"见素抱朴,少私寡欲"。《内经》主张"志闲而少欲",以为长生之道。葛洪强调调摄精神要"含醇守朴,无欲无忧,全真虚器,居平味澹",《遵生要旨》中说:"……人有三宝精气神。善养者不用太急,须要神全寡嗜欲、精全寡言语、气全寡思虑。"说明降低嗜欲,戒除杂念,才能气血调和,保精全神,使神气清静内守,邪不能害,以保持身体的健康。所以《类修要诀》提出"绝私念以养其心。"《红炉点雪》则强调说:"若能清心寡欲,久久行之,百病不生"。

要做到清心寡欲,必须注意以下 3 点:

1. 要以理收心,明确私心嗜欲对人的危害。《养生论》中有"清虚静泰,少私寡欲,知名位之伤德,故忽而不营,非欲而强禁也。识厚味之害性,故弃而弗顾,非贪而后抑也。"若欲而强禁,则欲不止,贪而后抑,则贪愈深,丝毫也达不到静神的效果。《医学入门》说"若不识尽天年度百岁乃去机括,虽终日闭目,只是一团私意,静亦动也;若识透天年百岁之有分限节度,则事事循理自然,不贪不躁不妄,斯可以却病而尽天年矣。……主于理,则人欲消亡而心清神悦,不求静而自静也",说明以理收心则私心杂念易除,而神易静。

2. 要除六害,正确对待个人的利害得失。《太上老君养生诀》云"且夫善摄生者,要先除六害,然后可以保性命延驻百年。何者是也?一曰薄名利,二者禁声色,三者廉货财,四者损滋味,五者除佞妄,六者去妒忌",六害不除,万物纠心,神岂能静。

3. 抑目静耳。眼耳为五官之一，是神接受外界刺激的主要器官，其功能受神的主宰和调节。目清耳静则神气内守而心不劳，若目驰耳躁，则神气烦劳而心忧不宁。老子主张用"不可见欲"的方法使"心不乱"。庄子也主张"无视无听，抱神以静，形将自正"，这种不视不听虽然是消极和脱离实际的，但适当的抑眼静耳，减少外界对神气的不良刺激，却是能够做到，而且是有益于健康的。故《千金翼方》说："养老之要，耳无妄听，口无妄言，身无妄动，心无妄念，此皆有益于老人也"。当然，目不可以不视，耳不可以无听，关键在于不要为了满足私欲而乱视妄听，使神气不宁。

此外，对于节制私欲，古人还提出了一些具体办法，如明理智，存敬戒，有决心及早觉速惩等，对于制欲宁神，做到清心寡欲，都是有积极意义的。

1.1.3 喜怒有节

喜怒人皆有之，唯太过则有害。《灵枢》云："喜乐者，神惮散而不藏。……盛怒者，迷惑而不治"，因此，古人多主张调和喜怒以安定神气，《内经》将"和喜怒"列为养生大法之一。《彭祖摄生养性论》"喜怒过多，神不归室"，说明喜怒太过能扰动神气，致使神气浮散不藏，躁动而不静。《灵枢》说："喜怒不节，则伤脏，脏伤则病起于阴也"。说明喜怒不节还能伤及人之脏腑阴阳而产生各种病证。

1. 少喜：喜本是一种欢快的情绪，但大喜或喜太过就会对身体造成危害。所以古人说"喜则气缓"，"喜伤心"。现实生活中遇有意料之外的喜乐之事，如果不能平静地对待，过分激动，超出了精神与人体本身的承受能力，就容易发生病变。如范进中举之后由大喜而疯癫就是很好的例子。过分的激动还可导致心脏病、高血压病等疾病的加重，甚或危及生命。如《养生延命录》所说："多乐则意溢，多喜则忘错昏乱"。因此，应当避免过分的情绪激动，要平静地对待日常生活中的事物，客观而理智地评价问题，做到心无大喜而有常乐，保持精神的稳定与协调。

2. 制怒：在七情之中，以暴怒伤人最烈，怒则气机逆乱而肝伤，故列为首忌之一。《红炉点雪》云："戒暴怒。夫气贵顺而不贵逆，顺则百脉畅利，逆则四体违和"。《摄生三要》说："嗔心一发，则气强而不柔，逆而不顺，乱而不定，散而不聚矣"。指出了怒的危害性。《摄生要录》说："大怒伤目，令人暗；多怒百脉不定，鬓发憔焦，筋萎为癃。好憎者使人心劳，弗疾去，具志气日耗，所以不能终其寿。"说明怒还是加速衰老，引起老年病的重要因素之一。暴怒还能引起危重症候，如《内经》所说："大怒则形气绝而血菀于上，令人薄厥"，在现实生活中，确有大怒而发生昏厥、休克甚至危及生命的。

怒的危害如此之大，要保证健康就应"戒怒"、"制怒"，减少情志刺激，防止过度的情绪波动。首先要加强自身的性情修养与文化修养，待人处事，心气平和，做到如孙思邈所主张的：众人大言我小语，众人多繁我小记，众人悖暴而我不怒，不以不事为累意，不临时俗之化，达到"淡然无为"的境界。清代名士曹庭栋说："事当值可怒，当思事身孰重，一转意向，可以焕然冰释"，这是说有些事既使真能令人发怒，也应当冷静下来，想想比起身体来，毕竟还是小事，思想转移一下，怒也就化为乌有了。

事实上，完全避免情志刺激是不可能的，但应当尽量减少或缓冲情志刺激带来的影响，孙思邈认为"凡人不可无思，当以渐遣除之，"遇有动怒时，应进行及时的自我宽慰和排解，使其对人体的危害减少到最低程度。

古人提倡"忍让"，把"忍让"视为美德。"忍让"也是制怒的重要方法。《养老奉亲书》说："百战百胜不如一忍，万言万当不如一默。"如能做到这一点，甚或达到"无故加之而不怒"的境界，注意忍让，敬人持己，趋利避害，自然可以制怒，从而不使形神受扰，收到延年益寿之效。

1.1.4 省思少虑

思虑是人的精神活动之一，人必有思，必有所虑，但少思则神活，多思则神败。过多思虑伤神气而损寿命。《灵枢》"怵惕思虑则伤神。"《彭祖摄生养性论》有云："切切所思，神则败。"《万寿丹书》指出"夫心者，神之舍也，心静则神安，心动则神疲。神者四肢之主，能少思虑，省嗜欲，扫除杂念，湛然不侵，则神自全。神全则身安，身安则寿永，是乃修身之大要也。"《养生肤语》中记有"人之致思发虑，致一思，出一神；注一念，出一神，如分火焉。火愈分油愈干火愈小，神愈分精愈竭神愈少。"说明思虑不可不节。所以《类修要决》主张"少思虑以养其神，"《千金要方》则要求"但能不思衣食，不思声色，不思胜负，不思曲直，不思得失，不思荣辱。心无烦，形无极……亦可得长年。"这里的少思和不思，主要应当理解为避免过分的、不正当的思虑。

过度思虑对人的健康危害极大，在实际生活中，人不可能无思无虑，但应当做到省思少虑，特别是对于个人得失，名誉地位，物质金钱等，不可以汲汲以求，处心积虑，以免失去心理平衡而影响健康，要做到这一点，就必须豁达达观，分析处理问题采取客观现实的态度和方法，一切从现实出发，不盲目追求。如思虑难以排解时，可以将注意力转移到另外的方面，将思虑暂时放置起来，随着时过境迁，自会迎刃而解。

1.1.5 忌忧伤悲

人有悲欢离合，月有阴晴圆缺，人生的道路难免会有悲哀伤愁，古人历来重视忧愁悲伤对人体健康的影响，《淮南子》云："忧悲多恚，病乃成积"，"心有忧者，筐床在席，弗能安也；菰饭犓牛，弗能甘也；琴瑟鸣竽，弗能乐也"，足见忧伤悲愁不但对人的精神产生巨大影响，还可以引起积证。《内经》说："忧悲思虑即伤人。"《摄生要录》说:"悲哀太甚,则胞络绝,而阳气内动,发则心下溃",《灵枢》则云:"愁忧者,气闭塞而不行",并认为"六十岁,心气始衰,苦忧悲",指出老年人精气衰退,心神不足,更易生忧悲之苦。忧悲不已,则易躁伤神气,损害健康,故《彭祖摄生养性论》说:"积忧不已,则魂神伤矣",《养性延命录》亦说:"多愁则心摄"。

忧愁悲伤对健康可产生巨大的危害,而人生在世又难免遇到,这就应当灭愁绪,去忧悲。首先应该养成豁达乐观的性格,具有宽广博大的胸怀,做到"不以物喜,不以己悲"。还应有坚强的意志,克服多愁善感。此外,世界上最令人愉悦的莫过于珍贵的友谊,友情可以填补往昔的遗恨,熨平精神上的创伤,充满友谊的真挚帮助、宽慰、鼓励等都是消除忧愁的法宝。患解忧除;然后食甘而寝宁,居安游乐,精神则可重新获得安宁,忧愁伤悲的不良影响亦可为之消除。

1.1.6 避免惊恐

惊和恐无论程度如何,都是异常的精神活动。惊和恐虽然都有害怕、恐惧的意思,但二者尚有区别。惊指惊吓,多从外至,即受外界的突然刺激而成,故惊则神气散乱;恐指恐惧,多自内生,乃内心的慌恐不安,恐则神怯气馁。《内经》曾谓"恐则气下",又说"惊则气乱"。惊恐不仅使人的精神和健康受到危害,导致气机逆乱,影响正常的生理功能,若遇大惊大恐时行房受孕,还会引起后代的先天性疾患。《内经》云:"人生而有病癫疾者,病名曰何?安所得之?岐伯曰:"病名为胎病,此得之在母腹中时,其母有所大惊,气上而不下,精气并居,故令子为颠疾也。"说明癫痫与在母腹中母受惊恐有密切的关系。可见惊恐对于养生保健和优生优育的危害甚大,应当尽力避免之。平素性格脆弱之人,应避夜间独行或独自涉于深山密林、荒冢人稀之处,同时应加强意志锻炼,自觉地消除不必要的恐惧心理,以保持精神的安宁与平静。

1.2 饮食保健

饮食是摄纳营养,维持人体生长发育的来源,是健康长寿的基本保证。中医在长期实践中积累了丰富的饮食保健经验,形成了完整的理论,提出了一系列关于饮食调理的正确原则和方法,为我国人民的健康长寿作出了宝贵的贡献。早在周代,我国就设有"食医"官职,负责以食治病。魏晋南北朝时,曾出现《食经》,系统阐发食物养生的功能。孙思邈认为饮食的医疗作用不容忽视,他说:"食能排邪而安脏腑,悦神爽志以资血气"。《养生论》提出"修性保神"和"服食养身"两类养生方法,而主张以"服食养生"为本,可见古人很早就已经认识到饮食保健对于健康长寿的重要意义。到宋代饮食养生逐渐形成专一学科,至明清两代以后,有关饮食养生法的著作相继问世,理论和方法更臻完善,受到普遍重视。

饮食保健作为长寿之道的一个重要环节,其内容十分广泛和丰富,其中许多原则和方法具有很高的科学性与实用价值,值得今人效法。

1.2.1 食宜清淡

提倡清淡饮食是我国古代养生家的一贯主张。古人认为清淡饮食能够防病强身,长寿延年,同时认为久食膏粱厚味、肥甘之品有生热、生痰、生湿之弊,极易引起病患,于健康极为不利。《内经》云:"膏粱之变,足生大疔",《吕氏春秋》说:"肥肉美酒,务以自强,命曰烂肠之食。"《韩非子》则云:"香美脆味,厚酒肥肉,甘口而疾形"。朱丹溪指出"因纵口味,五味之过,疾病蜂起",这些论述都说明膏粱厚味对人体的危害。嵇康在《养生论》中比较了南北居民所食肥淡不同,寿命的长短也不同。他说"关中土地,俗好俭啬,厨膳肴馐,不过菹酱而已,其人少病而寿；江南岭表，其处饶足，海陆鲑肴，无所不备，土俗多疾，而人早夭"。

正因为过食肥甘对健康无益而有害，所以历代养生学家都主张清淡饮食。孙思邈说："是以食最鲜肴务令减少。饮食当令节俭"，告诫人们少吃荤食，不要贪味。《医学心悟》主张："莫嗜膏粱，淡食为最"。《保养说》强调："能甘淡薄则五味之本，自足以养脏。养老慈幼皆然"。《吕氏春秋》指出"凡食无强厚味，无以烈味重酒"，还说"味众珍则胃充，胃充则中大鞔，中大鞔而气不达，以此长生可得乎"？孙思邈提倡老人的食物需"常宜轻清甜淡之物，大小麦曲，粳米为佳"，指出"善养性者常须少食肉，多食饭"。朱丹溪著《茹淡论》，主张少吃肉，多食"谷菽菜果，自然冲和之味"。

上述所谓清淡饮食实际上是指素食而言，素食可以防病，可以养生是古人在长期实践中发现的。现代研究证明：人体摄入脂肪过多，会使脂肪在体内堆积，附在血管壁上，会促使动脉硬化；动脉硬化最易导致高血压、冠心病，而这些病往往是老年人死亡的重要原因。所以控制动物脂肪及高胆固醇食物的摄入量是十分必要的，因而中医养生学强调素食是有一定科学道理的。另外据统计，世界各地所发现的长寿地区的人，多以蔬菜、谷物、瓜果为主食。

古人提倡的清淡饮食除素食外，还应提倡淡食，这里所谓淡食主要是从味道上讲的，饮食五味不要太过，特别是不要太咸，要严格控制食盐的摄入量.《内经》云"味过于咸，大骨气劳、短肌，心气抑"。《老老恒言》云："凡食物不能废咸，但少加使淡，淡则物之真味真性俱得。……血与咸相得则凝，凝则血燥。"《养生肤语》的作者陈继儒曾以自己的所见所闻，列举大量实例阐明咸多伤生，淡食延龄。他认为宫庭中人寿命多短，其原因之一，就是吃咸太过，五味太盛。他列举东光县村中三老，一生很少吃盐，以淡食为主，所以"俱年八十余，极强健"。孙思邈也曾提出过"咸少促人寿"的观点。现代研究发现,高血压、动脉硬化、心肌梗塞、肝硬化、中风及肾脏疾病与过量食盐有一定关系,国外有学者提出高血压即盐中毒。上述疾病对人们健康危害较大。因此,中医关于淡食延龄的认识是符合实际的,每一个希望自己健康长寿的人都应遵循之。

1.2.2 谨和五味

饮食五味是气血生化的来源,饮食五味调合则生气血,保健康;饮食五味不调,则损气血,减寿命。所以《内经》曾反复告诫人们要"食饮有节","谨和五味",并指出"是故谨和五味,骨正筋柔,气血以流,腠理以密,如是则骨气以精,谨道如法,长有天命"。

所谓五味,是指酸、甘、苦、辛、咸,这是食品主要的五种味道。谨和五味作为中医饮食调理的一个重要原则,在内容和含义上有广义和狭义之分。从广义上泛指饮食合理调配,狭义上主要指五味调和。

1. 合理调配

古人很早就认识到不同食物,所含营养成分也不同,只有全面而合理地进行搭配,才能使人体获得各种不同的营养,以满足人体各种生理功能的需要。《内经》提出:"五谷为养,五果为助,五畜为益,五菜为充,气味合而服之,以补益精气"的方案,并说"谷肉果菜,食养尽之"。谷物为主食,含有丰富的碳水化物,为人体提供了必须的热量和能量,五果、五畜、五菜为副食。五果指各种水果,五菜指各种蔬菜,为人体提供了多种维生素、纤维素及微量元素,这些在新陈代谢、生命活动中也是必不可少的。五畜,猪、牛、羊、鸡之类为人体提供了必须的蛋白质、脂肪和氨基酸。蛋白质是构成人体组织细胞的主要原料,脂肪也能提供热量,氨基酸更是新陈代谢所必需。这样各种食品齐全,主次配合合理,而且符合我国人民的饮食习惯,是一张科学的食谱。同时，由于防止了偏嗜，对人体健康是十分有益。每一个希望自己健康长寿的都应当乐于遵循之。

2. 五味调合

各种食品在气味上都有所差异，就其酸、甘、辛、苦、咸五种主要气味而言，对人体的作用和功效不同，应当谨慎调和不使太过或偏嗜，五味太过或偏嗜都会对人体产生不应有的危害，应当深以为戒。《内经》曾指出："味过于酸，肝气以津，脾气乃绝；味过于咸，大骨气劳，短肌，心气抑；味过于甘，心气喘满，色黑，肾气不衡；味过于苦，脾气不濡，胃气乃厚；味过于辛，筋脉沮弛，精神乃央"，说明饮食五味之偏嗜，易伤害脏腑，引起疾病，之所以如此，是五味各有归经的缘故。《内经》云："五味入胃，各归所喜，故酸先入肝，苦先入心，甘先入脾，辛先入肺，咸先入肾，久而增气，物化之常也，气增而久，夭之由也"。

五味太过不仅对相应的脏腑形成无形的危害，在临床上还可产生可见的病变，如《内经》所言："多食咸则脉凝泣而变色，多食苦则皮槁而毛拔；多食辛则筋急而爪枯，多食酸则肉胝䐢而唇揭，多食甘则骨痛而发落"。所以古人再三强调谨和五味，张子和说："五味贵和，不可偏盛"。

谨和五味，一是在食品选择上做到五味搭配合理，不使太过偏嗜；二是在烹调方法上人为地加以调整，充分利用五味的制约和生化作用，以保证营养，促进健康。

1.2.3 按时节量

按时节量是中医饮食调理的一个重要内容。所谓按时是饮食应有较为固定的时间规律，所谓节量是饮食应该节制数量并使之合理，无过饥过饱、不暴饮暴食等。

1. 按时

《吕氏春秋》云："食能以时，身必无灾"，在二千多年前，就提出了吃饭应当定时的问题。《尚书》中也有"食哉惟时"的记载，强调吃饭定时是保证身体健康的重要措施。饮食定时而有规律，是饮食调节的一个重要原则，因此，应适当安排饮食的时间，不使相距太远和太近，我国人民一般所习惯和沿用至今的一日三餐制，每餐间隔时间约为5小时，是很有道理的，因为一般性食物的消化吸收至少需要4～5小时，故早餐宜在早7时前后，午餐宜在中午12时前后，晚餐宜在下午6时前后，这样的时间安排既能使摄入的各种营养满足人体的需要，又符合于日常生活、工作与学习的安排，有利于健康，有益于养生。

　　此外，所谓食能以时还有一层含义，即应根据饥渴而决定饮食与否。《千金要方》说："是以善养性者，先饥而食，先渴而饮"。《遵生八笺》也说："当候已饥而进食，食不厌熟嚼；仍候焦渴而引饮，饮不厌细呷。无待饥甚而食，……时觉渴甚而饮"，这里将饮食的"时"定在饥渴之时，强调饥则食，渴则饮，而不要"饥甚"和"焦渴"时才进饮食。饥渴的产生受许多条件的影响，如剧烈运动、过劳、夜间值班等都会使饥渴的时间与常规的一日三餐时间有较大差别，这时选择饥则食、渴则饮，如夜餐等即是，这实际上也是在饮食时间上的合理调节。

2. 节量

　　合理的饮食原则不但要求在时间上进行适当安排，而且要求在数量上进行调节并使之适合人体的需要。

　　饮食在数量调节上总的原则是不过饱过饥，中医认为过饱过饥都会对身体造成危害。《内经》云："故谷不入，半日则气衰，一日则气少矣"，是指过饥；还说"饮食自倍，脾胃乃伤"，则是指过饱。《洞微经》曰："太饥伤脾，太饱伤气。盖脾借于谷，饥则脾无以运而脾虚；气转于脾，饱则脾过于实而滞气。故先饥而食，所以给脾；食不充脾，所以养气"。阐明了过饥过饱均可伤脾害气的道理。因此，孙思邈也认为"饱则伤肺，饥则伤气"，因此，他主张："食欲数而少，不欲顿而多，则难消也。常欲令如饱中饥,饥中饱耳"。这种似饱非饱、若饥非饥的饮食原则于人体健康是十分相宜的。在一日三餐的食量掌握上,古人主张应当区别对待,《内经》曰,日中而阳气隆,日西而阳气虚,故早饭可饱,午后即宜少食,至晚更必空虚。"后人在这些理论指导下,结合生活实践,总结出"早饭宜好,午饭可饱,晚饭宜少"的原则。

　　古代养生家认为少食可以延寿,老年人尤宜"食少"。《博物志》说:"所食逾少,心开逾益;所信逾多,心逾塞,年逾损矣",《老老恒言》也说:"凡食总以少为有益,脾宜磨运,乃化精液,否则极易之物,多食反致受伤,故曰少食以安脾也"。《东谷赘言》指出:"多食之人有五患,一者大便数,二者小便数,三者扰睡眠,四者身重不堪修养,五者多患食不消化",因此,《寿世保元》对饮食数量作了很好的概括"食惟半饱无兼味,酒至三分莫过频"。

　　古人关于少食可以长寿的主张符合饮食生理的实际,具有很高的科学性。现代医学认为,经常饱食,会使胃肠负担加重,消化液的分泌供不应求,以致引起消化不良。每餐过饱会使血液过多集中在肠胃,而使心脑等重要器官缺血,以致精神困乏,冠心病人还易引起心绞痛发作。长期饱食,摄入量超过身体的需要,就会变成脂肪贮存在体内而肥胖起来,从而诱发高血压、冠心病、糖尿病、胆石症等疾病。许多学者认为,连续长期饱食会使人未老先衰,折损寿命,因此平时不要过饱。老年人各项生理机能逐渐衰退,消化功能减弱,因而更应注意节饮食。

1.2.4　调适寒热

　　调节食物寒热,以使适得其宜,也是古人饮食调理的一个重要方面。《周礼》说:"凡食齐视春时,羹齐视夏时,酱齐视秋时,饮齐冬视时"。视是比如的意思,这句话的意思是饮食宜温,就比如春天的气候一样;汤类食品则易热,就好象夏天的气候一样;酱类食可凉吃,就好比秋天的气候;饮料类食品则可以冷用，就如同冬天的气候一样。说明食物种类不同，其宜寒宜热的特点也不尽相同，应当根据不同类别的食品进行恰当的调节。应当指出的是，这段论述所主张的食宜温、汤宜热、酱宜凉、饮宜冷的调节原则是合乎人的实际需要的，时至今日，人们对食品寒热的调节仍未离开上述原则。

对于饮食过寒过热可以损害五脏六腑，危及健康，古人也有明确的认识，《内经》谓："水谷之寒热，感则害于六腑"。《千金翼方》也说："热食伤骨，冷食伤肺"，所以应"热无灼唇，冷无冷齿"，指出了寒或热的适度。《寿养丛书》云："毋以脾胃热冷物"，意指不要给脾胃以太热太寒的食物，以免影响其正常的消化功能。

此外，也有人重点强调饮食以温热为主，《千金翼方》中就有这样的论述。《寿世保元》则认为："凡以饮食，无论四时，常令温暖，夏月伏阴在内，暖食尤宜。"《遵生八笺》则有"饮不厌温热"，"生冷勿食"之说。这些论述看起来似有所偏，但实际上所言温热，实质是暖食，皆非大热，因此，这些提法还是有一定道理的。

现代医学也认为，经常进食太热的食品，可以损害口腔及食道粘膜，引起相应的疾病；而过食生冷，则尤易损伤胃肠的消化功能，引起胃肠道疾病。由此可见，调适食物的寒热，对于维护人体健康具有重要意义，应当引起足够的重视。

1.2.5 清洁卫生

古人十分重视清洁卫生对健康的重要意义，主张忌食秽浊不洁食物。《论语》曾谓："鱼馁而肉败不食，色恶不食，嗅恶不食"，《金匮要略》云："秽饭、馁肉、臭鱼，食之皆伤人"，并专门论及禽兽鱼虫禁忌及果实禁忌问题，指出："诸肉及鱼，若狗不食，鸟不啄者，不可食之"，"肉中有朱点者，不可食之。"并说"生果停留多日，有损处，食之伤人"，"果子落地，经宿虫蚁食之者，人大忌食之"。说明古人视不洁之食物为大忌。尤其难能可贵者，已经认识到因瘟疫而死的动物可能有毒，应当禁食，张仲景说："六畜百死，皆疫死，则有毒，不可食之。"

临床上不少疾病特别是消化道疾病如菌痢、肠寄生虫等多由饮食不洁食物所致，古人虽然尚未认识到由口而入的一些病原微生物，但已经明确认识到不洁食物对健康的危害，主张忌食一切秽浊不洁之食物，丰富了饮食卫生的理论和实践，具有现实的指导意义。

1.2.6 饮食宜忌

饮食有所宜，亦有所忌。对于饮食宜忌，古人总结了丰富的经验。《养生录》指出："饮食六宜"，即"食宜早些，食宜缓些，食宜少些，食宜淡些，食宜暖些，食宜软些。"早些是指时间，缓些是指速度，少些是指数量，淡些是言味道，暖些是言寒热，软些是言质地。可见古人对饮食有多方面的要求与提倡，"六宜"十分合乎日常饮食的规律，这"六宜"之所反，即"晚些，""急些，""多些"，"咸些"，"冷些"，"硬些"则恰是"饮食六忌"。常记所宜而避免所忌，自然可以大有益于身体。

《千金翼方》曾说："不知食宜者，不足以全生"，了解饮食所宜与所忌，对于保健养生的意义和作用是不言而喻的。饮食宜忌的内容十分丰富，范围非常广泛，从广义上说，中医所有关于饮食调理之内容实际上都未越出"宜忌"的范畴。但是饮食宜忌也有其特定的含义与内容，主要包括进食宜忌和饮料宜忌。

1. 进食宜忌

进食宜忌主要是指在进食的所宜和所忌，即应当注意坚持和避免的问题。在时间上又主要指食时和食后。

(1) 食时宜忌

A. 食时宜专致忌分心：古人认为在进食时应当专心一致，不应思绪纷扰或言谈、看书或从事其他事情，这样既影响品味，又妨碍食物的消化与吸收，故古人提倡食宜专致而忌分心，《论语》云："食不语，寝不言，"《千金要方》也说："食无大言"，"及饥不得大语"，都是提倡进食应当专心致志。

B. 食时宜舒畅忌慎怒：良好的情绪有利于消化吸收，心情烦恼郁怒则对健康有害。《千金要方》云："人之当食，须去烦恼，如食五味必不得暴慎，多令人神惊，夜梦飞扬。"《达生要录》也说："怒后不可便食，食后不发怒，发怒多思多恐皆不食，倦时瞌睡时勿食，防食停于中而不下"，明确指出了心情不畅时进食的危害，告诫人们在进食时必须怀舒情畅。此外，古人还认为"胃好恬愉、脾好音声"，说明音乐对饮食的消化吸收大有裨益。《寿世保元》中说："脾好音声，闻声即动而磨食"，道家著作中也有"脾脏闻乐则磨"之说。说明柔和轻快的音乐乃至整个舒适整齐的环境，都可以作为一种良性刺激而通过中枢神经系统而调节人的消化功能，反之一切喧闹嘈杂的声音，混乱不堪的环境、污浊难闻之气味等都可影响情绪，使心情不畅，对消化和健康产生不利的影响。

C. 食时宜细嚼缓咽忌粗嚼急吞：进食时细嚼缓咽有利于促进消化吸收，故《千金要方》指出："食当熟嚼"，认为"美食须熟嚼，生食不粗吞。"《养病庸言》说："不论粥饭点心，皆宜嚼得极细咽下。"《医说》也主张："食不欲急，急则损脾，法当熟嚼令细"，这些论述都强调细嚼缓咽是饮食调理的重要环节，不可等闲视之。

(2) 食后宜忌

食后保养历来受到古人重视，积累了丰富的经验。有关论述切实可行，具有较高的科学性与普遍的意义。

A. 食后宜缓行忌急走

食后散步，有利消化吸收。《千金要方》指出："食毕当行步……令人能饮食，无百病。"《养性延命录》说："养性之道，不欲饱食便卧及终日久坐，皆损寿也。"《老老恒言》云："饭后食物停胃，必缓行数百步，散其气以输其食，则磨胃以腐化，……古之老人，饭后必散步为逍遥"，强调饭后散步活动，可以使气血流畅，脾胃功能健运，以促进消化吸收，减少疾病发生。

古人反对饭后急速行走或剧烈运动，认为这是食后保养之大忌。《寿世保元》谓："食饱不得速步走马，登高涉险，恐气满而激，致伤脏腑。"

B. 食后宜摩腹忌卧

食后摩腹有助于饮食消化，故《千金要方》提倡："平日点心饭讫，即自以热手摩腹，出门庭行五、六十步，消息之。""中食后，还以热手摩腹，行一、二百步，缓缓行，勿令气急，行讫，还床偃卧，四展手足勿睡，顷之气定。"《寿世保元》亦强调"食后常以摩腹数百遍，仰面呵气数百口，趑趄缓行数百步，谓之消化"。这些论述都说明食后摩腹对于促进食物的消化吸收具有重要作用。

饱后即卧可使宿食停滞，不利消化，有碍健康，古人认为食后忌卧。如《千金翼方》说："饱食即卧乃生百病。"饱后即卧妨碍食物的消化吸收，善养生者当忌之。

2. 饮料宜忌

饮料宜忌是饮食宜忌的主要内容。我国饮料主要为茶酒，茶酒的饮用数量、方法及时间等与健康关系十分密切，历来受到人们重视。

(1) 饮茶宜忌

我国是茶的故乡，早在公元四世纪，我国就将茶用来作饮料了，是世界上发现茶树和生产茶叶最早的国家。早在《诗经》、《尔雅》、《神农食经》等古代文献中就有关于茶的记载，唐代陆羽曾著《茶经》，成为世界上第一部茶叶专著。茶叶对人体的保健作用历来受到人们的重视，不仅我国人民普遍喜欢饮用，而且还与咖啡、可可一起成为世界三大饮料之一，日益受到世界人民的喜爱。

古人很早就认识到茶对人体的保健和医疗作用,《神农本草经》载:"茶味苦,饮之使人益思、少卧、轻身、明目。"《本草纲目》云:"茶主治喘急咳嗽,去痰垢。"《养生随笔》认为"饭后饮之,可解肥浓。"顾元庆在《茶谱》中谓:"人饮其茶,能止渴,消食除痰,少睡,利尿道,明目益思,除烦去腻,人固不可一日无茶。"足见茶具备多方面作用和功效。

现代医学研究表明茶叶除含有粗纤维、胶质、叶绿素外,还含有多种生物碱、多种维生素、黄酮类、鞣质、麦角甾醇、挥发油及少量的盐酸、硫胺、叶酸、蛋白质、矿物质等。因此具有醒脑提神,恢复疲劳,增强记忆力,预防龋齿,明目,降低血脂,预防高血压、利尿防结石及补充营养等功能,并能减少辐射伤害,所以适量饮茶对人体健康是有益的。

饮茶虽然好处很多,但如过量或不得法,不注意宜忌,也会对健康带来危害。

A. 不宜过量:古人很早就认识到过量饮茶的危害,《孙真人卫生歌注释》载:"茶能清心明目……,然茶有百损,虽独利于目,而四时皆不可多饮,深宵艰寐者,尤耗精神,瘦弱人脂液无多,岂堪消损!饥乏及房欲后尤禁之;若冷茶更大忌也。"《寿养丛书》载:"饮茶者宜热宜少,不饮尤佳,久饮去人脂,下焦虚冷,饥则尤不宜,令不眠。"这些论述都说明饮茶不易过量,饥乏时勿饮,冷茶忌饮。现代医学也认为过饮浓茶会使人兴奋过度,心跳加快,尿频、失眠,并可使体内水分增多,加重心肾负担。还可引起维生素 B_1 缺乏。

B. 饭前食后不宜饮:饮茶在时间宜忌上以白天工作之余,疲乏休息时饮用为宜,饭前不可饮,食后亦不可即饮,因茶含鞣质,能与食物中蛋白质结合成鞣酸蛋白,难以消化;还会使消化道粘膜收缩,影响食欲,消化和吸收,甚至可以出现便秘。李时珍曾谓:"茶苦寒,久饮茶每致腹胀少食。"《百药元铨》则认为:"中宫多湿,若更过饮茶汤……则以湿助湿,鲜有不败脾元而成中满之候者",都说明饮茶过量或时不相宜均可影响脾胃的消化功能。

C. 睡前不宜饮茶：因茶含有咖啡因，茶硷、柯柯碱等都有兴奋作用，影响入睡，同时茶硷的利尿作用也可使夜尿过多，不利休息。所以《博物志》："饮真茶，令人少睡眠。"《桐君录》也说："煎饮令人不眠"。

此外，高血压、心脏病、产妇、习惯性便秘、神经衰弱等病人均不宜饮茶。同时还应注意饮茶与某些食物如韭菜不宜同服等。

(2) 饮酒宜忌

酒在我国有悠久的历史，《内经》即有专篇《汤液醪醴论》，醪与醴都是酒类，用谷物经过酿制而成，随着历代劳动人民的不断创造，酒的品种不断增多，成为人们日常生活中重要的饮料。

中医认为少量饮酒有活血通脉，助药力，增进食欲，恢复疲劳，使人轻快的作用，不但可用于延年益寿，还可用于疾病防治，历代各类药酒不下数百种。《千金要方》曾说："冬服药酒两三剂，立春则止，此法终身常尔，则百病不生"。明确地肯定了药酒的保健作用。李时珍说："酒，天之美绿也。而曲之酒，少饮则和血行气，壮神御寒，消愁遣兴。"陈藏器说酒能"通血脉，厚肠胃，润皮肤，散湿气"，研究表明，每餐饮少量酒，可增进饮食，增强体质，并能预防心血管疾病。酒的种类不同，其作用也有差异，一般认为白酒可御寒或浸药用，米酒多作药引，黄酒则可活血止痛，葡萄酒可强心提神，有保护心脏的作用，啤酒富于营养，并可健胃消食，至于各种药酒，则能预防和治疗各种疾病。

饮酒的数量与方法宜根据各人不同的体质情况而定，但总的原则是少饮、淡饮、反对暴饮、杂饮。《养生要录》引阮坚之的话说："淡酒、小杯，久生细谈，非惟娱客，亦可养生。"《清异录》指出："酒不可杂饮，饮之，虽善酒者，亦醉。"说明宜饮淡酒，小量，缓缓饮之，不在同一时间饮用几种酒则有益于保健和养生。

有人认为饮酒要注意"三适"，即适量、适时与适情，实践证明，做到"三适"，则饮酒有益于健康，成为乐事，反之则遭祸于身心，百无一利。

A. 适量：主要指饮酒不可过量，不可暴饮。对于饮酒过量可以损害健康，导致疾病，甚至引起死亡，古人早有认识。《养生要录》云："酒者，能益人，亦能损人。节其分而饮之，宣和百脉，消邪却冷也。若升量转久，饮之失度，体气使弱，精神侵昏。宜慎，无失节度"，指出过量之危害，告诫人们要适度。《本草纲目》云："若夫沉缅无度，醉以为常者，轻则致败行，甚则丧躯损命，其害可胜言哉！"又说："过饮不节，杀人倾刻"，指出过量饮酒不仅可以导致疾病，甚至引起死亡。《饮膳正要》认为"少饮为佳，多饮伤形损寿，易人本性，其毒甚也。饮酒过度，丧生之源，"这些论述都强调了过量饮酒对健康和生命的危害。

现代研究证实，酒的有效成分是酒精即"乙醇"，白酒等烈性酒含醇量高达 40～60%，乙醇对人体损害极大，过量可引起急慢性酒精中毒。当人的血液中酒精达到万分之五到千分之二的浓度时，就会出现醉酒。达到千分之四时，就会造成急性中毒而死亡。长期的酒精刺激还可引起慢性胃炎，造成营养不良。由于酒精在肝脏分解，长期饮酒还会造成肝硬化和脂肪肝，肝硬化发病率在饮酒者比不饮酒者高七倍。此外，慢性酒精中毒还可引起心脏病及脑血管意外等多种疾病，直接危害人们的健康。

B. 适时：主要指空腹不饮酒。《养生随笔》说："古人饮酒每在食后。"空腹饮酒危害最大，在一小时就可被胃肠吸收 60%，一小时半吸收量达 90%，只有 10% 被水、汗和呼吸排出，而胃内容物内乙醇含量如超过 0.5% 即可产生危害。

睡前亦不可饮酒，汪颖反对夜饮，他说："既醉既眠，睡而就枕，热壅伤心伤目……停湿生疮，动火助欲，因而致病者多矣",这种提法是有一定道理的。

C. 适情:情指情绪与某些情形。情绪不佳,忧思恼怒时不宜饮酒,有人习惯以酒浇愁,但往往"借酒消愁愁更愁",饮酒虽可有短暂的欣慰感,但酒后往往更加惆怅,若有所失,此时饮酒最易醉,也最易损伤身体,应当戒之。

在某些特殊的情形,亦不宜饮酒,如性生活前不宜饮酒,此时饮酒万一怀孕,则会严重影响胎儿发育,遗患于后代。

此外,发烧、肝胆疾病、心脑血管疾病、肾病及严重胃肠疾病患者亦应戒酒,以免加重病情,不利康复。

1.3 起居保健

中医历来重视起居保健对于健康的重要作用,将起居调理作为养生学的一个重要内容。《千金方》说:"善摄生者,卧起有四时之早晚,兴居有至和之常制。"《寿亲养老新书》指出:"行住坐卧,宴处起居,皆须巧立制度",说明善自调理起居,作到有规律地生活与工作,对保持身心健康,延年益寿,实在不可或缺。起居保健的内容十分丰富,包括起居有常、安卧有方、衣着适宜、个人卫生等,其原则正确、方法合适,值得借鉴。

1.3.1 起居有常

《内经》曾将"起居有常"作"度百岁乃去"的重要一环,可见古人十分重视这个问题。起居指日常家居生活,有常即有规律,起居有常就是生活的规律化。古代养生学家认为,人的寿夭与起居的合理安排有密切的关系。《尚书》中即有"起居不节,用力过度,则络脉伤"的记载。《寿世秘典》中指出:"慎起居,谨嗜欲,守中实内,长生久视,道无逾此"。《养生要论》一书要求"慎节起卧,均适寒喧",如果违背了这些原则,生活不规律,不善于保养,就会损寿。

起居有常最重要的是要适应四时的变化。自然界的气候环境,在四时与昼夜之间都是在变化的,人的生理功能亦随之发生变化,因此,人们的日常起居生活就必须与之相适应。《内经》云:"阴阳四时者,万物之终始也,死生之本也,逆之则灾害生,从之则苛疾不起。"在起居调养方面,提出了"春夏养阳,秋冬养阴"的原则,同时还根据季节变化制定了与之相适应的作息制度:春季"夜卧早起,广步于庭";夏季"夜卧早起,无厌于日";秋季"早卧早起,与鸡俱兴";冬季"早卧晚起,必待日光。"不仅一年四季的作息时间因季节而异,就是昼夜晨昏亦应有所不同,《内经》云:"平旦人气生,日中而阳气隆,日西而阳气已虚,气门乃闭。"指出了一日之内,不同时间阴阳消长不同,人体的各种活动要顺应昼夜晨昏的变化。古人遵循的"日出而作,日入而息"的作息制度就是起居有常的实际反映。

1.3.2 安卧有方

睡眠既是消除疲劳、恢复体力的主要形式,又是调节各种生理机能,稳定神经系统平衡的重要环节,所以古人十分重视睡眠卫生,认为安卧有方与健康长寿关系极为密切。半山翁诗云:"华山处士如容见,不觅仙方觅睡方。"中医还用阴阳学说说明睡眠是调节人体阴阳平衡的需要,是生命活动过程的需要。《灵枢》说:"阳气尽阴气盛,则目瞑,阴气尽而阳气盛则寤"。

1. 睡前调理

(1) 睡前要思想安定,情绪平和

喜怒不节,悲忧不解,思虑过度,皆可影响心神而致睡眠不安。《睡诀》说:"早晚以时,先睡心,后睡眼。"只有"先睡心",才能"后睡眼",如果忧患重重、烦躁不安,往往难以入睡,甚至失眠,因此,睡前需摒除杂念,静神定志。《延寿药言》说:"临睡前宜用热水洗脚,将一切顾虑抛尽,宜思生平惬意赏心之事,或阅平和安慰静穆恬适之诗文,则心地光亮,神志安宁,入睡必易",实践证明睡前热水洗脚确能稳定情绪,有利于良好地睡眠。

(2) 睡前应节食

古人很早就认识到了"饱食即卧"的害处，强调"夜膳勿饱，……饱余勿便卧"。《内经》亦指出："胃不和则卧不安。"如睡前吃得过饱，必然会增加胃肠负担，影响睡眠，妨害健康。此外，睡前不宜用浓茶、烟酒、咖啡等刺激性食物，以免影响睡眠。

(3) 适量活动

睡眠前进行适量活动不仅可以放松肢体，而且有助于稳定情绪，《紫岩隐书》主张："每夜入睡时，绕室行千步，始就枕。……盖行则身劳，劳则思息，动极而返于静，亦有其理。……行千步是以动求静。"说明睡前稍事活动，散心、休闲，使精神舒缓，情绪稳定，则有助于睡眠，但不宜作剧烈活动。

(4) 诱导入静

对于辗转反思难以入眠者，古代养生家曾创造了许多诱导入静的方法。如《老老恒言》说："寐有操纵二法。操者，如贯想头顶，默数鼻息，返观丹田之类，使心有所着，乃不纷驰，庶可获寐；纵者，任其心游思于杳渺无朕之区，亦可渐入朦胧之境。"现代有人用默念数字来帮助入睡，其实就是该法的运用。

2. 睡时卫生

(1) 睡势

睡眠姿势是否正确，直接影响到睡眠的效果。古人主张的睡眠姿势是向右侧卧，双腿微曲，全身放松。《修龄要旨》说："侧曲而卧，觉正而伸。"《华山十二睡功总诀》指出："松宽衣带而侧卧之"，《老老恒言》则要求"卧宜右侧以舒脾气……，卧不欲左胁。……今宵敢叹卧如弓"。实践证明古人要求的这些睡眠姿势是合理的，一般认为睡眠的姿势以"右侧曲卧"为宜，而不采用仰卧和俯卧的姿势。

(2) 睡眠不可当风

睡眠不可当风而卧，风为百病之长，人在熟睡以后，易受风邪所袭。因此不得"乘月露外，乘便睡著，使人扇风取凉，一时虽快，风入腠理，其患最深，"《千金要方》曰："赤露眠卧，宿食不消，未逾期月，大少皆病，"《孙真人卫生歌》云："坐卧防风吹脑后，脑后受风人不寿。"都指出了当风而卧的危害，应当引以为戒。

(3) 睡眠不可对火炉

《琐碎录》说："卧处不可以首近火，恐伤脑"。卧时对火炉，最易火气蒸犯，夜间起身亦易受凉。

(4) 睡眠不可裹首掩鼻

睡眠切忌蒙头，一定要露首。《寿亲养老新书》所录之三叟长寿歌中即有"暮卧不覆首"的记载。一般认为睡眠时蒙头，呼吸不畅，还会吸入混浊之气，有碍身体健康。

(5) 衣被要温暖，枕头要舒适

《道林养生论》说："先安床暖席，"入睡前先安排好床，使床固定，被褥要松软温暖舒适，枕头高低适宜，质地松软有弹性，亦可根据需要选用药物枕，除可使人舒适外，还可防病治病。《老老恒言》在论枕头高低时指出："高下尺寸，令侧卧时恰于肩平，即仰卧亦觉安舒，"实践证明这种要求是合乎科学的，枕头过高和过低都对健康不利。孙思邈则强调"软枕头，暖盖足，"这些符合实际的主张，值得借鉴。

3. 醒后保养

古人对于醒后与晨起的保养也很重视，倡导了许多保养的方法。如《老老恒言》云："醒时当转动，使络脉流通，否则半身极重，或腰胁痛，或肢节酸者有之。"《遵生八笺》则要求醒来应叩齿、吐纳、咽津、按摩等，认为这些保养方法具有健身作用，又简便易行，可以广泛应用。

1.3.3 衣适寒温

衣服不仅是防寒保温、抵御疾病的人工屏障，同时又是反映物质和精神生活的外在表现。古人很早就知道穿衣与养生的密切关系，强调衣着要适体并应随四时气候的变化而增减。

1. 衣着应适体

古人认为衣着不在华丽，而在适体。《老老恒言》谓："衣食二端乃养生切要事。心欲淡泊，虽肥浓亦不悦口。衣但安其体所习，鲜衣华服与体不相习，举动便觉乖宜。所以食取称意，衣取适体，即是养生之妙药。"还说："长短宽窄，期于适体……其厚薄酌乎天时，""养老各异其衣……要之温暖适体，则一也。"这些论述都说明古人对于衣着强调其舒适、实用，而不追求华丽。总的原则以轻、软、宽大、舒适、式样简单，穿脱方便为原则。其内衣以棉织品为佳。

2. 随季节气候而增减

一年有春夏秋冬四时之别，一日有昼夜晨昏的不同，衣着也应根据季节和气候的变化而随时增减。《孙真人卫生歌》曰："春寒莫使棉衣薄，夏热汗多需换着，秋令觉冷渐加添，莫待疾生才入药。"说明衣着增减应随季节变化而异。《摄生消息论》云："正二月间乍寒乍热……天气暄寒不一，不可顿去棉衣。老人气弱骨疏体怯，风冷易伤腠理，时备夹衣，遇暖易之。一重渐减一重，不可以暴去。冬三月天地闭藏，……宜寒甚方加绵衣，以渐加厚，不得一顿便多。"指出春天天气虽然转暖，但忽冷忽热，易感时邪，衣着不可暴减。冬月虽然气寒冷，但秋令燥气未罢，不宜顿增厚褥重衾。陶弘景也说："绵衣不用频加添，稍暖又宜时暂脱。"

总之，人体若能顺应自然，根据四时季节气候的变化，随时增减衣着，对于防病健身是大有益处的。正如孙思邈所说："衣食寝处皆适，能顺时气者，始尽养生之道也。"

1.3.4 讲究卫生

古人历来重视个人卫生，认为只有讲究卫生才能预防疾病、保证健康，在漱口、刷牙、沐浴、洗脸、洗脚、叩齿等方面均有详细论述，至今看来，仍不失其科学性，具有其现实的指导意义。

1. 漱口刷牙

古代养生家很早就认识到保持口腔卫生对防止口腔疾病的重要性，认为应当坚持饭后漱口，每晚刷牙。《千金要方》说："食毕当漱口数过，令人口齿不败口香。"《老老恒言》云："食后微渣留齿隙，最为齿累……如食甘甜物，更当漱，每见年未及迈，齿即缺落者，乃甘味留齿，渐至生虫作蠹"，强调食后应当漱口，尤其在进甜食后，更当漱之，以免发生牙病。亦有不少医家主张临睡前漱口，《琐碎录》说："夜漱却胜朝漱，"《老老恒言》认为"早漱口，不若将卧内漱，"临睡漱口确比早漱有更重要的意义，值得提倡。

刷牙是我国古代的重要发明之一，宋代已有牙粉牙刷，《太平圣惠方》记载有制牙膏的方法。早在元代忽思慧著《饮膳正要》就记载："清旦用盐涮牙，无齿疾。"对于涮牙的时间，《金丹全书》作了精辟的论述："今人漱齿，每以早晨，是倒置也。凡一日饮食之毒，积于齿缝，当于夜晚刷洗，则垢污尽去，齿自不坏。故云晨漱不如夜漱，此善于养齿者。今观智者，每于夜后必漱，则齿至老坚白不坏。"元代罗天益的《卫生宝鉴》则提倡"早晚刷牙，"这是很有道理的，这种方法一直沿用至今。

2. 沐浴宜忌

清洁的身体是健康的保证，沐浴就是洗发、澡身，沐浴在我国有悠久的历史。《楚辞》中有"新浴者必振衣。"《史记》中有"新沐者必弹冠。"《孟子》更有"斋戒沐浴"等记载，说明我国古代劳动人民很早就有讲究卫生的习惯。《论语》中还有关于冷水浴的记载,"暮春者,春服即成,冠者五六人,童子六七人,浴手沂,风乎舞雩,咏而归,"说明古代养生家提倡用冷水浴来养生。

《老老恒言》说:"盖浴水不可太热,温凉须适于体,"并提倡"干浴"和"药浴",曰:"夜卧时,常以两手揩摩身体,名曰干浴……枸杞煎汤具浴,令人不病不老,纵无确效,犹为无损。"并认为如果春秋非浴之时入浴,需于"密室中大瓷缸盛及半,"以帐笼罩其上,然后入浴,浴罢急穿衣,衣必加暖,如少觉冷,恐即成感冒。"《摄生消息论》认为"冬月阳气在内,阴气在外,老人多有上热下寒之患,不宜沐浴,"《千金要方》主张:"不宜数数沐浴。"现代医学也主张老年人洗澡不必太勤,因老年人皮脂腺萎缩,洗澡过勤会使皮肤干燥,容易产生瘙痒,可以以干毛巾擦浴即"干浴"为宜。对于洗澡的时间,《泰定养生主论》认为"除夏日之外……十日一浴。若频浴则外觉调畅,而内实散气耗真也。"关于沐浴禁忌,《老老恒言》提出"饥忌浴","忌浴当风",这些主张都是合乎科学的,有参考借鉴的价值。

3. 手足卫生

手在人的感觉器官中是直接接触外界最多,而防护最差的,极易受到各种污染,因而手的卫生对人体健康关系极大,所以除经常洗手,保持手的清洁外,还应当经常剪指甲,《养生书》说:"甲为筋之余,甲不数截筋不替,"指出如果指甲经常不剪去,则筋不易更新。《延寿药言》认为"临睡前宜用热水洗脚"有助于稳定情绪,有利于睡眠。谚云"睡前一盆汤,勿用开药方,"形象生动地说明经常洗脚,特别是坚持睡前洗脚对健康大有益处,应当持之以恒。

此外,古人对个人卫生的其他方面如叩齿、咽津等也都有专门论述,具有一定的实用价值。

1.4 劳逸保健

劳即劳作，亦含疲劳之意，逸指闲适，或作安逸之释。人生存于自然界之中，就要与自然作斗争，就需要劳动与工作,而这种劳作必须在人体所能负荷的限度之内，这就需要适当的休息进行调节，也就是所谓有劳有逸。中医历来认为劳逸适度与否对健康的影响极为重大，反对过劳或过逸，提倡和主张劳逸适度。历代养生家也将劳逸失度视为养生之大忌。《养性延命录》说："养寿之法，但莫伤之而已"，这里所说的"伤"即指劳伤。孙思邈主张："不欲其劳，不欲其逸"，指出过劳或过逸都是有害于健康的，所以不应过劳，亦不应过逸。《老子养生要诀》也说："体欲少劳，但莫大疲,"亦指人体应当适量劳动而不至于过度疲劳。

劳逸失度有害人体，劳逸失度的范围十分广泛。以劳伤而言非单指形体之劳，还包括心神之劳，房劳等。以过逸伤人而言则包括精神过逸、形体过逸等。中医所强调的劳逸适度也体现在上述各个方面。

1.4.1 勿劳伤形体

中医认为过度劳累可损伤形体，轻则疲倦困顿，重则可引起相应的病变。《内经》曾指出："五劳作伤，久视伤血，久卧伤气，久坐伤肉，久立伤骨，久行伤筋，是谓五劳所伤。"说明无论行坐卧立过极，超越了人体所能承受的限度，都可以对形体带来损害。对于劳作对人造成损伤的程度，《彭祖摄生养性论》作了很好的解释："力所不胜而极举之则形伤也。"意思是体力达不到而勉强地去进行某种体力动作，即可损伤形体。

《内经》云："劳则气耗。"说明体力和精神过度消耗，最根本的是耗气，气不足则疲倦困顿、乏力、体力不支，在现实生活中这是很有道理的。长期的疾步奔走，身心处于紧张状态，精气大量消耗，真气逆于其里而不散，使人难以持久。静坐过久，可使脾胃气化运动减慢，因为脾主肌肉，脾气滞郁则肌肉瘦弱，所以久坐伤肉。站立过久，需要腰直骨坚，腰为肾之府，肾主骨，久立易于腰肾劳损，肾气损则骨易弱，所以久立伤骨。久卧之人则肺气出入较难，肺主全身之气，肺气郁滞则全身气缓，故久卧伤肺气。《养生书》说："久行伤筋劳于肝，久立伤骨损于肾，"说明了久劳对脏腑的损害。中医历来把"劳倦内伤"作为一个重要的发病原因。现代医学也认为当人体过度疲劳时，人体抵抗力明显下降，从而诱发各种疾病。

中医之谓劳伤除指劳作过度，而且也包括饮食、精神等方面的过劳。如《内经》曾说："饮食饱甚，汗出于胃；惊而夺精，汗出于心；持重远行，汗出于肾；疾走恐惧，汗出于肝；摇体劳苦，汗出于脾。故春夏秋冬，四时阴阳，生病起于过用，此为常也。"更明确地指出生病起于过劳，说明饮食、精神等方面的过劳亦能导致相应的疾病。

古人历来主张劳逸适度，即不可过劳，诸凡劳作，不使过极，以体力能够耐受并不感疲劳为度，劳后可进行适当调节，即稍事休息以消除疲劳。《养性延命录》说："是以养性之士，唾不至远，行不疾步，耳不极听，目不极视，坐不久处，立不至疲，卧不至懵；……不欲甚劳，不欲甚逸。"这种对人体活动的要求是十分科学和合理的。

《保生要录》曰："养生者形要小劳，无至大疲。故水流则清，滞则浊。养生之人，欲血脉常行，如水之流。坐不欲至倦，行不欲至劳，频行不已，然宜稍缓，即是小劳之术也。"这里则说明小劳无至大疲对养生的重要意义，并指出劳作中间的休息即是小劳的方法，值得借鉴。晋代著名医学家葛洪在《抱朴子》一书中提出一整套养生方法，其中有许多内容是讲劳逸的，他说："无久坐，无久行，无久视，无久听。不饥勿强食，不渴勿强饮。不饥强食，则脾劳，不渴强饮，则胃胀。体欲常劳，食欲常少，劳勿过极……早起不在鸡鸣前，晚起不在日出后。"对老年人外出步行,《内经》及《寿亲养老新书》主张老年人应在"四时气候和畅之日,量其时节寒温,出门行三二里,及三百二百步为佳。量力行但勿令气乏喘而已。亲故相访,间同行出游百步,或坐,量力谈笑,才得欢通,不可过度耳。"说明年老或体弱之人在行走或从事其他活动时应当量力而行,勿使过劳,以免影响健康,这是很值得借鉴的。

1.4.2 勿劳伤心神

中医历来认为七情过度皆可劳伤心神,妨碍健康与长寿。《灵枢》云:"怵惕思虑则伤神,"神伤则"破䐃脱肉,毛悴色夭;""愁忧而不解则伤意,"意伤则"四肢不举;""悲哀动中则伤魂,"魂伤"当人阴缩而挛筋;""喜乐无极则伤魄,"魄伤则"皮革焦;""怒而不止则伤志,"志伤则"腰脊不可以俯仰屈伸;""恐惧不解则伤精,"精伤则"骨酸痿厥"。充分说明七情过极,不仅损伤心神,而且可以伤及形体。神是人体生命活动的集中表现,彭祖曾说:"神强者长生",心神耗伤自然寿夭。古人还认识到心神劳伤往往是某些疾病发生的先导条件,孙思邈说:"怒甚偏伤气……气弱病相萦。"《养生论》也说:"喜怒悖其正气,"说明心神即伤,正气亦败,外邪易入,各种疾病也易于发生。

心神所伤对人的健康危害如此之烈,因此,古人历来重视保养心神,谨防七情过度,《琐碎录》说:"勿使悲欢极"。《摄生四要》提出:"少思以养神",以及中医一贯倡导的乐观、清心寡欲、无动喜怒、省思少虑、避免惊恐等精神调养方法,都是防止劳伤心神的有效措施。

1.4.3 勿房劳过度

房事即性生活,性生活是人类生活的重要内容之一,有人曾将性生活与物质生活、精神生活一起列为三大生活。我国在几千年前人们就开始了对性生活的研究与探讨,早在《内经》一书中，就有不少篇幅论述了房事与人体的关系，以后历代医家都从医学角度对房事对人体的生理影响、病理关系进行探讨，提出了许多科学的见解。

房劳过度即指无节制的性生活，对于房劳过度对人体健康的危害，古人论述颇多。《内经》曾提到："以酒为浆，以妄为常，醉以入房，以欲竭其精，以耗散其真，不知持满，不时御神，务快其心，逆于生乐，起居无节，故半百而衰也。"说明纵情声色，不自控制，必致精液枯竭，真气耗散，半百而衰。孙思邈说："姿其情欲，则命同朝露也。"也指出了房事不节可以损人寿命。他还淋漓尽致地写道："王候之宫，美女兼千，卿士之家，侍妾数百，昼则以醇酒淋其骨髓，夜则房室输其血气，耳听淫声，目乐邪色……或疾病而媾精，精气薄恶，血脉不充，……当今少百岁之人者，岂非所习不纯正也。"事实上，我国历代沉缅酒色的帝王往往早夭，说明上述论证是十分正确的。

房劳过度主要是消耗人的精气，而精为养身之本，"精少则病，精尽则死，"张景岳说："欲不可纵，纵则精竭；精不可竭，竭则真散。盖精能生气，气能生神，营卫一身，莫大乎此。"可见精气对生命的重要意义，房事过度耗精损神，则动摇了生命的根本，故难达长寿。彭祖说："服药百裹，不如独卧……夜接（性交）损一岁之寿，慎之。"这种说法似有些偏颇，但谨慎节制性生活的主张还是必要的。

至于老年人或病人，如不严格节制房事，则更是后患无穷。《寿世保元》说："年高之人，血气既弱，阳事辄盛，必慎而异之，不可纵心姿意。"说明老年之人，肾气已衰，更不能姿意妄为，房事不节。

如上所论，中医很早就已认识到房劳过度对人体的危害，因而提出了一系列戒房劳的主张和具体措施。

1. 勿早婚：祖国医学历来主张和提倡晚婚，认为未及成年而结婚，对身体是不利的。《养生医药浅说》记载："未及成年即为婚……戕伐元阳……而使精衰，气弱神散，而其结果则患滑精、阳痿、劳瘵、乏嗣者居多……。"《格致余论》亦说："男子十六岁而精通，女子十四岁而经行……古人必近三十、二十而后嫁娶，"从两性生理发展不同而阐述了不同的嫁娶时间，今天看来仍然是十分合理的。《冷卢医话》也提出："男子三十而娶，女子二十而嫁。"《寿世保元》主张："嬴女则养血，宜及时而嫁，弱男则节色，宜待壮而婚"，这些论述都说明晚婚对人体健康是有利的，指导人们要节制性欲，提倡晚婚。

2. 行房有度：度是适度的意思，即不能姿情纵欲，漫无节制。怎样才算适度呢？《春秋繁露》提出入房次数是："新壮者十日而一游于屋，中年倍新壮，始衰者倍中年，中衰者倍始衰，大衰者之月，当新壮之日。"孙思邈则主张："人年二十者（指二十到二十九岁），四日一泄；三十者，八日一泄；四十者，十六日一泄；五十者，二十日一泄；六十者，闭经不泄，若体力犹壮者，一月一泄。凡人气力超过人者，亦不可以抑忍，久而不泄，致生痈疽。"可见，对于性生活的频率与次数随年龄不同而有较大差别，总的趋势是随年龄增长而递减。在同年龄中，又应根据各人的体质及其他具体情况不同而有所差异。现代医学认为，衡量房事是否过度应以行房后第二天是否精神饱满，身心愉快为标准。多数人认为：一般人每周一、二次正常适度的房事，不会影响身体健康，可以达到性的愉快和满足。

3. 行房有禁：所谓行房有禁，就是说在某些情况下应当禁止房事。孙思邈曾说："凡新沐、远行及疲、饱食、醉酒、大喜、大悲、男女热病未瘥、女子月血（月经）、新产者，皆不可合阴阳。"《寿世保元》指出："饱食房劳，伤血气。……大醉入房，气竭肝肠。男人则精液衰少，阳痿不举；女子则月事衰微，恶血淹留，生恶疮。忿怒中尽力行房事，精虚气竭，发为痈疽。恐惧中入房，阴阳偏虚，自汗盗汗，积而成劳。远行疲劳行房，为五劳虚损，少子。月事未绝而交接生驳，又冷气入内，身痿面黄，不产。金疮未瘥而交会，动于血气，故令金疮败坏。忍小便而入房者，得淋病，茎中疼痛，面失血气，致胞转脐下，急痛死。时疾未复，犯病者，舌出数寸而死。"可见，在许多情况下，性生活都是在禁忌之列的，应当知其禁而避之。主要应避忌以下三点：

(1) 莫"醉以入房"：孙思邈说："醉不可以接房，醉饱交接，小者面黯咳喘，大者伤绝脏脉损命，"指出了醉后行房的危害性。醉后行房往往使人失去自制能力，易导致房事过度，伤肾耗精，损神折寿。同时易导致性生活不和谐，甚至伤害夫妻感情。还可严重影响后代的体质和智力。醉后入房偶然使妻子受孕，严重者可导致胎儿畸型，使出生后智力迟钝或呆傻，影响人口素质。此外，阳痿、早泄等疾病的发生也常常与醉后行房有关。

(2) 愤怒惊恐及疲劳时勿行房：中医十分重视七情劳伤对房事的影响。孙思邈说："人有所怒，气血未定，因为交合，令人发痈疽……"极言情绪不佳与劳伤时行房的危害。惊恐入房受孕后后代还易发生癫疾，《内经》云："人生而有颠疾者，病名曰何？安所得之？岐伯曰：病名为胎病，此得之在母腹中时，其母有所大惊，气上而不下，精气并居，故令子为颠疾也。"明确指出惊恐时入房时若受孕则胎儿易患颠疾之证，影响下一代健康，故应慎而避之。

(3) 气候异常时勿行房：气候异常指雷雨闪电之时，奇寒异热之中不可行房，否则不但影响成人健康，对胎儿也极为不利。孙思邈说："生而母子俱死者，雷霆霹雳日之子。"指出气候异常对母子的严重影响。因此，凡遇气候异常，均应避免入房。

此外，在妇女经期，妊娠头三个月和后三个月及新产后百天之内均应禁戒房事，新病之时勿入房，久病之后亦应慎之。

1.4.4　勿过度安逸

过劳伤人，过逸亦伤人。中医历来认为人欲健康，不可过劳，亦不可过逸。疲劳之后，暂时休息加以调节，这种逸是积极的，但如果过于安逸，就会成为消极的因素，而不利于健康。自古以来善养生者都劝告人们切勿过逸。孔子指出：以"佚游"为乐，则有损人体。葛洪说："是以善养生者，……调理筋骨，有偃卧之方；祛疾闲邪，有吐纳之术。"人体脏腑本处于不断运动之中，以发挥其生理作用，适当活动可以促进人体功能，相反，如果安闲好逸，就会使气血运行迟缓，经脉不畅，脏腑机能减退，四肢倦怠乏力，结果必然是体弱多病。伏尔泰曾说："生命在于运动，"他认为活动是冷静与自强的良剂。

勿过逸，一是要注意经常活动形体，《吕氏春秋》云："流水不腐，户枢不蝼，动也。形气亦然。"形体活动于外则气血流动于内。形体得到气血的营养则活动有力，气血由于形体的活动则运行通畅。手指臂肘常动则关节灵活，掌握自如；足胫股膝常动则骨骼坚强，行步矫健。在生活中应根据自己的不同情况，采取适当的活动措施，以保证身体的健康。二是勿久坐久卧，中医认为久坐伤肉，久卧伤气。以睡眠而言，古人认为："凡睡至适可而止，则神宁气足，大为有益。多睡则身体软弱，志气昏坠。"久坐之人则易使气血凝滞，从而导致疾病。所以人不宜久卧，不宜久坐，而应当经常进行适当活动以调节人体气血运行，从而保持健全的体魄。三是要勤动脑。勤动脑可以防止智力衰退。尤其是老年人，为防止大脑功能退化，就必须经常保持有足够的信息量来刺激大脑皮层，从而保证大脑血液的供应量，所以老年人应当经常读书看报，勤于思考问题。近年来科学家们用超声波测量不同生活方式的人的大脑，发现勤于思考的人，脑血管经常处于舒展的状态，使脑神经细胞得到良好的保养，从而使大脑不会过早衰老。

1.5 运动保健

运动作为一种有效的健身方法，自古以来受到人们重视，《易传·象辞·乾象》上说："天行健，君子以自强不息。"意思是说自然界在运动变化着,人也要运动不息才能保持健康长寿。清朝颜习斋在《言行录》说:"一身动则一身强,一家动则一家强,一国动则一国强,天下动则天下强,"充分说明了加强运动不仅可以每个人获得健康,也是民族兴旺发达、增强人民体质所必不可少的。

汉代名医华佗创"五禽戏",为我国古代体育健身运动的发展作出了卓越的贡献。1975年在湖南长沙马王堆三号汉墓出土的文物中,就有一幅画有静坐、伸臂、屈膝、抱腿、下蹲等各种姿势导引图的帛画,可见运动健身在我国有悠久的历史。

中医认为运动可以使精气流行不郁,《寿世保元》说:"养生之道,不欲食后便卧及终日稳坐,皆能凝结气血,久即损寿。"运动还可以增强脾胃的消化功能,华佗曾说:"动摇则谷气得销,血脉流通,病不得生。"孙思邈则反复强调:"食毕当行步踌躇,计使中数里来。行毕使人以粉摩腹上数百遍,则食易消,大益人,令人能饮食,无百病。"现代医学研究还表明,运动可加强心脏和血管功能,改善呼吸功能,对神经系统有良好作用,强筋壮骨,还能预防和治疗某些疾病,因此,运动是健康长寿所不可缺少的。

运动健身在方式上主要有主动和被动两种,劳动及各种体育运动等都属于主动运动,按摩则属于被动运动方式。运动保健方法甚多,诸如劳动、体育、舞蹈、导引、按跷等,均可据情选用之,若能持之以恒,自可收益身延年之效。

1.5.1 坚持参加劳动

劳动创造了世界,劳动是人类生存必不可少的内容。坚持适量劳动也是运动健身的重要方式。这里所说的劳动主要是指体力劳动。中医认为劳动可以运动形体,调剂精神,流畅气血,舒筋健骨等作用。华佗曾指出:"人体欲得劳动,但不当使极耳。"劳动对脑力劳动者和老年人来说,则具有更为重要的意义,它不仅能锻炼身体,促进健康,而且能够陶冶性情,培养高尚的情操。同时使大脑得到充分的休息，使精神畅悦，情绪稳定。孙思邈认为离开了劳动和运动，气机就会"不得安于其处，以致雍滞。"应当根据各自的具体情况，有意识地安排和参加一定的体力劳动。对于脑力劳动者来说，劳动作为一种休息和调节就显得尤为重要。

1.5.2　参加体育锻炼

体育是运动的最主要的活动方式，古人十分重视体育锻炼对健身的主要作用，创立过许多我们民族独特的锻炼项目，如太极拳、五禽戏、八段锦等，至今仍然风靡世界。及至现在，体育锻炼项目更是丰富多彩，比如跳、跑、行、举、射、游、投、拍等，门类众多，而且大部分项目简便易行，易于接受，均可据情选用。

1.5.3　常用运动方法简介

1. 散步：散步是最常用又最易进行的运动方法，古人历来主张在清晨、饭后、睡前或闲时散步，以运动形体，和畅气血，增进运化，调济精神，促进健康。《老老恒言》有散步专论。认为："散步者，散而不拘之谓，且行且立，且立且行，须得一种闲暇自如之态。"并指出散步可以舒筋使四肢健、助消化及养神等多种功能。实践证明散步确是益身强体、简便易行的运动方法。

2. 舞蹈：舞蹈也是一种运动形体的有效方法之一。《吕氏春秋》有作："舞以宣导之，"来预防"民气郁阏而滞着，筋骨瑟缩而不达"之类病证的记载。《红炉点雪》亦云："舞蹈所以养血脉，"并强调"食后宜稍动作舞蹈。"现代研究也表明一些轻松活泼的舞蹈确锻炼形体，有益身心。

3. 导引：导引是古代流传下来的一种以肢体运动与呼吸运动相结合的运动健身方法，如华佗五禽戏、婆罗门导引十二法等都在导引的范畴之内。古人认为导引的作用，主要是斡旋气机，周流荣卫，行气活血，舒筋健骨，除劳去烦等方面。如《老老恒言》说:"导引之法甚多,……不过宣畅气血,展舒筋骸,有益无损。"

4. 太极拳: 太极拳也是最常用的运动方法,它是明末民间流行的某些拳势同古代呼吸导引相结合的产物,所以,太极拳亦属气功中动功一类,而且内外兼修,动静结合。太极拳以阴阳环抱之太极图而命名,人体同宇宙万物由对立统一的阴阳两方面组成一样,人体要健康无病,必须阴阳和调,处于不断运动的平衡状态之中,太极拳就可达到这样的目的。解放后,国家体委公布了简化太极拳,简便易行,尤为人们所喜爱。

除以上几种方法,其他如按跷(按摩)、天竺国按摩法、跑步、武术等也都是行之有效的运动健身方法。若能掌握要领,持之以恒,必可大有益于身心。

1.6 顺应自然保健

人生存于自然界之中,自然气候的变化和环境的差异与人体健康有十分密切的关系。古代医家在"天人相应"学说指导下,认为人与自然界是统一的整体,自然界包括四时气候和环境是在不断变化的,而这些变化不仅与人类生理功能改变有关,在一定条件下,还影响着病理过程的发生和发展。《灵枢》说:"天暑衣厚则腠理开,故汗出。天寒则腠理闭,气涩不行,水下流于膀胱,则为溺与气。"这是说气候条件不同,人体水液排泄的方式亦不同。风寒暑湿燥火六气按一定的规律变化,方不致害,若气候发生反常变化,则成六淫,成为致病的因素。地理环境的突变若超出了人的适应能力,如由高原居处迁至平原湿地,由炎热之南方移至寒冷之塞北等,亦能引起人体相应的病变。

人体要获得和保持健康,就必须与自然环境条件的变化相适应,主要是顺应四时变化,调适环境,避免秽浊之气等。

1.6.1　顺应四时

四时者，春夏秋冬，人应当顺应四时气候的变化，《内经》谓："夫四时阴阳者，万物之根本也。所以圣人春夏养阳，秋冬养阴，以从其根，故与万物沉浮于生气之门。逆其根，则伐其本，坏其真矣。故四时阴阳者，万物之终始也，死生之本也。逆之则灾害生，从之则苛疾不起，是谓得道。道者，圣人行之，愚者佩（背）之。"《灵枢》也说："智者之养生也，必须四时而适寒暑，和喜怒而安居处，节阴阳而调刚柔，如是则僻邪不至，长生久视。"强调人体必须适应四时气候的变化，才能健康长寿。

1. 春季养生：中医认为春天为发陈之季，万木萌发，欣欣向荣，人在起居、饮食衣着等方面均应与之相适应。《内经》云："春三月，此为发陈，天地俱生，万物以荣，夜卧早起，广步于庭，被发缓形，以使志生。"这是指春天是富于生气、万物欣欣向荣的季节，人们应该入夜即睡，早些起身，披发解衣，使形体舒缓，放宽步子在庭院中漫步，以使精神愉快、胸怀开畅。《千金要方》主张："春欲晏卧早起，"并指出"虽云早起，莫在鸡鸣前。"这是言春天的起居调摄的，《内经》认为如果违背这些原则就会损伤肝脏，而且到夏季还易发生寒性病变。

在饮食方面，《孙真人卫生歌》认为应该："春月少酸宜食甘。"《云笈七签》说："春气温，宜食麦以凉之，禁吃热物。"《摄生消息论》也指出："饭酒不可过多，米面团饼不可多食，致伤脾胃，难以消化，"这些都说春天宜食甜软易消之食，避免过食醇味、辛燥之物，以防影响消化功能。

在衣着方面，《孙真人卫生歌》主张："春寒莫使棉衣薄。"《摄生消息论》指出："天气寒暄不一，不可顿去棉衣。老人气弱骨疏体怯，风冷易伤腠里，时备夹衣，遇暖易之，一重渐减一重，不可暴去。"由于春天天气由寒转暖，时有变化，故应谨避风寒。

此外,《摄生消息论》还主张:"春日融和,当眺园林亭阁,虚敞之处,用摅带怀,以畅生气。不可兀坐,以生抑郁。"春天主生发,人应当调畅情志,避免精神抑郁,实践证明,这些论述都是符合实际的。

2. **夏季养生**:夏季是一年之中最炎热的季节,万物生长茂盛,人体阳气也最易发泄。在起居调摄方面,《内经》认为:"夏三月,此为蕃秀。天地气交,万物华实;夜卧早起,无厌于日;使志无怒,使华英成秀,使气得泄,若所爱在外,此夏气之应,养长之道也。逆之则伤心,秋为痎疟,奉收者少,冬至重病。"指出在起居作息方面应当是在夜晚睡眠,早早起身,不要厌恶长日,应当保持精神愉快而切莫发怒,使气机宣畅,通泄自如,这是适应夏季的气候,保护长养之气的方法,如果违逆了这些方法,就会损伤心脏,秋冬时则会患疟疾或其他疾病。

在饮食调摄方面,《千金要方》说:"夏七十二日,省苦增辛,以养肺气。"就是说夏天应少食苦味,多食辛味,以免心火过旺而影响肺气的宣发。《养生论》还主张:"夏气热,宜食菽以寒之,不可一予热也,"这是指夏天宜食杂粮以寒体,而应避免过热的食物。《养生书》认为肥腻之品亦不易食,指出:"夏季后秋分前,忌食肥腻饼臛油酥之属,此等物与酒浆瓜果,极为相妨,夏月多疾以此。"《养老奉亲书》也说:"生冷肥腻,尤宜减之。"

在穿着方面,《孙真人卫生歌》说:"夏月汗多须换著,"指夏天天热汗多,衣服要薄一些,勤洗勤换。

古人对夏月纳凉也有严格要求,《养老奉亲书》说:"夏月天暑地热,若檐下过道,穿隙破窗,皆不可纳凉,以防贼风中人。"《摄生消息论》说:"檐下、过廊、弄堂、破窗、皆不可纳凉,此等所在虽凉,贼风中人最暴,惟宜虚堂、净室、水亭、木阴洁净空敞之处,自然清凉更宜调息净心,常如冰雪在心,炎热亦于吾心少减。"还说:"不得于星月下露卧,兼使睡著,使人扇风取凉。"《理虚之鉴》还提出:"又防因暑取凉,长夏防湿。"这些都是我国人民长期生活经验的总结，至今仍有教益。

3. 秋季养生：《内经》云："秋三月，此为容平。天气以急，地气以明。"是说秋天万物成熟平定，天高风急，地气清肃，所以在起居方面就应当"早卧早起，与鸡俱兴；使气安宁，以缓秋刑；收敛神气，使秋气平；无外其志，使肺气清。"《内经》认为这是"秋气之应，养收之道也。逆之则伤肺，冬为飧泄，奉藏者少。"这些论述说明了秋季的气候特征，人应早睡早起，神志安宁，以收敛神气，保持肺气的清肃，这是适秋令特点而保养人体收敛之气的方法，违逆则会伤及肺脏，冬天还要发生泄泻。

在饮食调摄方面，《饮膳正要》指出："秋气燥，宜食麻以润其燥。"麻是芝麻。还有的主张秋天宜食生地粥以滋阴润燥。在食物性味上应减少辛味而增加酸味食物，以免肺气太过而使肝气抑郁。

在衣着方面，《孙真人卫生歌》云："秋令觉冷渐加添，莫待疾生才入药。"是说秋天天气转凉，应及时添衣以免受凉伤身。

4. 冬季养生：冬季气候寒冷，宇宙万物都处于收藏状态。人类在冬季则应注意防寒保暖，使阴精潜藏于内，阳气不致妄泄，而与冬季的自然气候相适应。如《内经》所言："冬三月，此为闭藏。水冰地坼，无扰乎阳；早卧晚起，必待日光；使志若伏若匿，若有私意，若已有得；去寒就温，无泄皮肤，使气亟夺，此冬气之应，养藏之道也。"这段话阐述了冬季气候特点和起居，精神调养的原则，如果违背了这些原则，就会："逆之则伤肾，春为痿厥，奉生者少。"邱处机指出："宜居处密室，温暖衣衾，……不可冒触寒风。"

在饮食调摄方面，邱处机指出："饮食之味，宜减酸增苦以养心气"。在穿衣方面，邱处机指出："寒极方加绵衣，以渐加厚，不得一顿便多"。对于冬季取暖，古人也有明确要求，邱处机主张："帷无寒即已，不得频用大小烘炙，尤其损人；手足应心，不可以火炙手，引火入心，使人烦躁。"这些观点是符合实际的。

总之，古代医家对四季摄生的论述，至今仍有其现实的指导意义，对人类健康作出了巨大贡献。

1.6.2 调适环境

自古以来，人们就认识到地理环境与人的健康密切相关。不同的自然和水土环境条件可对人体产生不同的影响。《内经》云："一州之气，生化寿夭不同，其何故也？歧伯曰："高下之理，地势使然也。崇高则阴气治之，污下则阳气治之。阳胜者先天，阴胜者后天，此地理之常，生化之道也。……高者其气寿，下者其气夭，地之小大异也，小者小异，大者大异。"充分阐明了地势高低对人的健康和寿命的影响，对于气候对地理的影响，古人也有明确认识，《内经》曾说："燥胜则地干，暑胜则地热，风胜则地动，湿胜则地泥，寒胜则地裂，火胜者地固矣。"说明自然界气候的变化与地理环境的改变是紧密相联的。

大量研究资料表明，长寿与地域有密切关系，居住在空气清新，气候寒冷的高山地区的人多长寿，而居住在空气污浊，气候炎热的平原地区的人则多短寿，当然地势高低都是相对的。我国著名的长寿地区—广西都安、巴马的调查表明，51位百岁老人全部住在农村而且绝大部分住在山腰以上的地方，湖北地区调查也发现90岁以上的125位长寿老人中，有96%住在农村。这当然不是绝对的。这些调查研究的结果证实古人的论述是符合客观实际的。

既然环境对人体健康关系密切，人类就应当对环境进行调适，以使之有利于人的健康和长寿。环境调适主要是对生活环境的选择和改善。

1. 环境选择

古人历来重视居处环境的选择，认为居处低凹潮湿，污秽肮脏，可致疾病丛生。居处高亢无潮，清洁卫生，则体泰延寿。《释书》曾记载："宅，择也，择吉处而营之也"。《博物志》亦说:"居无近绝溪、群冢、狐蛊之所,近此则死气阴匿之处也"。指出居处应远离积淤死水和墓地等处而营造,而应当"背山临水,气候高爽,土地良沃,泉水清美"。空气新鲜,阳光充足,水源清洁;依山临水,绿树成荫是最佳的养生环境,而最忌浓烟污雾、沙尘黑粉、污泥浊水、噪音喧嚣等,故一般说来,山区优于平原,乡村优于城市。除乡村营建住宅应尽可能遵循上述原则外,作为城市职工在退离休后,若条件允许下迁居农村为宜。城市住宅也应尽量避开车马喧嚣、烟雾迷漫的市中心和工业区。

2. 环境调适

生活环境的选择固然重要,但在实际上常常是可供选择的机会和条件较少,有的根本不可能,特别是在人口稠密集中的城市,则受到更大的限制,因此,在可能的条件下,对生活环境进行必要的调适和改善,还是可行而大有益于健康的。

(1) 改善居室环境:居室是人们抵御外界风雨寒暑侵袭,维护人体正常生理功能的建筑设施,它造成一种良好的房室微小气候,从而保证人们休息、睡眠和恢复体力。人的一生有一半时间是在住室中度过的,所以住室结构是否合理,卫生条件是否良好将直接影响着人们的健康。孙思邈曾说:"凡人居止之室,必须周密,勿令有细隙,有风气得入。"陈直亦说:"栖息之室,必常洁雅,夏则虚敞,冬则温密,其寝寐床榻,不须高广,比常之制,三分减一,低则易于升降,狭则不容漫风,裀褥厚藉,务在软平,三面设屏以防风冷"。这些论述都对居室内这一小环境的安排和布局提出了合理的要求,指出居室宜冬暖夏凉,防风防潮,床铺、被褥应当安置合理等。

古人对于居室朝向、床铺位置、窗户开关、居室明暗度、房屋高低等也都各有讲究。如《天隐子养生书》说:"何为安处?曰非华堂邃宇,重裀广榻之谓也。在乎南向而坐,东首而寝,阴阳适中,阴暗相半。屋勿高,高则阳盛而明多;屋无卑,卑则阴盛而暗多。故明多则伤魄,暗多则伤魂。人之魂阳而魄阴,苟伤明暗，则疾病生焉。……吾所居室四边皆窗户，迅风即阖，风息即开。吾所居坐，前帘后屏，太明则下帘以和其内映，太暗则卷帘以通其外曜。内以安心，外以安目。心目皆安，则身安矣。"这些主张和要求符合实际需要，很有借鉴价值。

现代研究也表明，居室的面积、容积、高度和进深十分重要，不可太小，每人居室体积不应少于 15 立方米，以保证有足够的呼吸空间。居室高度应为 2.6~3.5 米，不宜太低。居室进深度一般不应超过地板至窗上缘高度的 2~2.5 倍。居室的适宜温度冬季为 17~22℃，夏季 17~25℃。相对湿度最好为 40~60%。若条件许可，均应参照上述要求对居室进行改造，以使之适宜于人的养生和保健。

(2) 改善周围环境

居室周围环境包括庭院环境对于人体健康也有极为密切关系，应当予以美化和改善。

古代养生家很重视美化居住环境，住宅多座落在山青水秀、阳光充足之处。我国大部分地区的住宅是坐北朝南，门窗面向太阳，既光线充足，空气流通，又冬暖夏凉。而且住宅周围多广种竹木花草，既美化环境，又能防风防尘、调节空气。这样的环境对人们的健康长寿无疑是大有裨益的。清代著名养生家曹慈山对住宅环境非常讲究，他虽然住在城里，却能因地制宜："辟园林于城中，池馆相望，有白皮古松数十株，风涛倾耳，如置身岩壑……至九十余乃终"。他在《老老恒言》中提倡老人要亲自在"院中植花木数十种，不求名种异卉，四时不绝便佳"，"阶前大缸贮水，养金鱼数尾"。这既美化了环境，又陶冶性情，实在有益于健康长寿。

美化周围环境，主要是绿化，广种树木植物花草，现代研究表明，绿化可以调节气温和湿度；调节空气中的二氧化碳浓度以净化空气；能防风防尘杀菌；能消除噪音；对人体各器官也有良好的作用。

改造周围环境还包括消除噪音,消除工业废气污染等,以创造良好的居住环境,促进人体健康和长寿。

(3) 保持清洁卫生

保持居处的环境卫生也是防病保健的一个重要因素。在我国最早的甲骨文中就有大扫除的记载。《礼记》中有"凡内外,鸡初鸣……洒扫室堂及庭"的记事,说明在两千多年前我们的古人就很重视环境卫生。《梦梁录》说:"十二月,不论大小家,俱洒扫门闾,去尘秽,净庭户。"这是指春节前的大扫除。其他还有端午节以雄黄酒挥洒床帐间等,都是十分必要的民俗卫生措施。古人还注意到通过沟渠通峻,消除污水以防止瘟疫,如《周书秘奥造册经》曰:"沟渠通峻,屋宇洁净,无秽气,不生瘟疫病。"指出了屋宇洁净可以减少疾病,提高健康水平。对于空气消毒法古人亦有论述,《居家宜忌》谓:"卧榻前,宜烧苍术诸香,以辟秽气及诸不译",指出了以烟熏法进行空气消毒,以达到预防疾病的目的。这些认识与方法至今仍不失其指导意义。

2 实用保健方药

2.1 常用保健中药

保健中药是指能补充人体物质、增强机能、提高抗病能力、促进人体健康或康复、以延年益寿的一类中药。因其具有补养作用，又称补益药或补养药。保健中药依作用和应用范围的不同而分为补气药、养血药、助阳药、滋阴药和其他保健中药五类。

2.1.1 补气药

凡具有补气功能，消除或改善气虚症状的药物称为补气药。人体的生长发育、新陈代谢等一系列生命活动，无不依赖于气的作用。气的生成和运行又赖于脾肺等脏器的功能正常。因脾为后天之本，气血生化之源；肺主一身之气。各种原因导致脾肺等脏器功能失常而出现气虚证时，则机体活动能力不足，表现为疲乏无力、精神不振、食欲不佳、少气懒言、易出虚汗等衰弱症状。服用补气药，便可消除或改善气之不足，使身体康复。有些补气药，如人参、大枣、蜂王浆、刺五加、饴糖、蜂蜜等，在没有明显气虚而体质偏弱的情况下少量服用，也可起到养生防病、延年益寿的作用，但以中老年人且秋冬季服用为宜。

服用补气药应根据不同的气虚症状选择相应的药物，并应根据兼症辨证施治。补气药不可过量服用，以防气滞。

1. 人参

人参按加工方法的不同可分为生晒参、糖参（白参）、红参；按产地不同可分为吉林参、高丽参（朝鲜参）等。其中以产于吉林省抚松县者质量最好。人参味甘微苦，性微温，能大补元气、补脾益肺、生津止渴、安神增智，是冬令进补的佳品，其主要有效成分为人参皂甙类。年老体弱,或过度劳累之后,不思饮食,周身无力,疲倦欲睡但久久难眠时,服用少量人参,能补气安神、增进食欲、恢复体力。临床上多用于久病气虚以及各种休克病人,因能生津,又用治气阴两亏者。

药理证实,人参具有强壮作用,有助于改善机体各脏器,特别是循环、神经和内分泌系统的功能,改善机体的免疫状态和对自然环境的适应能力,有利于延长寿命。

人参适于虚证,体质强壮者不宜滥用。常用量5~10克,水煎服,反藜芦,畏五灵脂,恶皂荚。服时忌萝卜、茶叶。

2. 西洋参

西洋参味苦、微甘、性寒,能补气养阴、清火生津,其主要有效成分为人参奎酮、人参皂甙。本品药效比较缓和,最宜于治疗小儿高热、烦渴、泄泻脱水以及肺结核之虚热燥咳者。又可用于各种原因导致的气阴两伤。年老体弱者适量服用,能改善人体功能,提高抗病能力。西洋参具有解热作用,能促进人体抗体形成,改善免疫功能,补益强壮。

本品常用量为3~6克,水煎服。忌铁器火炒,反藜芦。

3. 太子参

太子参味甘性平,能补气生津,其主要有效成分为皂甙、果糖、淀粉等。太子参为清补之品,有近似于人参的益气生津、补益脾肺作用,但药力较弱,常用于病后体虚。因能生津,又常代替西洋参而用于热病后期气阴两亏、邪未尽去但有气虚津少口渴者。体弱年老、疲倦乏力、食欲不振者也可服用。

常用量10~30克,水煎服。

4. 刺五加

刺五加味辛、微苦,性温,能益气健脾、补肾安神、祛风除湿,其主要有效成分为多种刺五加甙、有机酸及数十种微量元素。本品为滋补强壮、扶正固本的重要药物,其药理作用与人参十分相似或高于人参。对各种不明原因的体虚、老年病、更年期综合征、原发性高血压、低血压、麻痹性或兴奋性阳萎、毒物中毒等均有较好疗效。又适于高空作业人员、运动员、潜水员等服用。药理表明，刺五加对中枢神经系统和血压有双向调节作用，具有明显的抗疲劳作用，能提高脑力和体力劳动的效率，延长寿命。能改善免疫功能，增强人体对有害因素的抵抗力，能兴奋性腺、肾上腺，降低血糖，抗利尿、抗炎，抑制肿瘤的生长。又能调整人体功能而有"适应原"样作用。

常用量9～30克，水煎服。也可入其他剂型。

5. 党参

党参原产于山西上党。野生者称野台党，栽培者称潞党参。味甘性平，能生津养血、补中益气。主要含有皂甙、蛋白质、维生素等。本品无毒，属补益类长寿药，适用于各种气虚病人，如各种原因引起的衰弱症、各种贫血等。与解表药、泻下药同用，可扶正祛邪，治体虚外感或里实正虚之证。党参对中枢神经系统有兴奋作用，可减轻疲乏感。能降压、升血糖、增加红细胞和血红蛋白量，改善免疫机能，提高抗病能力。

常用量10～30克，水煎服。忌萝卜、茶叶，反藜芦。

6. 黄芪

黄芪味甘微温，能补气升阳、益卫固表、托毒生肌、利水退肿，其主要有效成分为香豆素、黄酮、皂甙等。本品为常用补气药之一，适用于脾肺气虚或中气下陷、表虚自汗、痈疽不溃或溃久不敛以及尿少浮肿等症。如胃下垂、子宫脱垂、脱肛、久泻久痢、小便失禁、慢性肾炎等。黄芪能降压、强心、抑菌，保护肝脏，减轻肾脏病变。能兴奋中枢神经系统，有类似性激素样作用，具有强壮作用。

常用量10～30克，水煎服。

7. 白术

白术味苦、甘，性温，能补气健脾、燥湿利水、止汗安胎，其主要有效成分为苍术醇、苍术酮和维生素A。白术为健脾佳品，每多用于慢性消化不良、慢性非特异性结肠炎、脾虚水肿、肾性水肿、营养不良性水肿及妊娠水肿等，又常用于安胎或治疗体虚自汗及慢性风湿性关节炎。白术具有强壮、降低血糖作用，能改善血凝状态，促进肠蠕动，改善内外环境的协调，抑制细胞突变，从而促进人体健康。

常用量5～15克，水煎服。

8. 甘草

甘草味甘性平，能补脾益气、润肺止咳、缓急止痛、缓和药性，其主要有效成分为甘草甜素、甘草次酸、甘草黄碱酮、甘草甙等。甘草临床应用相当广泛，可用于胃及十二指肠溃疡、传染性肝炎、阿狄森氏病、支气管哮喘、肺结核、血小板减少性紫癜、血栓性静脉炎等病症。因能缓和药性，调和百药，又多用于各种方剂的配伍中。本品对消化性溃疡有良效，能改善消化系统功能，具有肾上腺皮质激素样作用，并有解毒、解热、止咳平喘、抗炎及抗过敏作用，体外实验有抗菌作用。另能降低胆固醇，改善动脉粥样硬化。

常用量3～15克，水煎服。大剂量服用易引起水肿及血压升高。反海藻、大戟、甘遂、芫花。

9. 山药

山药以产于河南新乡地区者为佳，称为怀山药。山药味甘性平，能益气养阴、补脾肺肾，其主要有效成分为皂甙、粘液质、胆碱、糖蛋白、多种氨基酸、维生素C、多巴胺等。本品为滋养性平补脾胃药，多用于脾虚泄泻、肺虚咳嗽、糖尿病、遗精、小便频数、慢性肾炎、虚劳羸瘦等症。山药具有诱生干扰素，增强机体的免疫功能，改善冠状动脉及微循环血流、镇咳、祛痰、平喘、滋补强壮等药理作用。

常用量10～30克，水煎服。

10. 黄精

黄精味甘性平，能补脾益气、润肺滋阴，为补益类长寿药。

常用于病后体弱、慢性病营养不良、肺结核、肾虚精亏、脾胃虚弱等症，又可作为年老体弱者的滋补强壮剂。黄精具有降低血糖、降压、抑菌、抗结核，防止动脉粥样硬化，增强 T 细胞的数量和功能，延长体细胞寿命，滋补强壮而抗老益寿等药理作用。其主要有效成分为蒽酸、醌类、粘液质、糖类、生物碱等。

常用量 10~20 克，鲜者 30~60 克，水煎服。

11. 大枣

大枣味甘性温，能补中益气、养血安神、缓和药性，其主要有效成分为蛋白质、糖类、有机酸、维生素等。本品属补益类长寿药，适用于脾胃虚弱者。无病服用也可固护脾胃，充养后天。因其味甘，兼有缓和药性和矫味作用。大枣可以增强肌力，具有强壮作用。又能保护肝脏，改善过敏性和原发性血小板减少性紫癜的症状。另有镇静和利尿作用。

常用量 3~12 枚，或 10~30 克，水煎服。

12. 饴糖

饴糖味甘性温，能补脾益气、缓急止痛、润肺止咳，其主要有效成分为麦芽糖和少量蛋白质。饴糖为滋补强壮、健胃补虚之佳品，无病服用也为益品。适于治疗胃及十二指肠球部溃疡、慢性胃炎、肺虚咳嗽、慢性支气管炎、肺结核等，也可用于解毒。本品具有滋补强壮、健胃、润肺止咳等药理作用。

常用量 30~60 克，入汤剂分二三次溶化服。

13. 蜂蜜

蜂蜜味甘性平，功能补中缓急、润肺止咳、滑肠通便，其主要有效成分为糖类、无机盐、酶、蛋白质、色素、花粉粒等。本品具有多种医疗保健价值，适用于老年体弱、病后津亏、肠燥便秘、虚劳久咳、溃疡病、慢性肝炎等。又可外敷疮疡、烫伤、内服解乌头、附子等药物毒性。另多用于中药材的加工炮制及制剂中。老年体弱者常服有益于健康。本品有抑菌和滋补强壮等药理作用。

常用量 15～30 克，冲服。

2.1.2 养血药

凡能补血养血，改善或消除血虚证症状的药物称为养血药。

衰老的机制相当复杂，血虚无疑是其重要原因。血虚的基本症状是：面色萎黄、唇舌色淡、头晕眼花、手足发麻、心慌心悸等。此时服用养血药物，可促进周身血液循环，使脏器功能协调而推迟衰老。

养血药质多粘腻，过服常影响食欲。

1. 阿胶

阿胶以产于东阿（今山东省东阿县及平阴县东阿镇）而得名，以山东、浙江、江苏等地产量较多，其中山东平阴阿胶厂和山东东阿阿胶厂生产的阿胶，均为驰名中外的优质产品，近年来山东定陶阿胶厂生产的阿胶也获奖。

阿胶味甘性平，功能补血止血、滋阴润肺，其主要有效成分为多种氨基酸、钙、硫等物质。阿胶为治血虚之要药，其补血作用甚佳，兼有强壮作用，具有广泛的适应症。多用于各种贫血、出血症，又常用于务种妇科疾病，尤为产后血虚之补益佳品。年老体弱者适量服用，可起到营养强壮的作用。药理证实，阿胶能升高红细胞和血红蛋白，防治进行性营养障碍症，改善体内钙平衡和免疫功能，并有升压作用。

常用量 5～10 克，开水或黄酒化服，入汤剂应烊化冲服。

2. 当归

当归主产于甘肃省东南部的岷县（秦州）。味甘辛，性温。功能补血、活血、止痛、润肠，其主要有效成分为糖类、多种氨基酸、数十种无机元素、多种维生素等。当归为养血的首选药，临床应用相当广泛，血虚诸症、月经不调等妇科疾患每多选用。也可用于高血压病、冠心病、脑动脉硬化、各种贫血、血栓闭塞性脉管炎、大便秘结等。本品具有多种药理作用，能强心、扩冠、降压、降低胆固醇、缓解动脉粥样硬化。具有抗恶性贫血、镇静、镇痛、抗菌和保护肝脏的作用，对子宫有双向调节作用。

常用量5～15克，水煎服。补血用当归身，破血用当归尾，和血（即补血活血）用全当归。酒制能加强活血之功效。

3. 熟地黄

熟地黄味甘微温，功能养血滋阴、补精益髓，其主要有效成分为 β-谷甾醇、甘露醇、地黄素、生物碱、脂肪酸、葡萄糖、氨基酸、维生素 A 等。本品属补益类长寿植物药，常用于治疗血虚萎黄、眩晕、心悸、失眠、月经失调、崩漏以及肝肾阴虚之症，又可治疗糖尿病、传染性肝炎、风湿或类风湿性关节炎等。熟地黄能抗炎、抗菌、保肝、利尿，并有性激素样作用，能改善循环系统之功能，降低血糖，防止化疗所致之白细胞减少。

常用量10～30克，水煎服。

4. 何首乌

何首乌味苦、甘、涩，性微温，功能补益精血、截疟、解毒、润肠通便，其主要有效成分为大黄酚、大黄素、大黄酸、大黄素甲醚、卵磷脂等。何首乌是补血养精、强筋健骨、乌须黑发、延年益寿之良药，多用于精血亏虚、须发早白、久疟、肿毒、疮疡、肠燥便秘、高血压、冠心病、高胆固醇血症等。本品能降低血脂，缓解动脉粥样硬化，有类似肾上腺皮质激素样作用，并能强心、泻下、抑菌。

常用量10～30克，水煎服。补益精血用制首乌。

5. 白芍

白芍味苦、酸，性微寒，功能养血敛阴、柔肝止痛、平抑肝阳，其主要有效成分为芍药甙、牡丹酚、β-谷甾醇、挥发油、树脂、脂肪油、糖、淀粉、粘液质、蛋白质、三萜类等。白芍是补阴血的常用药，多用治血虚引起的四肢肌肉痉挛抽搐、血虚月经不调、肝气郁滞之腹痛、血虚肝旺、自汗盗汗、溃疡病、胃肠炎等。药理表明，白芍能抗炎、抗溃疡、解痉、抗菌、镇静、镇痛、扩冠、增强机体抵抗力，并有止汗、利尿作用。

常用量10～30克，水煎服。

6. 龙眼肉

龙眼肉味甘性温，功能补心脾、益气血，其主要有效成分为皂甙、脂肪油、脂肪酸、糖类、维生素、胆碱等。本品是一种香甜可口、味道鲜美的果品，宜于年老体弱者作为调补益寿之品。常用于治疗心脾两虚之神经衰弱、气血不足、体虚慢性出血、血虚月经过多、产后水肿、肺结核、高血压、冠心病等。本品具有抑菌、抗癌、镇静、降低血脂、增加冠脉流量、增强体质等多种药理作用。

常用量10～15克，煎汤、熬膏、浸酒或入丸剂。

7. 桑椹

桑椹味甘性寒，功能滋阴补血、生津、润肠，其主要有效成分为芸香甙、花青素甙、胡萝卜素、维生素、鞣酸、糖类、脂肪油等。桑椹为养血滋阴佳品，适用于血虚阴亏之眩晕、耳鸣、失眠、须发早白、肠燥便秘、糖尿病、高血压、动脉硬化、各种贫血、神经衰弱等。本品能提高T细胞的数量和功能，改善免疫功能，从而起到滋补强壮、延年益寿之作用。

常用量10～15克，水煎服，也可熬膏、浸酒或生食。

2.1.3 助阳药

凡能扶助人体之阳气，改善或消除阳虚证症状的药物称为助阳药。

阳虚证包括心阳虚、脾阳虚、肾阳虚，由于肾阳为元阳，对人体脏腑起着温煦生化的作用，故阳虚诸证往往与肾阳不足有着十分密切的关系。肾阳虚主要表现为：畏寒肢冷、腰膝酸软、体质虚弱、精神不振、性欲淡漠、夜尿增多、白带清稀等。助阳药具有补肾阳、益精髓、强筋骨之作用，能调节肾上腺皮质功能，调整能量代谢，促进性腺机能，促进生长发育，增强机体抵抗力，故可以改善或消除阳虚症状，延缓衰老。

助阳药性多温燥，体格健壮者慎用。

1. 鹿茸

鹿茸味甘咸、性温，功能补肾阳、益精血、强筋骨，其主要有效成分为鹿茸精、磷酸钙、碳酸钙、胶质、蛋白质、磷、镁、胆固醇、维生素 A 等。鹿茸是名贵药材之一，为峻补元阳之要药。多用于治疗阳萎、遗精、不孕、小儿发育不良、严重贫血、风湿性心脏病、神经衰弱、疮疡久溃不敛等症。本品具有较强的雄性激素作用，能促进蛋白质合成，升高白细胞，增强人体机能。能促进造血和生长发育，促进骨折和溃疡的愈合。又可强心、利尿，增强子宫张力及收缩，改善阳虚病人之能量代谢。

常用量 1～3 克，研细末，一日三次分服。

2. 蛤蚧

蛤蚧味咸性平，能补肺气、助肾阳、定喘嗽、益精血，其主要有效成分为蛋白质、脂肪、淀粉。蛤蚧为动物类滋补助阳药，主产于广西。多用于肺结核引起之喘咳带血、支气管哮喘、肺气肿、阳萎、尿频、神经衰弱等症。蛤蚧具有性激素样作用，能直接或间接地兴奋性腺，并可增强人体机能，促进生长发育。

常用量 3～7 克，水煎服。研末服每次 1～2 克，一日三次；浸酒服每浸 1～2 对。

3. 巴戟天

巴戟天味辛甘、性微温，功能补肾助阳、祛风除湿，其主要有效成分为橄树素甙、维生素 C、糖类、树脂等。巴戟天为补肾要品，具有补肾培元、抗老延寿之作用。适于阳萎、小便失禁、尿频、女子不孕、月经不调等病症。药理证实，巴戟天具有肾上腺皮质激素样作用，能强心、扩冠、降压，具有较强的抗菌作用和一定的祛痰、镇咳、平喘作用，能调节机体的免疫功能，防止化疗所致之白细胞减少。

常用量 10～15 克，水煎服。

4. 杜仲

杜仲味甘性温，能补肝肾、强筋骨、安胎，其主要有效成分为杜仲胶、树脂、糖甙、有机酸、维生素 C 等。杜仲为中医传统的助阳药，又是一种安全的天然降压药，实为补益强壮、延年益寿之佳品。适用于肝肾不足、腰膝酸痛、高血压、小儿麻痹后遗症、先兆流产、习惯性流产等。本品具有良好的降压、利尿作用，可以减少胆固醇的吸收，松弛子宫，抑制中枢神经系统而起镇静作用。

常用量 10～15 克，水煎服。炒用比生用疗效为佳。

5. 冬虫夏草

冬虫夏草味甘性温，功能益肾补肺、止血化痰，其主要有效成分为冬虫夏草酸、冬虫夏草素、蛋白质、脂肪、维生素 B12、多种氨基酸、虫草多糖、尿嘧啶、腺嘌呤核苷等。冬虫夏草是名贵的滋补药材，为年老体弱者的扶正固本良药。适用于病后体弱、贫血、阳萎遗精、腰膝酸软、肺结核之虚喘咳血以及体虚易感冒者。本品对中枢神经系统有抑制作用，能镇静、解痉、抗炎、抗菌、祛痰、镇咳、平喘、抗肿瘤，又可降压、扩冠、降低血脂，增强常压缺氧耐受力，从而具有补虚固本、延年益寿之功效。

常用量 5～10 克，煎汤服；或与鸡、鸭、鱼、猪肉等炖服；或入丸散剂。

6. 紫河车

紫河车为人的胎盘，甘咸而温，功能补精、养血、益气，其主要有效成分为多种氨基酸、免疫因子及多种激素。紫河车是温肾壮阳、滋补强壮的良药，适用于肾气不足、精血衰少之不孕、阳萎、遗精、气血亏虚之消瘦乏力、面色萎黄、产后乳少、肺肾两虚之气喘等。也可用于肝炎及流感的预防或作为年老体弱者之补品。本品能促进性腺及生殖器官的发育，防止化疗所致之白细胞减少，激发免疫，兴奋机体机能，促进生长发育。

常用量 1.5～3 克，研末装胶囊吞服，一日二三次。鲜胎盘每次半个或一个，水煮服食。

7. 菟丝子

菟丝子味辛甘、性平，能补阳益阴、固精缩尿、明目止泻，其主要有效成分为树脂甙、β-谷甾醇、糖类、淀粉酶、维生素 A 等。本品为补肾壮阳之常用药，具有延年益寿之功效，适用于肾虚腰膝酸软、遗尿、尿频、遗精、习惯性流产、高血压、视力减退、糖尿病等。菟丝子具有降压、强心、抗菌、兴奋子宫的药理作用，又可调节免疫功能，增强人体机能，调整和提高人体代谢功能。

常用量 10～15 克，水煎服。

8. 胡桃仁

胡桃仁即核桃仁，味甘性温，功能补肾、温肺、润肠，其主要有效成分为脂肪油、蛋白质、碳水化合物、钙、磷、铁、胡萝卜素、核黄素等。胡桃仁为人们所喜爱的食品，适于老人和体弱者作滋补用。可用于治疗慢性喘息性支气管炎、肾虚腰痛、腿软、习惯性便秘、尿路结石等。本品具有良好的降压、抗炎作用，能滋养强壮、扶正固本，具有较高的营养价值。

常用量 10～30 克，水煎服。也可生食。

9. 阳起石

阳起石味咸微温，能温肾壮阳，其主要有效成分为硅酸镁、硅酸钙。本品为矿物类壮阳药，适用于肾阳虚衰之男子茎头寒、阳萎不起、女子宫冷、阴部湿痒以及腰膝冷痹之症。

常用量 3～6 克，入丸散剂。本品不宜久用。

10. 补骨脂

补骨脂苦辛大温，功能补肾壮阳、固精缩尿、温脾止泻，其主要有效成分为皂甙、树脂、有机酸、补骨脂素、补骨脂乙素、异补骨脂素等。本品为温肾壮阳的常用药，适用于阳萎遗精、遗尿、尿频、腰膝冷痛、阳虚腹泻、子宫出血、银屑病、白癜风等。补骨脂有雌激素样作用，能扩冠、强心、镇静、解痉，能兴奋平滑肌，抗菌，促进皮肤色素新生，提高人体免疫功能。

常用量 5~10 克，水煎服。孕妇禁用。

11. 淫羊藿

淫羊藿辛甘而温，功能补肾壮阳、祛风除湿，其主要有效成分为淫羊藿贰、黄酮贰、甾醇、挥发油、维生素 E 等。本品是一味很有潜力的强壮保健药，适用于阳萎、遗精、尿频、腰膝酸软、风湿痹痛、四肢麻木、小儿麻痹症、妇女更年期高血压、冠心病、慢性支气管炎等。淫羊藿具有雄激素样作用，能降压、强心、扩冠、抑菌、抗病毒、降低血糖，能调节免疫功能，提高肾上腺皮质功能。

常用量 10~15 克，水煎服。也可浸酒、熬膏或入丸散剂。

2.1.4 滋阴药

凡能滋养阴液、生津润燥，改善或消除阴虚症状的药物称为滋阴药。

阴虚可分为肺、胃、肝、肾等阴虚，是年老体弱者的常见症候，又多见于热病后期及若干慢性疾病。一般表现为：津少口渴、干咳少痰、潮热、盗汗、心烦、失眠、遗精、头晕、两目干涩等。滋阴药可通过改善机体内的糖分解代谢，使亢进的能量代谢恢复正常，提高机体的免疫功能，调节体液代谢等机理，起到生津润燥、滋补强壮之作用。

滋阴药大多甘寒滋腻，脾胃虚弱、痰湿内阻、腹胀便溏者不宜使用。

1. 沙参

沙参有南沙参和北沙参两类。南、北沙参均味甘微寒，能清肺养阴、益胃生津，以北沙参功效更佳。其主要有效成分为皂贰、挥发油、三萜酸、豆甾醇、β-谷甾醇、生物碱等。沙参具有较好的滋补营养作用，适用于肺热阴虚之干咳少痰、劳嗽咯血以及热病伤津之口干舌燥、食欲不振者。本品具有解热、祛痰、镇痛等药理作用。

常用量 10～15 克，鲜者 15～30 克，水煎服。忌与藜芦同用。

2. 天冬

天冬甘苦大寒，功能清肺降火、滋阴润燥，其主要有效成分为天冬酰胺、谷氨酸等 19 种氨基酸、葡萄糖、甾体皂甙等。本品属补益类长寿药，有强骨健体、防老之效。适于热病伤阴、肺虚燥咳、老年性慢性支气管炎、肺结核、百日咳、乳房肿瘤、便秘、遗精等病症。天冬具有多种药理作用，能镇咳、祛痰、抗菌，抑制肿瘤生长，改善心肺功能和人体适应环境的能力，减少体细胞的突变。

常用量 10～15 克，水煎服。便溏者不宜服用。

3. 石斛

石斛味甘微寒，功能养胃生津、滋阴除热，其主要有效成分为石斛碱、粘液质、石斛酮等。石斛为滋养胃阴的常用药，属滋补强壮之品。适用于热病伤津、胃阴不足、阴虚津亏、虚热不退、慢性胃炎、糖尿病等。本品能解热镇痛，帮助消化、强心、降压，防止化疗所致之白细胞减少，增强人体免疫功能，改善体内代谢，调节体液平衡。

常用量 6～15 克，鲜者 15～30 克，水煎服。入汤剂宜先煎。

4. 麦冬

麦冬味甘、微苦，性微寒，功能润肺养阴、益胃生津、清心除烦，其主要有效成分为多种甾体皂甙、β-谷甾醇、氨基酸、葡萄糖和维生素 A 样物质。麦冬有防老之效，属补益类长寿药。适用于肺燥干咳、胃阴不足、心烦失眠、肠燥便秘、吐血、衄血、慢性咽炎、冠心病等。本品可改善胰岛细胞和心血管系统的功能，增强机体适应环境的能力，减少体细胞突变，明显提高常压及减压耐缺氧能力,并有较强的抗菌作用。

常用量10~15克,水煎服。

5. 玉竹

玉竹味甘性平,功能滋阴润肺、生津养胃,其主要有效成分为铃兰苦甙、铃兰甙、山柰酚甙、槲皮醇甙、维生素A、蒎酸等。本药为清补之品,可作为年老体弱者的一般补品,但效力较弱。适用于肺胃阴伤、心力衰竭、冠心病、肺结核、糖尿病等。玉竹药理作用广泛,能强心、扩冠、降低血糖、抗菌,有类肾上腺皮质激素样作用,能增强人体免疫能力,提高心肺功能和适应环境能力,改善胰岛细胞和血管运动中枢功能,从而起到补益作用。

常用量10~15克,水煎服。

6. 百合

百合味甘微寒,能润肺止咳、清心安神,其主要有效成分为秋水仙碱、淀粉、蛋白质、脂肪、糖、钙、磷、铁等。百合作为常用滋阴药而具有抗老延寿之作用,适用于肺热咳嗽、虚烦惊悸、失眠多梦、慢性肾炎、肺结核、高血压、支气管哮喘、慢性支气管炎等。本品具有一定的祛痰、镇咳、平喘作用,能提高或改善免疫功能和心肺功能,防止化疗引起的白细胞减少。

常用量10~30克,水煎服。鲜用30~50克,煮粥或作菜食。

7. 枸杞子

枸杞子味甘性平,能滋补肝肾、明目、润肺,其主要有效成分为甜菜碱、胡萝卜素、玉蜀黍黄素、烟酸、多种维生素等。枸杞子为滋阴补肾、防病益寿之佳品,适用于肝肾阴虚、阴虚劳嗽、慢性肾炎、慢性肝炎、肝硬变、糖尿病、肿瘤等。枸杞子具有降低血糖,降低血脂,改善免疫功能,保护肝脏等多种药理作用。并能明显改善化疗所致之白细胞减少症,降低血压。

常用量5~10克,水煎服。

8. 女贞子

女贞子味甘苦性凉，功能补益肝肾、清热明目，其主要有效成分为三萜类齐墩果酸、甘露醇、葡萄糖、油酸、亚油酸、女贞子甙、脂肪酸等。女贞子为常用滋补强壮之品，有预防早衰、推迟老化、延年益寿之作用。适用于肝肾阴虚、头晕目眩、腰膝酸软、须发早白、视力减退、慢性肾炎、慢性肝炎、冠心病、中心性视网膜炎、白细胞减少症等。女贞子具有强心、利尿、保肝、抑菌、增加白细胞和降低血脂等多种药理作用，又能增强人体免疫功能而起强壮作用。

常用量10～15克，水煎服。

9. 黑芝麻

黑芝麻味甘性平，能补益精血、润燥滑肠，其主要有效成分为蛋白质、脂肪油、糖、纤维素、钙、磷、铁、维生素B_2、E、芝麻素、芝麻酚等。黑芝麻既是祛病强身的良药，又是味道鲜美的食品，适用于高血压、冠心病、动脉硬化、神经官能症、肠燥便秘、肝肾阴虚、头晕目眩、须发早白、贫血、乳汁缺乏等。药理证实，本品能抗衰老，降血脂，降血压，降低血糖，通便，是老少皆宜的保健佳品。

常用量10～30克，水煎服，或炒熟食用。

10. 鳖

鳖又名甲鱼，鳖肉味甘性平，鳖甲味咸性寒，功能滋阴潜阳、凉血、软坚散结，其主要有效成分为蛋白质、脂肪、碳水化合物、钙、磷、铁、维生素、动物胶、角蛋白、碘等。鳖为血肉有情之品，是滋阴养血之佳品，滋补作用以鳖肉为佳。适用于肝肾阴虚、病后体虚、骨蒸潮热盗汗、阴虚风动、高血压等。尤宜于年老体弱者作为滋补之用。健康人服食也有益处。现代研究表明，本品对增加营养，增强体质有重要作用，是较理想的滋补品。

每次一只，烹食。鳖甲10～30克，水煎服。

11. 银耳

银耳味甘、淡，性平，功能滋阴润肺、益气和血，其主要有效成分为蛋白质、树胶质、酶、多糖、无机盐、维生素B等。银耳是珍贵的滋补佳品，适用于年老体弱者，健康人服食于身体有益。可用治肺结核咳血、高血压、动脉硬化、白细胞减少症、癌肿、慢性病体虚等。本品具有滋补强壮之药理作用，能提高人体免疫力，兴奋造血功能，促进蛋白质和核酸的合成，并能抗癌，改善呼吸系统病变。

常用量3～10克，炖食。或与其他食品做成羹。

2.1.5 其他保健中药

凡在《中药学》中分类不属于补益药，但具有补益作用，可用于治疗人体虚弱、预防疾病、养生益寿的一类中药，均归于此。

随着现代药理研究的深入广泛，许多中药的保健作用不断被开发出来，这类药物的共同特点是：保健效果好，可食性强，毒副作用极小。

1. 酸枣仁

酸枣仁味甘性平，功能养心安神、敛汗，其主要有效成分为枣仁皂甙、甾醇、三萜化合物、大量植物油、维生素C、蛋白质等。酸枣仁传统归属安神药，现代药理证实，本品能镇静、催眠、镇痛、镇痉、抗惊厥、降温，具有降压、改善心血管系统和免疫系统功能、兴奋子宫、抗休克、减轻局部水肿之作用，并有滋补强壮作用。现多用作年老体弱者之营养滋补品。

常用量6～15克，水煎服。酸枣也可生食，或入其他剂型，或制成各种营养品（酒、饮料等）。

2. 山楂

山楂酸甘微温，功能消食化积、活血散淤，其主要有效成分为三萜类、黄酮类、β-谷甾醇、硬脂酸、维生素C、胡萝卜素等。山楂营养丰富，酸甜可口，是一种理想的果品。本品具有持久的降压作用和强而持久的强心作用，能降低血脂，增加冠脉流量，抗心律失常，并有较强的抑菌作用和助消化功能，是高血压、冠心病患者以及年老体弱者的补益佳品。

常用量6～15克，鲜者30～50克，水煎服。或生食，或制成片、糕、酱、汁、晶、酒等。

3. 莲子

莲子味甘而涩，性平，功能补脾止泻、益肾固精、养心安神，其主要有效成分为淀粉、棉子糖、蛋白质、脂肪、碳水化合物、钙、磷、铁等。本品传统用作收涩剂，适用于夜寐多梦、遗精、滑精、肾虚尿频、脾虚久泻、心悸、虚烦不眠等。莲子具有抗癌、降压等药理作用。年老体弱及健康人常食之，能增强体质、延年益寿。

常用量6～15克，水煎服。也可煮粥熬羹或入其他剂型。

4. 灵芝

灵芝味淡、微苦，性温，能滋补强壮、安神定志、补中健胃，其主要有效成分为赖氨酸、亮氨酸等15种氨基酸、生物碱、肽、糖类、甾醇类、三萜类、挥发油、树脂和13种无机元素等。灵芝是扶正固本、滋补强壮的珍贵药品，药理作用相当广泛，适用于冠心病心绞痛、传染性肝炎、白细胞减少症、神经衰弱、贫血等，又是体弱年老者的滋补佳品。灵芝能强心、扩冠、对抗动脉粥样硬化的形成，具有镇咳、祛痰、平喘、抑菌等作用，能提高机体免疫能力，保肝，镇静，镇痛，抗癌，兴奋造血系统。

常用量1.5～3克，水煎服；或0.9～1.5克，研末吞服；或浸酒，或入其他剂型。

5. 茯苓

茯苓味甘、淡，性平，功能利水渗湿、健脾和胃、宁心安神，其主要有效成分为茯苓酸、β-茯苓糖、胆碱、蛋白质、脂肪、麦角甾醇、钾、钠、卵磷脂，等。茯苓是最常用的中药之一，因含有多种营养物质，又为保健益寿之佳品。适用于水肿、小便不利、脾胃虚弱、慢性腹泻、心悸失眠、美尼尔氏综合症等。本品具有利尿、镇静、抑菌、抗癌、强心、降低血糖、改善消化系统功能，提高免疫能力等多种药理作用。

常用量10～15克，水煎服。也可制成丸、散、粥、点心服用。

6. 薏苡仁

薏苡仁味甘、淡，性微寒，功能利水渗湿、健脾、除痹、清热排脓，其主要有效成分为蛋白质、脂肪、碳水化合物、维生素B_1、薏苡素、薏苡酯等。薏苡仁适用于小便不利、水肿、脾虚泄泻、风湿性关节炎、肺脓疡、肺结核、癌肿等。常食本品可以轻身益气，故可作为年老体弱者尤其是兼有行动不便者的保健营养品。本品能解热镇痛、强心、抗肿瘤，并可改善呼吸功能。

常用量10～30克，水煎服。或煮粥食用。

7. 芡实

芡实味甘、涩，性平，功能益肾固精、补脾祛湿止泻，其主要有效成分为蛋白质、淀粉、糖、脂肪、维生素B_1、B_2、C、尼克酸、胡萝卜素、钙、磷、铁、等。芡实是健脾益肾之良药，延年益寿之上品。可用治脾虚泄泻、日久不止、肾虚遗精、小便失禁、白带过多等。现代研究表明，芡实含有对人体有益的五大营养素，并且容易消化，确为祛病强身、滋补益寿之佳品。

常用量10～15克，水煎服。或煮粥食用。

8. 香菇

香菇味甘性平，能益气补虚、健胃、透疹，其主要有效成分为蛋白质、脂肪、碳水化合物、维生素、钙、磷、铁、尼克酸等。香菇可用于食欲不振、吐泻乏力、小便淋浊、痘疹不透、癌肿、高脂血症、佝偻病、贫血等。近来，香菇的保健营养价值日被重视和应用，并已成为滋养强体、祛病延年之上品。本品具有抗肿瘤、降血脂、提高免疫功能、防治佝偻病等药理作用。

常用量6~9克,水煎服。或与肉、鸡、鱼炖食。

9. 木耳

木耳味甘性平,具有益气、凉血、止血之功效,其主要有效成分为蛋白质、糖类、脂类、甾醇类、无机盐和维生素,等。木耳既是宴席上的佳品,又是保健防病、延年益寿之良药。可用于治疗高血压、冠心病和各种出血症等。本品有止血、防治动脉粥样硬化、轻身强志、抗衰老等作用。

常用量15~30克,为菜食用,或作羹食。

10. 菊花

菊花味甘、苦,性凉,能疏风清热、平肝明目、消炎解毒,其主要有效成分为挥发油、菊甙、胆碱、氨基酸、维生素、腺嘌呤、微量元素等。菊花历为辛凉解表药,适用于外感风热证及痈疖肿毒等,近用治冠心病、高血压等。现代研究发现,菊花能改善心血管功能,降低血栓形成,防治心脑血管疾病。又可解热、镇静、抑菌、抗病毒,并具有抗衰老、延年益寿之作用。

常用量6~9克,水煎服。或浸酒、泡茶服。

11. 丹参

丹参味苦微寒,功能活血祛瘀、凉血消痈、养血安神,其主要有效成分为丹参酮、隐丹参酮、丹参新酮、β-谷甾醇、维生素E等。丹参属活血祛瘀药,用于瘀血腹痛、癥瘕积聚、月经不调、血瘀经闭、疮痈肿毒、热入营血等。现用治冠心病、血栓闭塞性脉管炎、慢性肝炎、肝脾肿大、小儿迁延性肺炎等效果良好。药理表明,丹参具有抗衰老作用,能提高免疫功能,扩冠、强心、降压,抑制血小板功能,抗肿瘤、抗菌、镇静。故现又用作却病健体、抗老益寿之品。

常用量5~15克,水煎服,或入其他剂型。

12. 三七

三七味甘、微苦,性温,功能滋补强壮、止血活血、散瘀定痛，其主要有效成分为皂甙类、止血活性物质、黄酮类、生物碱、蛋白质、糖类、脂肪油、挥发油、树脂、核苷、胡萝卜素，等。三七传统归作止血药，用于各种出血症和跌打损伤、瘀血肿痛，现又用于贫血、体虚、冠心病、高脂血症、运动过度综合征等。现代研究发现，三七与人参在化学成分和药理作用等方面有许多相似之处。三七具有明显的补血强壮作用，能改善心血管系统的功能，具有免疫调节作用，对血糖有双向调节作用，又可止血、抗炎、镇静、止痛，是一味很有前途的滋补保健药品。

常用量3~10克，研粉吞服，每次1~1.5克（熟三七粉每次3~5克）。三七花可浸酒或泡茶。

13. 天麻

天麻味甘性平，功能息风止惊、平肝潜阳、镇静安神，其主要有效成分为天麻素、香荚兰醇、琥珀酸、β-谷甾醇、维生素A样物质、甙类、生物碱等。天麻传统属平肝息风药，用于治眩晕、肢麻、半身不遂等。药理表明，天麻除有良好的镇静、镇痛、抗惊厥作用外，尚能增强机体的免疫功能，改善心肌的营养血流，提高实验动物的耐缺氧能力，故有延年益寿之效。

常用量3~10克，水煎服，或研末每次1~1.5克吞服。亦可浸酒或制成其他剂型。

14. 花粉

花粉是指群蜂采集植物花的雄蕊上的生殖细胞，授粉于雌蕊而生长发育的蜜源花粉。能滋补强壮、美容、抗衰老，其主要有效成分为20种氨基酸、14种维生素、24种无机元素、18种天然活性酶、脂肪、激素、芳香类物质等。花粉具有滋补强壮、兴奋造血功能、调节心血管功能、抗菌、抗癌、抗衰老等多种药理作用，是年老体弱以及健康人防病强身、抗老益寿的理想之品。尤宜于神经衰弱、贫血、前列腺肥大、糖尿病、心血管疾病、溃疡病、更年期综合征患者及运动员服用。

花粉多为成品，可按说明服用。

2.2 常用保健中成药
2.2.1 补气成药

1. 补中益气丸

补中益气丸主要成分为黄芪、党参、甘草、当归、陈皮、升麻、柴胡、白术。蜜丸每丸重9克,水丸每袋重18克。口服,蜜丸每次1丸,日2次;水丸每次9克,日2次。方出自《脾胃论》。

本药能补中益气,升清降浊,适用于脾肺气虚引起的头痛懒言、阴虚自汗、恶风厌食、劳疟寒热、久泻久痢、胃下垂、子宫脱垂、多种虚证、各种贫血、慢性胃炎等。

2. 参苓白术丸

本药主要成分为人参、茯苓、白术、白扁豆、山药、甘草、莲子、桔梗、砂仁、薏苡仁,方出自《太平惠民和剂局方》。水丸,每袋重18克,每服6~9克,日1~2次,口服。

本药能调补脾胃,适用于脾胃虚弱引起的饮食不化、或吐或泻、形瘦色萎、神疲乏力、慢性肾炎、肺结核等。

3. 四君子丸

四君子丸出自《太平惠民和剂局方》,药由党参、白术、茯苓、甘草组成。水丸,每袋重18克,每服6克,日3次。

本药能健脾益气,适用于脾胃虚弱引起的食少便溏、面色萎黄、头晕乏力,如慢性胃肠炎、溃疡病、迁延性或慢性肝炎、贫血、白细胞减少症等。也可作为年老体虚者的调补品。

4. 十全大补丸

本方出自《太平惠民和剂局方》,药由党参、黄芪、肉桂、熟地黄、白术、当归、白芍、川芎、茯苓、甘草组成。蜜丸,每丸重9克,每服1丸,日2次。

本药能补中益气、养血和营,适用于气血两虚引起的体弱、面色萎黄、虚劳喘嗽、精神倦怠、遗精失血、腰膝无力等。

5. 两参精

本方由延吉市制药二厂设计研制，主要成分为人参精、五加参精。口服液，每安瓿 10 ml，每服 1 支，日 1 次，早饭前服。

本药能益气养血、滋补强壮，适用于神经衰弱、年老体弱、病后虚羸、食欲不振、心力衰竭、肝炎、贫血等。常服能增强机体功能，提高抗病能力。

6. 人参蜂王浆（双宝素口服液）

本品由北京东风制药厂及杭州第二中药厂等生产，主要成分为人参、蜂王浆、蜂蜜等。蜜浆剂，每支 10 ml，每服 1 支，日 2 次。

本品能滋补强壮、益气健脾，适用于体质虚弱、病后体弱、营养不良、神经衰弱、疲乏无力、食欲不振、神经代谢机能衰退症等。久服可促进生长发育，增强智力、体力，预防疾病，延年益寿。双宝素口服液由杭州第二中药厂生产，成分、功效与人参蜂王浆基本相同。

7. 北京蜂王精

本品由北京营养补剂厂研制生产，主要成分为蜂王浆、人参、党参、枸杞子、五味子等。口服液，每安瓿 10 ml，每服 1 支，晨起或睡前服。

本药能补中益气生津，适用于食欲不振、神经衰弱、贫血、胃溃疡、未老先衰、肝炎、关节炎、脉管炎等，是一种高级滋补营养品。

8. 延年益寿精

本品系武汉中联制药厂按清朝太医院秘方"延年益寿丹"之处方，遵古炮制，提取精炼而成。口服液，每支 10 ml，每服 1 支，日 1～2 次，晨起或睡前服。

本品能调节人体新陈代谢，促进组织细胞迟缓老化，改善老年人衰老现象。适用于衰老体弱者。

9. 五加参冲剂

本品由哈尔滨中药一厂研制生产,主要成分为刺五加。冲剂,每块12.25克,每服1块,日2次。

本品能扶正固本、宁神益智,适用于神经衰弱、病后体弱、体倦乏力、失眠多梦、食欲不振、冠心病、白细胞减少症等。

10. 大力士补液

本药由黑龙江中医研究院实验药厂研究生产,主要成分为刺五加、黄芪、丹参等。糖浆剂,每瓶500 ml,每服20 ml,日3次。

大力士补液能滋补强壮、益智宁神,可用于素体虚弱、病后体弱、神疲乏力、腰膝酸软、头目眩晕、心悸怔忡、失眠等。

11. 人参Vit C滋补片

本药由北京制药厂生产,主要成分为人参、维生素C。片剂,每服3~5片,日3次。

本药能补气健体,适用于年老体弱、病后失调、肺虚喘促、脾虚泄泻、神衰健忘、食欲不振、慢性肝炎、糖尿病、贫血、高血压、维生素C缺乏症等。

12. 青春宝

本品由杭州第二中药厂研制生产,主要成分为人参、天冬、熟地黄等。

青春宝能益气、养阴、补精血,适用于中老年人精气不足、阴血亏少、身体衰弱者以及病后体弱等。

13. 万年春滋补浆

万年春滋补浆由无锡市中药厂生产,主要成分为人参、太子参、党参、蜂皇浆、麦冬、制首乌、枸杞子、当归等。口服液,每支10 ml,每服1支,日1次。

本品能补中益气、滋阴养血,适用于气虚血亏、肝肾阴虚、津液不足、病后体弱、食欲减退、神经衰弱、老年体衰等。

2.2.2 养血成药

1. 八珍丸

本方出自《瑞竹堂经验方》,药由人参(党参)、熟地黄、当归、白芍、川芎、茯苓、白术、甘草组成。蜜丸,每丸重9克,每服2丸,日2次。

本品能调补气血,适用于气血亏虚引起的形容憔悴、食欲不振、四肢无力、头晕目眩、月经不调等。也可用于各种贫血、原发性血小板减少性紫癜、风湿性心脏病等。

2. 复方阿胶浆

本品由山东东阿阿胶厂研制生产,其主要成分为阿胶、人参、山楂等。蜜浆剂,每服20 ml,日3次。

复方阿胶浆能益气补血,适用于气血两虚、各种贫血、白细胞减少症等,年老、体弱及运动员服用,可强身壮体、抗病益寿。

3. 康宝

康宝由山东烟台中药厂研制生产,主要成分为刺五加、蜂王浆、淫羊藿、枸杞、黄精、熟地、黄芪、山楂等。蜜浆剂,每瓶100 ml,每服5～10 ml。

本品能补气养血、温肾益精、抗衰老,适用于气血两虚、各种贫血、年老体弱、病后体虚等,亦可作为健康人之防病保健品。

4. 参芪王浆养血精

参芪王浆养血精由吉林省延吉市制药二厂生产,主要成分为蜂王浆、人参精、北芪精等。口服液,每支10 ml,每服1支,日1次,早饭前服。

本品能养血益气、强心健脾,适用于贫血、身体虚弱、年老体弱、神经衰弱、肝炎、脱发等症。

5. 人参首乌精

人参首乌精主要成分为红参、何首乌等。口服液，每支50 ml，每服 10 ml，日 3 次。

本品能养血益气、宁神益智，适用于气血两亏、健忘失眠、食欲不振、肢体倦怠及阳萎早泄等症。

6. 阿胶滋补精

阿胶滋补精的主要成分为阿胶、党参、熟地等。冲剂，每服20 克，日 2 次，开水冲服。

本品能养肝滋肾、大补气血，适用于气血两亏、身体虚弱、年老体弱等症。

7. 两仪冲剂

两仪冲剂主要成分为党参、熟地等。冲剂，每筒 250 克，每服 20 克，日 2 次，开水冲服。

本品能补益气血，适用于气血两亏、身体虚弱、病后体弱等症。

8. 益寿滋补浆

益寿滋补浆的主要成分为人参、何首乌、全当归、白茯苓、金樱子等。糖浆剂，每瓶 300 ml，每服 20 ml，日 2 次。

本品能益气养血、健脾补肾，适用于气血两亏、身体虚弱、须发早白等症。长期服用能补血养心、强筋壮骨、乌须黑发、调经和血。

9. 补血宁神片

补血宁神片系广州红卫制药厂研制生产，主要有效成分为首乌藤、鸡血藤、熟地等。片剂，每服 5 片，日 3 次。

本药能养血安神、滋阴补肾，适用于失眠健忘、夜梦遗精、小便频数、腰膝酸软、月经不调等症。

10. 参归枣汁

参归枣汁系安徽蚌埠中药厂研制生产，主要成分为红枣、太子参、当归等。蜜浆剂，每服 10～20 ml，日 2～3 次，温开水冲服。

本品能养血生津、益气健脾，适用于气血不足、神疲体弱、纳少乏力、诸虚劳损症。

2.2.3 助阳成药

1. 金匮肾气丸

金匮肾气丸出自《金匮要略》，药由熟地、山药、肉桂、丹皮、茯苓、附子、山萸肉、泽泻组成。蜜丸，每丸重9克，每服1丸，日2次。

本药能温补肾阳，适用于肾阳不足、脾胃虚寒、腰酸足软、小腹拘挛、遗精、大便溏泻、小便频数、下肢浮肿等症。

2. 海龙蛤蚧精

海龙蛤蚧精由山东济南中药厂研制生产，其主要成分为海龙、蛤蚧、北芪、人参、首乌、当归、杞子、沉香等。口服液，每瓶10ml，每服1瓶，日1～2次。

本品为一种高级强壮滋补剂，功能补身益气、补血强心、养颜明目，适用于神经衰弱、疲劳过度、气血两亏、腰酸背痛、四肢无力、头晕目眩等症，尤为年老体弱者的滋补佳品。

3. 男宝

男宝（补肾胶囊）由山西省侯马中药厂生产，主要成分为驴肾、狗肾、海马、人参、鹿茸、阿胶、黄芪、山萸肉等。胶囊剂，每粒0.3克，每服2～3粒，日2次。

本药能温肾壮阳、益气健身，适用于肾阳虚衰、阳萎滑泄、腰膝酸痛、肾囊湿冷、精神萎靡、食欲不振等症。

4. 参茸鞭丸

参茸鞭丸由大连中药厂生产，主要成分为人参、鹿茸、貂鞭、海马、杜仲、枸杞、肉桂等。水丸，按该药说明服。

本品能补肾助阳、强精增髓，适用于肾虚气弱、神经衰弱、阳萎、早泄、遗精及男女一切肾虚性疾患。

5. 阳春药

阳春药的主要成分为水貂鞭、梅鹿鞭、广狗鞭、鹿茸、淫羊藿、巴戟天、黄芪、飞阳起石、菟丝子、何首乌、肉苁蓉、山药。胶囊剂，每服2粒，日2次。

本药能健腰助阳、补虚强壮，适用于体质虚弱、身亏遗精、四肢乏力、头晕耳鸣、惊悸健忘、腰膝酸软、记忆减退、神衰失眠、食欲不振等。

6. 益肾糖浆

益肾糖浆由天津第一中药厂研制生产，主要成分为枸杞子、覆盆子、五味子。糖浆剂，每服5~10ml，日服2次。

本品能益肾扶阳、填精补髓，适用于身体虚弱、肾亏阳萎、梦遗滑泄、小便混浊等。

7. 参茸大补丸

参茸大补丸（浙江方）主要由生晒参、鹿茸、肉苁蓉、鹿角胶、锁阳、沉香、肉桂、附子、菟丝子、枸杞子、杜仲、首乌、山药、茯苓、远志等组成。蜜丸，每丸重3.2克，每服1丸，日1~2次。

本药能补肾壮阳、生精益髓，适用于阳虚胃寒、腰膝酸痛、阳萎遗精、早泄、滑精、小便频数等。

8. 雏凤精

雏凤精是由山东济南中药厂研制生产的一种高级强力滋补剂，主要成分为鸡胎、羊鞭、人参、砂仁、黄芪、枸杞、淫羊藿、鹿茸、肉桂、当归、肉苁蓉等。口服液，每瓶10ml，每服1瓶，日2次。

本品能补肾助阳、强腰壮身、益气养血，适用于气血不足、肾阳亏虚引起之贫血、腰酸背痛、四肢乏力、头晕耳鸣、神衰失眠、心慌、用脑过度、记忆减退、食欲不振、性机能减退或妇女子宫寒冷、月经不调等。

9. 海马补肾丸

海马补肾丸由天津第三中药厂根据名医处方研制生产，主要成分为海马、人参、花龙骨、枸杞子、黑驴肾、补骨脂、茯苓、黄芪、核桃仁、鹿茸、蛤蚧尾、海狗肾、鲜对虾、虎骨、花鹿肾、山萸肉、当归等。丸剂，每10粒重2.7克，每服10粒，日2次，空腹服。

本品能补肾壮阳、健脑强身，适用于身体虚弱、气血两亏、肾气不足、面黄肌瘦、心慌气短、腰酸腿软、阳萎遗精等症。

10. 梅花鹿茸血

梅花鹿茸血的主要成分为鹿茸血、梅花鹿茸、刺五加等。口服液，每支10 ml，每服1支，日1次，早饭前服。

本品能温肾壮阳、生精补血，适用于男子性机能衰退、女子月经不调、子宫寒冷、赤白带下、病后及产后虚弱、年老体弱、心脏衰弱、营养不良、贫血、用脑过度、记忆力减退、腰膝酸软、头晕失眠等症。

11. 海参丸

海参丸主要由海参、胡桃肉、羊腰子、猪脊髓、鹿角胶、龟板、杜仲、牛膝、巴戟天、菟丝子、补骨脂、枸杞子、当归组成。蜜丸，每丸重9克，每服1丸，日2次。

本药能补肾壮阳、养血益精，适用于肾阳不足、阳萎遗精、腰膝酸软、头晕耳鸣、四肢乏力等症。

2.2.4 滋阴成药

1. 六味地黄丸

六味地黄丸方出自《小儿药证直诀》，药由熟地黄、山药、山萸肉、茯苓、泽泻、丹皮组成。蜜丸，每丸重9克，每服1丸，日2次。

本药能滋补肝肾，适用于肝肾阴虚之腰膝酸软、眩晕耳鸣、失眠梦遗、消渴口干、潮热盗汗、五心烦热等症。

2. 人参固本丸

人参固本丸由人参、山药、熟地黄、天冬、麦冬、山茱萸蜂蜜、茯苓等药组成。蜜丸，每丸重9克，每服1丸，日2次。

本药能滋阴养血、益气生津，适用于阴虚气弱引起的身体虚弱、心慌气短、腰痛耳鸣、四肢酸软、虚劳骨蒸等。

3. 健脑冲剂

健脑冲剂主要成分为枸杞子、酸枣仁等。颗粒冲剂，每袋14克，每服1袋，日1次，每晚睡前服。

本药能滋肾养阴、健脑养心安神，适用于肝肾阴虚、神经衰弱、失眠健忘、头晕耳鸣、腰膝酸软等症。

4. 参杞蜂皇浆

参杞蜂皇浆由蜂乳、蜂蜜、党参、枸杞子等组成。蜜浆剂，每支10 ml，每服1支，日1～2次。

本品能滋补肝肾、益气明目，适用于肝肾阴虚、头晕目眩、腰膝酸软、食少体倦、年老体弱、病后体弱等症。

5. 滋阴百补丸

滋阴百补丸主要成分为当归、茯苓、远志、牛膝、麦冬、知母、肉苁蓉、枸杞子、女贞子、菟丝子、锁阳、巴戟天、柏子仁、山萸肉等。蜜丸，每25丸重约3克，每服6～9克，日2次。

本药能补肾滋阴、固涩安神，适用于阴虚内热、头晕神疲、腰酸肢软、盗汗遗精、年老体弱等。

6. 康复丸

康复丸为西安国药制药厂研制生产的一种滋补强身成药，主要成分为太子参、当归、五味子、珍珠母、山药、熟地、川断。丸剂，每服10粒，日3次。

本品能益肾补虚、养血固精、强身健体，适用于病后体虚、肝肾阴虚、头晕耳鸣、腰酸乏力、失眠健忘、遗精、盗汗等症。

7. 清宫寿桃丸

清宫寿桃丸是天津达仁堂制药厂根据清宫保健秘方研制生产的一种滋补强壮成药。蜜丸，每丸重6克，每服1丸，日2次。

本药的主要成分为益智仁、大生地、枸杞子、天冬、人参、当归、核桃肉等。

清宫寿桃丸能补肾益元、滋阴助阳、补气养血、延年益寿，是年老体弱、病后体虚以及各种虚弱症患者却病强身、抗老益寿之佳品。

2.2.5 其他保健成药

1. 灵芝片

灵芝片（冲剂）是广西中医学院药厂研制生产的保健品，主要成分为灵芝。片剂每片1克，每服1~2片，日2次；冲剂每块13克（含生药3克），每服1块，日1次。

本品能补心安神、健脾和胃、滋补强壮、延年益寿，适用于神经衰弱、头晕失眠、食欲不振、冠心病、高脂血症等，又是年老体弱者的保健佳品。

2. 益脑复健丸

益脑复健丸主要成分为三七、西红花、川芎等。胶囊剂，每粒0.3克，每服6~8粒，日3次。

本品能益脑健神、舒经通络、活血化瘀、豁痰开窍，适用于急性缺血性中风引起的口眼歪斜、半身不遂、舌蹇语涩等症。

3. 脑灵素

脑灵素由佳木斯中药厂、山东临沂健康药厂等生产，主要成分为人参、鹿茸、龟板、鹿角胶、酸枣仁、枸杞子、五味子、茯苓、远志等。糖衣片，每片重0.5克，每服2~3片，日2次。

本品能补气血、养心肾、健脑安神，适用于神经衰弱、健忘失眠、头晕目眩、心悸气短、倦怠无力、体虚自汗、阳萎遗精等。

4. 优康平

优康平是山东威海制药厂参照古方研制生产的一种保健成药，其主要成分为银耳、五加参、五味子、丹参、板蓝根、甘草等。饴糖剂型,每块 5.2 克,每服 1~2 块,日 2~3 次。

本品能扶正固本、养血安神、清热解毒,增强机体抵抗力。对流感、肝炎有抵抗和预防作用。能促进机体发育,成人、老年人久服可大补元气、增强体质。

5. 安神补心丸

安神补心丸由上海中药一厂生产,主要成分为丹参、五味子、石菖蒲、合欢皮、墨旱莲、女贞子、首乌藤、生地、珍珠母等。丸剂,每服 15 粒,日 3 次。

本品能滋阴养血、补心安神,适用于心悸、失眠、头晕耳鸣等。

6. 益春宝口服液

益春宝口服液的主要成分为鹿茸提取物、蜂王浆、刺五加浸膏等。口服液,每支 10 ml,每服 1 支,日 1 次,晨起或睡前服。

本品可强心健脾、补肾安神、益气养血,适用于神经衰弱、精力不足、食欲不振、发育不良、年老体弱、产后病后体弱等,并可用于运动员及少年儿童保健。

7. 灵芝强体片

灵芝强体片主要成分为人参、灵芝等。片剂,按该药说明服。

本品能益气养血、补益强壮,适用于神经衰弱、头晕耳鸣、心烦失眠、食欲不振、贫血萎黄、少气乏力等症。

8. 丹七片

丹七片由北京同仁堂制药厂研制生产,主要成分为三七、丹参。片剂,每服 3 片,日 3 次。

本药能强心扩冠、活血化瘀,并有一定的强壮滋补作用。适用于冠心病心绞痛、神经衰弱等。

9. 女宝

女宝是长春中医学院与吉林省东丰制药厂联合研制的一种妇

科新型保健药，主要成分为人参、鹿胎、鹿茸、红花、丹参、丹皮、川芎、阿胶等。胶囊剂，每粒0.3克，每服4粒，日3次。

本品能益气活血、滋阴助阳、调经止带，适用于妇女月经不调、痛经、闭经、带下、宫冷不孕、产后诸疾等，也可用于男子虚劳精衰、腰膝酸软等症。

10. 更年安

更年安由天津第三中药厂生产，主要成分为熟地、何首乌、泽泻、茯苓、五味子、珍珠母、夜交藤、玄参、浮小麦等。片剂，每片0.3克，每服6片，日2~3次。

本品能滋阴清热、除烦安神、健身养神、益寿延年，适用于男、女更年期综合征以及各种阴虚阳亢之老年性疾病。

2.3 保健药酒

药酒是一种中药与酒相结合的液体剂型。一般用白酒、黄酒或米酒浸泡或煎煮中药，去除药渣而成；或者用中药和糯米、粳米或秫米之类谷物一起，加酒曲发酵酿制，去糟渣而得。药酒既有口服者，也有外用的；既可用以治疗疾病，又可用于预防疾病、保健养生。用于滋补保健、养生延寿、预防疾病或病后康复调理的口服药酒，在药酒中占有很大比例，常称作保健药酒。运用药酒作保健，是中医传统的有特色的保健方法之一。

药酒古称醪醴。在《内经·汤液醪醴论》中论述了汤液醪醴的制法和治疗作用。后至东汉末年张仲景《金匮要略》载红蓝花酒，治妇人腹中刺痛。唐代以来，临床上广泛应用药酒，如唐代孙思邈《备急千金要方》、《千金翼方》和王焘《外台秘要》均载多种药酒方，后世的方药著作中收载药酒方更加丰富，明代李时珍《本草纲目·酒》中就介绍69种药酒。解放后大量生产的三鞭酒、龟龄集酒等，深受国内外欢迎。随着精神文明、物质文明的发展，药酒，特别是保健药酒，将进一步得到发展和广泛应用，为人民健康作出更大贡献。

2.3.1 药酒的保健作用

酒是广受人们喜爱的饮料,药酒是药以饮料的形式出现,服用方便,宜于长久坚持。服用药酒已成为一种许多人乐于接受的保健养生方法。恰当地选服药酒,可发挥以下几方面的保健作用。

1. 协调阴阳

人体的健康长寿,有赖于阴阳平衡,阴平阳秘。阴阳平衡失调,则易患疾病,或加速衰老。保健药酒有的偏于补阳,有的偏于滋阴,亦有阴阳双补。根据不同机体阴阳平衡失调的具体情况,常服相应的药酒,有助于协调阴阳,保持阴阳动态平衡,而保持健康长寿。

2. 补益气血

气血是人体生命活动的重要物质基础。气表现于脏腑组织的功能活动,生命活动的维持依赖于"气"的温煦、推动、气化、防御、营养和固摄等功能,又依赖于"血"内养五脏六腑、外濡皮毛筋骨的作用。气血亏虚,则百疾易攻,早衰易老。凡有气虚、血亏者,服用有益气或养血作用的保健药酒,使气旺血盛,则生命力旺盛,祛病抗老。

3. 滋补五脏

肝、心、脾、肺、肾五脏具有化生和储藏精、气、血和津液等精微营养物质的生理功能。人体的生、长、壮、老,在很大程度上取决于五脏功能的正常与否,取决于脏腑之气(特别是肾气)的盛衰。五脏虚衰是许多内伤杂病的原因,又可导致和加速衰老。各脏器分别专司不同的功能,根据有关的脏腑虚损证候可确定何脏虚衰。若根据脏腑所虚的具体情况,服用相应的滋补药酒,就能使脏腑机能恢复正常,从而使身体强健。祖国医学认为肾为先天之本,脾胃为后天之本,两者与健康长寿关系最密切。所以滋补保健药酒中以补肾固本药酒和补脾健胃药酒较多,也较常用。心为"五脏六腑之主",主神明,主血脉,养心安神药酒也属常用。

4. 祛病驱邪

除各类滋补药酒之外,自古就流传和应用许多祛风湿、散寒邪或温经通络活血的药酒。这些药酒不仅用于疾病的治疗,也有一定的保健作用。如平素易感受风寒湿邪,或有血瘀络阻倾向者,服用相应药酒,有祛邪防病的作用。若患风寒湿痹、中风偏瘫或胸痹心痛等病证,经汤剂、丸散剂治疗之后,康复阶段适量服用适当的药酒,则有利于加快康复,恢复功能和预防复发,从而做到祛病健身或带病延年。

5. 延年益寿

分析衰老的原因,多与阴阳失调、五脏虚衰、气血亏虚,精耗神伤有关,故各类滋补保健药酒多兼有补益抗衰、延缓衰老的作用。在几千年的抗老延寿探索中,也发现不少确有延缓衰老作用的保健药物和药酒,经常服用就有强身体、壮筋骨、乌须发、明耳目、泽肌肤、悦容颜等作用,使人老而不衰,延长寿命。

2.3.2 药酒保健的机理

许多中药的有效成分可以溶解于酒(乙醇)中,这是药酒发挥作用的物质基础。几千年的临床经验和现代实验研究证明,保健药酒常用的中药及其有效成分确可从各方面发挥保健延寿作用。如:人参有较好的临床抗衰老作用,提高免疫功能,调节内分泌功能,促进蛋白质合成,增强抗疲劳能力,抗心肌缺血,降血糖,增强造血机能;黄芪延长体外培养细胞株寿命,提高免疫力,增强肌力和应激能力,促进蛋白质合成,扩张血管,降血压;灵芝提高免疫功能和耐缺氧能力,抗心肌缺血,调节核酸、蛋白质代谢,清除羟自由基从而抗衰老;当归增强造血机能,提高免疫能力,增加肌力和耐寒力,保护肝脏,增加心肌营养性血流量,抗心肌缺血和心律失常,抑制血小板聚集,防止血栓形成，通过抗氧化作用延缓衰老；何首乌抗动脉粥样硬化和抗心肌缺血，提高细胞免疫，抑制过氧化脂质，促进过氧化物歧化酶活性而抗衰老；枸杞子降血糖、降胆固醇，减轻动脉粥样硬化，保护肝脏；山楂降血压，降血脂，抗心肌缺血，促进消化；菊花增加冠脉流量，抗心肌缺血，抗血栓，并富含具有抗衰老作用的微量元素硒，等等。这些中药制成的药酒，如人参酒、灵芝酒、首乌酒、枸杞酒、菊花酒、当归酒和许多复方药酒，就能通过上述机理发挥滋补保健、抗衰防老的作用。

近年来，对某些复方保健药酒进行了基础实验研究和机理探讨。上海医药工业研究院对十全大补酒的研究表明，能增强非特异性免疫，增进胃肠蠕动，增加冠脉流量，提高耐缺氧能力，可以部分解释该药酒补气健脾强身临床疗效的机理。山西中药厂等研究了龟龄集酒，证明可使巨噬细胞活性显著增加，网状内皮系统清除异物的能力明显提高，抗体产生的水平显著增加，提示促进特异性与非特异性免疫功能；还具有增强中枢神经功能，提高识别和记忆能力的作用，还具有强心、镇静等作用，提示对大脑皮层功能有促进兴奋和抑制的双向调节作用。第一军区大学的研究表明，人参王浆酒含有多种游离氨基酸和水溶性维生素等营养物质，有增强和促进机体性机能作用，有显著的抗疲劳和强壮作用，能增强正常和免疫功能低下机体的细胞免疫、体液免疫、特异性免疫和非特异性免疫功能。这一类工作还有待更广泛、深入地进行。现代科学研究将不仅充分肯定保健药酒的作用，还将深入认识其作用机理，指导对药酒的应用。

2.3.3 药酒保健的特点

1. 酒助药势，提高药效

酒有通血脉、御寒气、助药势之效。如《本草纲目》所说："少饮则和血行气，壮神御寒"。《名医别录》则曰："主行药势"。酒性温热，宜和百脉，可使滋补、散寒、温通、活血等药物更好地发挥功效，提高治疗效果。酒的主要成分是乙醇，是一种良好的有机溶媒，又有良好的穿透性，易于进入药材组织细胞中，发挥溶解作用。中药的许多有效成分，如生物碱及其盐类、挥发油、甙、鞣质、有机酸、树脂、糖类及部分色素等，都较易溶解于酒中，使中药的效果更好地发挥。有人以对小鼠免疫功能影响为指标，对比观察龟龄集酒与龟龄集原始粉、龟龄集升炼药粉，证明以龟龄集酒的作用最好。

2. 作用广泛，应用灵活

保健药酒的作用很广泛，一般人服用可强身健体防病；中老年人服用可抗衰延寿；因脏腑阴阳气血失调所致各种慢性病患者服用，有辅助治疗和促进康复的作用。由于配制方便，可以根据个体的实际状况以及季节、药源等，灵活调整组方，随时配制服用。

3. 药性稳定，服用方便

酒有一定的防腐作用，若含乙醇 40% 以上，还可延缓许多药物有效成分水解，增强了稳定性。药酒适合长期存放，也方便经常服用。保健药酒中常常选用药食两用之食疗中药，如龙眼、山楂、桑椹、枸杞、薏米、菊花等，所用其他滋补保健中药也大多为药性平和之品，适量服用一般保健药酒也是较安全的。

2.3.4 保健药酒的适用范围

1. 补气药酒

适用于有气虚见证者。气虚的表现为：神疲乏力，少气懒言，肢体倦怠，饮食减少，自汗，舌质淡胖或有齿印，脉虚无力。

2. 养血药酒

适于血虚者服用。血虚的见证：面色苍白或萎黄，头晕眼花，起立时眼前昏暗，唇舌色淡，指甲淡白，手足发麻，舌质淡，脉细。

3. 滋阴药酒

适用于阴虚者。阴虚表现为：五心烦热，午后升火，口干咽燥，虚烦不眠，头晕目眩，盗汗，便秘尿赤，舌红或少苔、无苔，脉细数。

4. 助阳药酒

适用于有阳虚证候者。阳虚见证：全身或局部畏寒或肢冷，面足浮肿，阳痿精冷，夜尿频多，便溏而尿清长，舌淡胖苔润，脉沉微迟。

5. 补五脏药酒

分别适用于某脏虚损者。

心虚见证：心悸胸闷，失眠多梦，健忘，脉结代或细弱。

肝虚见证：头晕目眩，急躁易怒或情志抑郁，喜叹息，双目干涩，肢体麻木，脉弦细。

脾虚见证：食欲减退，食后腹胀，喜按，面色萎黄，肌瘦无力，大便溏泄。

肺虚见证：喘促气短，久咳，痰白，易患感冒。

肾虚见证：腰脊酸痛，胫酸膝软或足跟痛，耳鸣耳聋，发脱齿摇，尿后有余沥或失禁，性功能减退，不育、不孕。

6. 延年益寿药酒

适用于一般中老年服用。这类药酒多兼有补肾健脾、补养气血等功效。

7. 防治疾病的保健药酒

适用于某些特定疾病的预防、辅助治疗和病后康复调理。

另有气血双补药酒，适用于既有气虚见证，又有血虚表现者；阴阳双补药酒，适用于兼有阴虚、阳虚证候者。

2.3.5 药酒的制作方法

药酒的制作方法有多种，如冷浸法、热浸法、酿制法、渗漉法、回流加热法等。家庭制作保健药酒主要用前两法，后两法主要用于工业化生产,不作详细介绍。欲制出高质量的药酒,必须注意原料、配制方法和工具。

1. 原料

(1) 酒

酒是配制药酒的溶媒,本身亦有一定功效,所以应有适当选择。最常用的是白酒和黄酒。

白酒,又称烧酒,市售各种大曲、二曲、老窖等皆为白酒,属于蒸馏酒,一般酒精含量较高,在 40~60% 左右。用白酒配制的药酒稳定性较好,平素有一定酒量者多喜饮用。由于含酒精量较多,过量饮入酒精有害于健康,平素不喜爱饮酒者宜少饮,或用低度白酒(含乙醇量 40% 左右)配制,或改用黄酒配制。

黄酒,是一种发酵酒,如绍兴酒即属黄酒,含酒精量较低,一般在 20% 以下,尚含有葡萄糖、麦芽糖、氨基酸等,有一定营养保健价值。黄酒配制的药酒,较适合于不喜爱饮酒者,年老体弱者。由于含酒精量低,稳定性可能较差,配制后应及时饮用。葡萄酒也属于含酒精量低的(一般 7~8%)发酵酒。

配制药酒所选用的白酒或黄酒,都应该用质量较好者。

(2) 药材

按照处方和规定的用量备好中药材后,应作适当加工炮制。凡规定应该炮制者,均应以传统正规的方法认真炮制,以保证药效和减少副作用。应注意去除杂质,必要时适当清洗。药材应适度切制或粉碎,以扩大药材和酒的接触面,有利于有效成分浸出。但也不宜粉碎过细,以免药酒混浊。

有时药酒中还可加适量冰糖或蜂蜜以调味。

2. 制法

(1) 冷浸法

将适当切制或粉碎的药材,置于适宜容器内,按处方规定加入适量酒,密封浸泡,每日搅拌或振荡 1 次,7 日后可适当减少搅拌振荡次数,浸泡 15~20 天左右(冬季可适当延长时间),取上清液，与药楂压榨液合并，静置过滤即得。

(2) 热浸法

方法与冷浸法基本相同，要将盛有药材和酒的容器隔水加热，至液面出现泡沫时（有称鱼眼沸），取下容器，密封，或换注于另一适宜容器内密封，继续浸泡半月以上，取上清液，与药渣压榨液合并，静置过滤即得。

以上两法均可将适度粉碎的药材装于布袋内，悬于酒中，依法制取。

另外，也可将药材加水煎煮，滤药汁，加热浓缩成稠膏，冷却后加入适量酒，置容器内密封，若干天后取上清液过滤而得。药材含芳香挥发性成分时不宜用本法。

(3) 酿制法

将糯米（或秫米、粳米）加水浸泡，蒸煮成饭，冷却至30℃左右，加入酒曲和加工好的药材（或药材煎煮滤汁浓缩的药汁）拌匀，置适当容器内，密封，保持适当温度，经1~2周发酵即成，压榨过滤得澄清酒液，盛入存贮容器，隔水加热至75°~80℃，杀灭酵母菌及杂菌，以便贮存和保证质量。此法所制药酒药性作用较和缓，宜于老年人和身体虚弱者长期服用。

3. 工具

制备药酒应选用适当的容器。以保证不与药材成分起化学反应为原则。多用陶瓷、玻璃或不锈钢器具。家庭多用瓷坛、瓷瓮、砂锅、玻璃瓶等。容器应有盖，以便密封，防止酒挥发。不可使用铁、锡器具。

2.3.6 服用药酒注意事项

1. 掌握适应范围，辨证服用药酒

中医讲究辨证论治，服用药酒也要掌握辨证用酒的原则。根据不同个体的体质特点和证候表现，辨其虚实、寒热及脏腑、气血、阴阳等，服用相应对证的药酒，才能有较好的效果。对于每种药酒,都要按照其功效和适用范围来使用。并不是任何人都可随便服用滋补或延年益寿的药酒。

2. 注意酒精毒性,掌握禁忌、用量

药酒中含有一定量的酒精。少量饮酒,摄入酒精量不多,尚有益而无大害。有研究资料表明,每日饮酒不超过相当于白酒30克的量,有助于减少冠心病所致死亡的危险性。有人提出,为了安全,每日酒精的摄入量须限制在45克以下。长期过量饮酒对肝脏、心脏、神经系统等都有危害,还有致畸作用。对于过量饮酒的危害,祖国医学早有论述,《本草纲目》指出:"面曲之酒,少饮则和血行气,壮神御寒,消愁遣兴;痛饮则伤神耗血,损胃亡精,生痰动火。……若夫沉缅无度,醉以为常者,轻则致疾败行,其则丧邦亡家而陨躯命,其害可胜言哉?"所以,服用药酒有一定的限制和禁忌,还要掌握适当用量。一般说来,患肝脏疾患,严重心脏病或心功能不全,消化性溃疡,活动性肺结核,慢性肾炎,慢性肠炎,严重高血压,妇女孕期、哺乳期,儿童及对酒精过敏者,都不宜服用药酒。有些药酒因所含药物的关系,有特殊的禁忌规定,如有的在妇女月经期禁用,有的阴虚火旺者禁用等。服用量一般根据药酒的性质、服用者体质及病情等确定。对于规定的服用量,一般不要超过。若含有药性猛峻甚至有毒性的药物,尤宜慎用,服量宜小,并从小量开始,无明显不良反应时适当逐渐加量。若药性平和,年轻力壮,或病情较重时,用量可稍大;年老、体弱、妇女,或病情轻者,用量宜稍小。不喜爱饮酒或酒量小者,用量宜小,或用黄酒、低度白酒配制药酒。长期服用药酒滋补或抗衰老者。每次服用量也宜较小些。

3. 其它注意事项

服用药酒要注意时令。酒性温热,尤其是温补性药酒,最适于冬季服用,若夏季服用则宜减量。

疾病的部位不同,服用药酒的适宜时间也不同。病在胸膈以上者,一般在饭后服用;病在腹部以下的,宜在进饮食前服用;

养心安神药酒或调经种子药酒，应在晚上服用。

药酒的贮存，应注意密封，存阴凉干燥处。

2.3.7 常用保健药酒

我国古今记载和应用的保健药酒甚多，这里只能选介一小部分。选介的原则是：1. 适于家庭自制；2. 药效较可靠；3. 药性较平和；4. 药材较易购买；5. 药味较少。大部分药酒方出自古今医籍及临床报道，有的对剂量等略作调整，有的根据作者经验有所修改，亦有作者经验方。一般配制方法已于前述，除需特别说明者外，不再详述制法。

1. 补气药酒

(1) 人参酒

人参 30 克，为粗末，装瓶中，加白酒 500 克，冷浸法或热浸法配制。每日早、晚各服 10～15 ml。不必去除药渣，饮完后可再加适量白酒浸泡 1 次。待酒服尽，可食药渣。

有大补元气，补益脾肺，生津固脱，安神益智之效。适用于气虚诸证。凡元气不足，久病气虚，劳伤虚损所致气短乏力，倦怠神疲，食欲不振，眩晕心悸，津伤口渴，自汗虚脱，阳痿，消渴等症皆可服用。有抗衰老效果。

(2) 参芪益气酒

黄芪 45 克，党参 45 克，陈皮 9 克，大枣 10 枚，白酒 1000 克，冷浸法或热浸法配制。每日早、晚各温服 10～20 ml。

有益气健脾开胃之效。适用于一般气虚乏力，少气懒言，神疲倦怠，食欲不振等症。药性平和，但作用逊于人参酒。

(3) 三圣酒

人参 21 克，山药 21 克，白术 21 克，白酒 500 克，冷浸法或热浸法配制。每日早、午、晚各空腹温服 10～20 ml。

有补元气，健脾胃之效。适用于体虚气弱，神疲纳呆，面黄肌瘦之症。方出《圣济总录》。

(4) 黄芪生脉酒

人参 30 克，黄芪 60 克，麦冬 18 克，五味子 12 克，白酒 1000 克，冷浸法或热浸法配制。每日早、晚各服 10～20 ml。

能大补元气，兼滋阴生津，固表敛汗。用于气虚为主而兼阴虚津伤之症，如心肺气阴不足，喘咳自汗，口渴，舌红干少苔，脉虚无力者，或热伤元气，气短自汗，口渴，舌红少苔，脉虚者，皆可服用。本方系著名的生脉散方增入黄芪，加强了益气固表作用。

(5) 长生固本酒

人参 60 克，枸杞子 60 克，山药 60 克，五味子 60 克，天冬 60 克，麦冬 60 克，生地黄 60 克，熟地黄 60 克，诸药切制成片，以生绢袋盛之，浸于 15kg 酒中，坛口以箬竹叶封固，将酒坛置于锅中，隔水加热，约半小时，取出酒坛，埋土中数日出火毒，取出静置，滤出药酒。每日早、晚各服 10～20 ml。

本方出自《寿世保元》，有益气养阴，滋补肝肾之效。适用于气阴两虚所致疲倦乏力，腰酸腿软，心烦口干，头晕目眩，心悸多梦，须发早白等症。家庭配制时可酌减药、酒之量，热浸法或冷浸法制备。

2. 养血药酒

(1) 阿胶酒

阿胶 75 克，黄酒 500 克，将阿胶细块置入小坛内，加入适量黄酒，以淹没阿胶为准，将坛置文火上煮沸，边煮边续添黄酒，至酒添尽，阿胶化尽，取下小坛候冷，收贮于瓶中。每日早、午、晚各空腹温服 20～30 ml。

有补血滋阴，止血，清肺润燥功效。适用于阴血亏虚，面色萎黄，头晕目眩，心悸心烦，虚烦不眠，阴虚燥咳及各种出血证，妇女崩漏，月经过多，妊娠下血，小产后下血等的病后调理。

(2) 龙眼桑椹酒

龙眼肉30克,桑椹30克,加白酒500克,冷浸法制备。用黄酒配制亦可。也可用酿制法制备。不加白酒,另用适量粳米、酒曲。每日早、晚各服15～20 ml。

有养血滋阴,补益心脾,安神生津等功效。适用于血虚阴亏、心脾不足所致头晕目眩,心悸失眠,食少体倦,记忆减退,须发早白等症。两药均为果品,即便无明显症状亦可适量服用,有养心益脾、滋补益智之效。

(3) 归圆酒

菊花250克,枸杞子500克,当归250克,龙眼肉1500克,白酒15公斤,酒酿5公斤,冷浸法或热浸法配制。每日早、晚各服10～20 ml。

有养血益精,补益心脾肝肾,安神明目之效。适用于血虚精亏,心脾肝肾不足,面色萎黄,头晕目眩,视物昏花,心悸失眠,体弱健忘等症。本药酒方载《集验良方》、《惠直堂经验方》等,又称养生酒、归圆杞菊酒。另有《食鉴本草》归圆仙酒只用当归、龙眼肉,专于补血养心。

(4) 圆肉补血酒

龙眼肉250克,制首乌250克,鸡血藤250克,米酒1500克,冷浸法制备。每日早、晚各服10～20 ml。

有补血益精,滋补肝肾,养心安神,活血通络之效。适用于心血不足,肝肾亏虚,面色无华,头晕目眩,心悸失眠,须发早白等症。

(5) 胶艾酒

阿胶30克,当归30克,艾叶9克,生地15克,川芎15克,白芍21克,甘草9克,黄酒250克,将黄酒倒入砂锅,加入温开水250克,放入粗碎的各药(阿胶除外),置文火上煮百沸,取下待温,滤渣,将滤得的药酒倒入砂锅,加入阿胶细块,置文火上煮,注意搅拌,待阿胶化尽即成。若用于治疗,以上为1日量,早、午、晚分3次空腹温服。用于保健及病后调理,服量酌减。

有养血活血、止血、调经、安胎之效。适用于妇女血虚、冲任虚损引起的月经过多、崩漏不止，或妊娠下血，胎动不安，或产后下血，淋漓不断。胶艾汤为《金匮要略》方，《千金方》始用酒剂。

3. 滋阴药酒

(1) 女贞子酒

女贞子 90 克，黄酒 500 克，冷浸法配制。每日早、晚各空腹温服 20 ml。

能滋阴血，补肝肾，清虚热，强筋骨，乌发明目。适用于肝肾阴虚，头晕目眩，视物不明，腰膝酸软，筋骨无力，须发早白等症。《医便》记载该酒有延年之功。

(2) 二冬酒

天冬 60 克，麦冬 60 克，米酒 500 克，冷浸法制备。每日早、晚空腹服 20～30 ml。

有养阴清肺，滋肾益胃，清心除烦，生津润燥等功效。适用于肺燥咳嗽，痰粘咯血，津亏口渴，心烦不安，肠燥便秘等症。

(3) 银耳香菇酒

白木耳 30 克，香菇 30 克，米酒 500 克，热浸法制备。可加适量冰糖调味。每日早、午、晚各空腹服 20 ml。

能滋阴益气，润肺养胃。该酒性甚平和，一般体弱多病的中老年人皆可服用，偏阴虚气弱者服之尤佳。肺热阴亏，咳嗽咯血及肿瘤患者可作辅助治疗或康复调理之用。白木耳、香菇的提取物有提高免疫力，，抗癌和降血脂作用。

(4) 枸杞药酒

枸杞药酒的主要成分为枸杞子、熟地黄、黄精、百合、远志、白酒等。药厂生产的药酒剂，每服 10～15 ml，日 2～3 次，温服。

本品能滋肾益肝，适用于肝肾不足、体弱羸瘦、腰膝酸软、失眠、年老病后体虚等。

(5) 洋参固本酒

西洋参 21 克，天冬 30 克，麦冬 30 克，生地 30 克，熟地 30 克，白酒 1500 克，热浸法配制，其中隔水煮沸的时间宜适当延长。每日早、晚各空腹服 10～20 ml。

有养阴益气，滋补精血功效。适用于阴亏气虚精衰所致形体消瘦，精力衰减，骨蒸烦热，口干咽燥，短气干咳，腰膝酸软，面容憔悴，须发早白，精亏不孕等症。该酒之中药方系人参固本丸方易人参为西洋参，更偏专滋阴。《瑞竹堂经验方》认为人参固本丸能使"髭发不白，颜貌不衰，延年益寿"。

(6) 春寿酒

天冬、麦冬、熟地、生地、山药、莲子肉、红枣各 30 克，加酒 2500 克，热浸法制备。每日早、晚各空腹服 20 ml。

有滋养阴血，益肾健脾之效。适用于阴精不足，脾肾亏虚所致面容憔悴，须发早白，口燥咽干，心烦不宁，胃纳减少，肢倦乏力等症。该酒与洋参固本酒相比，加强了益肾健脾之力，而后者滋阴益气之效更著。本药酒方出《万氏家传养生四要》。

(7) 固精酒

枸杞子 120 克，当归 60 克，熟地 180 克，白酒（或黄酒）3000 克，热浸法配制，隔水加热时间宜适当延长。每日早、晚各空腹饮 20 ml。

该酒养阴益精补血，滋补肝肾。宜于阴虚血少精亏之头晕目眩，视物不明，腰膝酸软，须发早白，遗精早泄，男性不育等症。据其功效应用，《惠直堂经验方》所载该药酒称之固精酒。

4. 助阳药酒

(1) 仙灵脾酒

淫羊藿 60 克，白酒（或米酒）500 克，冷浸法配制。每日早、晚各空腹服 10～15 ml。

有壮阳益肾补肝，强筋骨，祛风湿之效。适用于肾阳不足之男子阳痿、女子不孕,及腰膝酸软,畏寒乏力,四肢麻木,筋骨挛急,风湿痹痛等症。

(2) 蛤蚧酒

蛤蚧1对(去头足,粗碎),黄酒1000克,冷浸法制备。每日早、晚各空腹服10~20 ml。

可助肾阳,补肺气,益精血,定喘嗽。适用于肾阳不足之阳痿,肾虚作喘,肺虚咳嗽,虚劳喘咳及久病阳气虚弱,神疲气短诸症。

(3) 鹿茸酒

鹿茸9克,山药30克,白酒500克,冷浸法配制。每日早、晚各空腹饮服10~15 ml。

有补肾阳,益精血,强筋骨,调冲任等功效。适用于阳虚精亏之神疲乏力,筋骨无力头晕目眩,耳聋健忘;男子阳痿,阴囊湿冷,滑精遗尿;女子白带清稀,宫冷不孕等症。该方为《普济方》等收载。

(4) 复方鹿茸虫草酒

鹿茸6克,冬虫夏草30克,枸杞子30克,白酒500克,冷浸法制备。每日早、晚各空腹服10~15 ml。

功效应用与鹿茸酒相似,更有补肺,补肝肾,平喘止咳化痰之所长,又可用于肺肾亏虚之痰饮喘咳等症。

(5) 羊肾二仙酒

羊外肾(睾丸)1对,淫羊藿150克,仙茅150克,枸杞子150克,菟丝子150克,白酒10 kg,冷浸法制备。每日早、晚各空腹10 ml。

有壮阳补肾益肝,强筋壮骨之效。适用于阳虚体弱,肝肾不足,神疲乏力,畏寒倦怠,腰膝酸软,筋骨不健,阳痿精冷,宫冷不孕等症。

(6) 三鞭补酒

三鞭补酒系山东烟台中药厂研制生产的一种高级滋补品,它的主要成分为海狗鞭、梅鹿鞭、广狗鞭、人参、鹿茸、大海马、大蛤蚧、上肉桂、上沉香、飞阳起石、五花龙骨、覆盆子、补骨脂、菟丝子、淫羊藿、何首乌、桑螵蛸、巴戟天、山萸肉、丹皮、黄芪、牛膝、杞果、生地、熟地、黄柏、川椒、杭芍、当归、白术、云苓、肉苁蓉、泽泻、菖蒲、小茴香、甘松、山药、杜仲、远志、高粱酒等。本品为药酒剂，每服 30 ml，日 2 次。

本品能生精补血，健脑补肾，适用于体质虚弱，未老先衰，腰背酸痛，贫血头晕，自汗盗汗，面色苍白，肾亏遗精，神经衰弱，用脑过度，惊悸健忘，畏寒失眠，气虚食少等症。长期服用可强身壮体，防病抗老，益寿延年。

(7) 东北三宝酒

东北三宝酒由吉林中药厂生产，主要成分为人参、鹿茸、貂鞭。药酒剂，每服 10～30 ml，日 2 次。

本品能温肾壮阳，益气健脑，适用于肾阳虚衰、阳痿早泄、腰膝酸软、阴囊湿冷等。

(8) 琼浆

琼浆由北京中药厂研制生产，主要成分为人参、鹿茸、龙眼肉、陈皮、狗脊、枸杞子、补骨脂、黄精、金樱子、淫羊藿、冬虫夏草、怀牛膝、灵芝、当归、佛手、雀脑。药酒剂，每服 9～15 ml，日 2～3 次。

本品能温肾壮阳，滋补气血，适用于体质虚弱，精神倦怠，腰酸腿软，四肢无力，阳痿不举，遗精早泄等症。

5. 气血双补药酒

(1) 芪归双补酒

黄芪、党参、当归、龙眼肉、桑椹子各 30 克，陈皮 9 克，白酒（或黄酒）1500 克，热浸法或冷浸法配制。每日早、晚各空腹服 10～20 ml。

有益气补血，养心健胃之效。适用于一般身体虚弱，气血不足所致精神不振，面色萎黄，疲乏无力，少气懒言，头晕目眩，心悸健忘，食欲不振等症。

(2) 八珍酒

人参9克（或党参30克），茯苓21克，白术21克，当归21克，白芍21克，熟地24克，川芎12克，甘草9克，生姜9克，大枣10枚，白酒（或黄酒）3000克，热浸法制备。每日早、晚各空腹服10～15 ml。

主要功效是补益气血，适用范围与芪归双补酒相似。该酒又有健脾行血之所长，脾胃不足，气虚血少，心肺亏损等症皆宜。

(3) 十全大补酒

黄芪45克，党参45克，茯苓30克，白术30克，熟地45克，当归30克，白芍30克，川芎15克，肉桂15克，甘草15克，白酒5000克，冷浸法或热浸法制备。每日早、晚各空腹服10～15 ml。

该酒比八珍酒补力更大，药性偏温，适用于气血双亏而见症偏于虚寒者。

6. 阴阳双补药酒

(1) 虫草酒

冬虫夏草30克，白酒500克，冷浸法制备。每日早、晚各空腹服10～20 ml。不必去除药渣，饮完后可再加适量白酒浸泡1次。

虫草酒既补肾阳，又补肺阴，兼止血化痰，平喘止咳。一般病后体虚不复，神疲乏力，食欲不振或自汗畏寒者均可服该酒以保健。阳痿遗精，腰膝酸软，或久咳虚喘，痨嗽咯血亦可服之作辅助治疗或促进康复。

(2) 二仙酒

仙茅30克，淫羊藿30克，巴戟天30克，当归30克，黄柏21克，知母30克，白酒2000克，冷浸法配制。每日早、午、晚各空腹饮服10～20 ml。

有补肾阳，滋肾阴，泻肾火，调冲任之效。适用于更年期高血压、更年期综合征或妇女月经不调、闭经以及其他慢性病见有阴阳两虚而虚火上炎者。

(3) 滋阴百补药酒

熟地、生地、制首乌、枸杞子、沙苑子、鹿角胶各90克，当归、胡桃肉、龙眼肉各75克，肉苁蓉、白芍、人参、牛膝、白术、玉竹、龟板胶、白菊花、五加皮各60克，黄芪、锁阳、杜仲、地骨皮、丹皮、知母各45克，黄柏、肉桂各30克，以上药粗碎，绢袋盛之，适量热酒冲入，密封坛口，浸15～20日，滤出药酒可用。药渣可再加适量酒浸泡。每日早、晚各空腹随量热饮。以上药量，首次用酒量以25～30 kg左右为宜，以后复浸时酒量减半。每次饮服10～20 ml。

该酒见于《林氏活人录汇编》。有滋阴补阳，养血益精补气，补益五脏，强健筋骨等多方面功效。适用于阴阳两虚，气血不足，五脏虚衰所引起的虚损诸证。有阴阳气血虚弱表现的中老年人经常适量服用，可增强体质，可望获延缓衰老之效。

7. 补益五脏药酒

前述几类药酒都有对某脏或几脏的补益作用，补益五脏药酒对气血阴阳也有调补作用。下面只举例简介。

(1) 茯苓酒

茯苓60克，白酒500克，冷浸法制备。每日早、中、晚饭前空腹饮服10～20 ml，亦可睡前饮服。

有健脾补虚，养心安神之效。适用于脾虚体弱，食欲不振，倦怠乏力，肌肉麻痹消瘦，心悸失眠等症。

(2) 神仙药酒丸

木香9克，丁香6克，檀香6克，茜草60克，砂仁15克，红曲30克，共研细末，炼密和丸，以作泡酒用。每丸约重9克，1～3丸泡酒500克，饮服适量。《清太医院配方》收载此方，称有"开胃健脾，快膈宽胸，顺气消食"之效。用茜草量较大，是为使白酒转红，应用时可酌减。脾胃不健，不思饮食，食后腹胀者宜服。

(3) 养心安神酒

龙眼肉 30 克，酸枣仁 30 克，茯神 30 克，柏子仁 15 克，五味子 15 克，麦冬 15 克，白酒 2000 克，冷浸法制备。每日早、午各服 10 ml，睡前服 20 ml。

有养心安神，滋阴补血之效。适用于阴血不足，心神失养所致的心悸心烦、失眠多梦、倦怠健忘等症。

(4) 参蛤虫草酒

人参 30 克，蛤蚧 1 对（去头足），冬虫夏草 30 克，胡桃仁 30 克，白酒 2000 克，冷浸法制备。每日早晚各空腹温服 10～20 ml。

该酒补肺肾，助阳气，益精血，纳气定喘。适用于阳气虚弱，久病体虚，神疲乏力，健忘失眠，腰膝酸软，虚性喘咳等症。

(5) 复方海马酒

海马 2 只，明虾 30 克，淫羊藿 15 克，白酒 500 克，热浸法或冷浸法制备。每日早、晚各饮服 10～20 ml。

有补肾助阳，强壮筋骨，开胃调气之效。适用于肾阳虚衰之阳痿，神疲乏力，纳少气短，腰酸腿软，夜尿频数等症。

(6) 首乌杞菊酒

何首乌 30 克，枸杞子 30 克，菊花 30 克，当归 21 克，龙眼肉 21 克，胡麻仁 30 克，白酒 2000 克，热浸法或冷浸法配制。每日早、晚各空腹服 10～20 ml。

有滋补肝肾，补益精血，明目安神之效。凡肝肾精血不足之头晕目眩，视物不明，精神不振，腰膝无力，须发早白，遗精带下，健忘心悸等症，均宜于服用，并可延缓衰老。

(7) 补血顺气药酒

天冬、麦冬各 120 克，生地、熟地各 250 克，人参、茯苓、枸杞子各 60 克，砂仁 21 克，木香 15 克，沉香 9 克，上药为粗末,装入绢袋,放入盛有 15 公斤白酒的瓷坛,隔水煮沸,改文火煮半小时,以酒转黑色为宜,取下候冷,继续浸数日即成。每日早、晚各空腹服 10~20 ml。

有益气补血滋阴,调养五脏,健胃行气之效。五脏亏虚,气血不足所致精神不振,面色无华,体倦乏力,少气懒言,须发早白,头目晕眩,腰膝无力,食欲不振,健忘心悸等症均宜服用。

8. 延年益寿药酒

这类药酒多通过协调阴阳,补益气血,滋养五脏以抗衰延寿。前述某些药酒,如坚持长期服用,可以延缓衰老。下面另介绍几则。

(1) 百岁酒

蜜炙黄芪、茯神各 60 克,当归、熟地、生地各 36 克,党参、麦冬、茯苓、白术、枣皮、川芎、龟板胶、防风、枸杞、陈皮各 30 克,五味子、羌活各 24 克,肉桂 18 克,红枣 1000 克,冰糖 1000 克,泡高粱烧酒 10 公斤,煮烧 1 柱香的时间,或埋土中 7 日更好。随量饮之。

此方载于《药方杂录》,称授方者谓:"可治聋、明目、黑发、驻颜","此方名周公百岁酒,其方得之塞上,周翁自言服此方四十年,寿已逾百岁,翁家三代皆服此酒,相承无七十岁以下人。"该药酒补益气血,滋养阴精,助命门之火,而又行气祛风,能补五脏虚损,故有黑发驻颜延寿之效,可作为一个较为平和的补益长寿药酒,宜一般中老年体虚者服用。

(2) 延寿九仙酒

人参、炒白术、茯苓、炒甘草、当归、川芎、熟地、酒炒白芍各 60 克,枸杞子 250 克,生姜 60 克,大枣 30 枚(去核),煮好酒 17.5 公斤,不拘时随量饮之。具体制法可参考热浸法。

《明医选要济世奇方》所载此方谓:"治诸虚百损,返老还童。"所用药物为八珍汤加枸杞子,故有补气血、益肝肾之效,宜于气血亏虚、肝肾不足者。所增入大剂量枸杞子,有补肾养肝、益精明目之效，单味枸杞子浸酒即有补虚损、益颜色等功效，故该药酒对中老年人的补益作用较前已介绍的八珍酒更强，更全面，并有延寿抗衰之效。

(3) 疗百疾延寿酒

黄精60克，天冬45克，松叶90克，苍术60克，枸杞子75克，白酒5公斤，冷浸法制备。每日早、晚各饮服10~20 ml。

该酒原载《中藏经》。该药酒滋肾润肺，益肝补脾，养阴精，补心气，明眼目，祛内湿，健筋骨，适用于诸脏虚损，阴精不足之体倦乏力，饮食减少，头晕目暗，筋骨不利，心烦失眠，须发早白等症。对中老年偏于阴精亏虚、脏气不足者，是一种养生延寿的较为平和的药酒。

(4) 精神药酒

人参、生地、枸杞子各15克，淫羊藿、沙苑子、母丁香各9克，沉香、远志肉各3克，荔枝核7枚，高粱白酒1公斤，冷浸法45天后可饮用。每日饮1次，徐徐呷服10 ml。

这是近代名医吴棹仙先生研制的利于延年益寿的药酒，由其门人在《四川中医》杂志介绍。该药酒益气助阳养阴，益肝肾，健脾胃，安神益智，散寒止痛，故有助于趋于衰老的中老年人恢复旺盛的精力，而延缓衰老，由此得名。

9. 防治疾病保健药酒

纯属治疗性药酒在这里不作介绍，只简介几种常见病预防、辅助治疗和病后康复调理的保健药酒，供参考。

(1) 菊楂益心酒

菊花30克，山楂45克，白酒500克，冷浸法配制。每日服3次，每次饮服10~20 ml。

有平肝明目，疏风清热，健胃消食散瘀之效。现代研究表明两药均有降血压，增加冠脉流量，抗心肌缺血，抗衰老等作用，菊花有抗血栓作用，山楂有降血脂、健胃作用。故该酒适用于高血压病、高脂血症、动脉粥样硬化、冠心病的预防和辅助治疗，久服可延年益寿。

(2) 健心灵酒

黄芪 30 克，丹参 30 克，川芎 12 克，桂枝 6 克，白酒 500 克，冷浸法制备。每日服 3 次，每次饮服 10～20 ml。

山东中医学院附院研究的"健心灵"为益气活血通阳方，治疗冠心病有较好疗效，实验证明有抗心肌缺血，增强抗疲劳能力和耐缺氧能力等作用。配制为酒剂，可用于冠心病、缺血性脑血管病的预防和辅助治疗、病后康复调理。

(3) 屠苏酒

麻黄、川椒、细辛、防风、苍术、干姜、肉桂、桔梗各同等分量，研粗末，装绢袋，浸于适量的酒中，密封容器，3 日后可饮用。据药物浓度及饮者酒量，从小量开始酌量服用。

屠苏酒是我国传统的预防瘟疫等传染病的药酒，历代有多种配方。上方为《景岳全书》所载，有祛风散寒、温中健脾之效，适量饮服有助于防治风寒感冒和胃寒疼痛。其他数方中含有个别有毒性的或猛峻之药，不作介绍，若用之宜慎。

(4) 独活寄生酒

生地、白芍、桂心、茯苓、杜仲、牛膝各 9 克，桑寄生 15 克，独活、秦艽、川芎、人参、防风各 6 克，细辛、当归、甘草各 3 克，白酒 1000 克，冷浸法制备。每日服 1～2 次，每次饮服 20～30 ml。

该药酒原载《万病回春》，有人据此改为上述用量制法。有补肝肾，益气血，祛风湿，止痹痛之效，是一种扶正祛邪的药酒。可用于肝肾不足，气血两虚的风寒湿痹的治疗和康复调整。风湿性、类风湿性关节炎，慢性腰腿痛，坐骨神经痛等有上述见证者可以服用。

(5) 参茸酒

人参 60 克，鹿茸 30 克，当归、秦艽、红花、枸杞子各 6

克,防风、鳖甲、萆薢、羌活、川牛膝、独活、杜仲、白术、玉竹各 3 克,丁香 2.4 克,用多年存性烧酒 10 公斤,将药料入酒内封妥;再存数年,将药料滤出,入冰糖渣 120 克,烧酒 1 公斤,兑妥用之。

《清太医院配方》所载该药酒以益气温阳为主,兼以补肝肾,滋阴精,强腰膝,祛风,除湿,活血。亦属扶正祛邪的药酒,凡因气血不足,肝肾亏虚,而感受风寒湿邪所致诸症,均可用本方辅助治疗或康复调理。《清太医院配方》称该酒"治男妇左瘫右痪,半身不遂,口眼歪斜,手足顽麻,下部痿软,筋骨疼痛;一切三十六种风,七十二般气;并寒湿诸痛,及虚损劳伤,真火不足,饮食不化,肚腹不调,十膈五噎,气滞积块,泻痢痞满,肚腹冷痛;男子阳衰;女人血虚,赤白带下,久无子嗣,一切男妇虚损杂症。久服则气血充足,百病不生,益寿延年,老当益壮。"具体配制可按一般冷浸法,不必拘于存数年,每日可服 2 次,每次饮服 10~20 ml。

2.4 保健膏滋

膏滋又称煎膏剂,是中药材加水煎煮,去渣取液浓缩后,加蔗糖或蜂蜜等制成的稠厚状半流体制剂。膏滋是属于中药传统膏剂的一种内服剂型,在我国应用的历史十分久远。大约成书于春秋、战国时的医书《五十二病方》中已载有膏剂方。唐代《千金要方》、《千金翼方》载黄精膏、陆抗膏、仙方凝灵膏等补益延寿膏滋多首。其后历代都创制许多养生祛病的膏滋,如宋代《洪氏集验方》琼玉膏等,不仅在民间广泛应用,而且深受宫廷医药的重视。至今仍保留着有效的传统膏滋成药,江南等地区更是把补益类膏滋视为冬令进补的佳品,不少著名药店也自制膏滋,深受欢迎。

纵观膏滋的古今应用,既可防治各种疾病,又常用于养生抗老。由于膏滋功专效宏,药力缓和而持久,贮存、携带和服用方便，制备也较为简便易行，又能节省中药材，具有经济实用的特点。因而，十分适合平素扶弱补虚，救偏却病和抗衰延寿，是用于自我保健的好药。

膏滋处方大多为复方，也有单味药组成者，其组方和应用十分讲究辨证。作为防病养生、抗衰延年的保健膏滋，大多通过调节阴阳、补益气血、滋养五脏、填补精髓等功效，发挥扶正固本、整体调整的作用，而增强体质，延缓衰老；也有通过祛邪防病，而有益于某些疾病的预防保健和康复保健。这样可把保健膏滋分为若干类，每一种又都有其功效和适应症。在应用保健膏滋时，一定要根据不同个体的具体情况，辨证选用相应的膏滋。

膏滋的服用，一般是以温开水冲服，亦有视病情的需要而以温热的黄酒冲服的，治疗咽喉疾病者可含在口中噙化。滋补膏滋宜在空腹时服，养心安神类宜睡前服，病在下焦者可于饭前半小时左右服，病在上焦者宜饭后半小时左右服。服用膏滋的剂量，一般根据膏滋药物的性质、病情和体质等因素确定。药性平和无毒者，特别是药食两用之品加工的膏滋，服量较大无妨；含有猛峻、有毒药物者，服量宜小，并从小剂量开始，视服药反应而适当增减。体质壮实，急病、重病者，服量可适当增加；体弱、年老者，无病或轻病、慢性病者，服量宜偏小些。下面诸方中介绍的用量，为一般情况下成人用量，可在上下一定幅度内适当增减。

下面介绍适合家庭自制保健膏滋的一般方法：

备料　　包括处方规定的中药，蔗糖或蜂蜜。中药材要去除杂质、尘土，使之清洁，按规定炮制，必要时粗碎。糖大多为白糖，白沙糖或冰糖，亦有用红糖者。糖要预作处理，有炒糖与炼糖两法。炒糖，系将糖置铜锅中干炒至全溶，色转黄，开始发泡至冒清白烟即可。炒时要勤翻动，使受热均匀。炼糖，即制转化糖，取糖10公斤，加水5~6公斤，加热煮沸半小时左右，加入0.1%酒石酸适量，搅拌均匀，微沸2小时即成。此法使蔗糖转化为葡萄糖或果糖。蜂蜜要选用优质者,并要经过炼制。炼蜜,是将蜂蜜置锅内加热,使之溶化,捞去浮沫,至蜜中水分大部蒸发,翻起大泡,呈老红色,酌加约10%的冷水,继续加热使沸,乘热倾出,以绢筛滤去杂质而得。炼蜜要适当,不要过嫩、过老,一般500克生蜜可炼制400克左右炼蜜为宜。

制备清膏 将药材加适量清水浸泡数小时至半天。煎煮药数小时,滤汁,药渣加水再煎,反复3次,将几次滤出的煎汁及药渣中的压榨汁合并,静置沉淀,以多层纱布过滤。将滤液再置锅中,以大火加热至沸,捞去表面浮沫,药汁转浓后改用小火保持微沸,使徐徐蒸发,并不断搅拌以防止局部过热而焦化结底。若用棒挑起所制得的稠膏,呈薄片状流下,为较适度,夏天可略稠些,冬天略稀些。此称清膏。

收膏 浓缩制成清膏后,加入已炼制过的糖或蜜,边加边不停地搅拌使均匀,即得。也可在炒糖即成之时,加入预留的药汁,使糖化薄,倾出用绢筛过滤,与已浓缩制得的清膏混合,在锅内以文火煎熬,浓缩即得。煎药、浓缩和收膏均宜用砂锅、铜锅或搪瓷锅,铝锅亦可用,但不可用铁锅。

贮藏 宜分装于玻璃或搪瓷、陶瓷容器内,应密封,置阴凉处。

下面分别举例介绍各类保健膏滋,大多数出自古今文献,但对药物剂量、制法、功用分析等,结合现代认识和经验而有所斟酌和调整。有的未注明出处,系作者经验方。

2.4.1 补气膏滋

1. 人参膏

人参(去芦)250克,粗碎,煎煮3次,浓缩,兑炼蜜250克收膏。每日早、晚各服15克。

《景岳全书》载有此方。有大补元气,健脾益智之效,并有抗衰老作用。适用于有气虚诸证者和年老体衰者服用。

2. 代参膏

党参、黄芪、白术、龙眼肉各 250 克,煎煮,浓缩,加经过炼制的冰糖 250 克收膏。每日早、晚各服 15 克。

此方出自《中药成方配本》。有益气健脾养心之效。适用于一般有气虚见证者和老年体虚者,尤以心脾气虚者为宜。

3. 益气开胃膏

人参 30 克,茯苓、黄芪、炒麦芽、山楂各 250 克,砂仁 15 克,煎煮,浓缩,酌加炼蜜收膏。每日早、晚各服 15 克。

本方系益气健脾与消食化积、行气开胃相结合,补消兼施,可免纯补滋腻呆胃之弊。一般体弱气虚、脾胃不健,纳呆食少者均可服用。

2.4.2 养血膏滋

1. 桑椹膏

桑椹 1000 克,捣绞取汁,煎熬成膏,或酌加炼蜜收膏。每日服 2~3 次,每次服 30 克。

《素问病机气宜保命集》载有桑椹膏。有养血滋阴,乌须发,润大肠之效。可用于须发早白,肠燥便秘者。中老年人偏于阴血虚者服用此膏甚宜。

2. 杞圆膏

枸杞子、龙眼肉各 500 克,煎熬成膏,或酌加炼蜜收膏。每日服 2~3 次,每次服 15~30 克。

本方见于《摄生秘旨》。有补益精血,养心安神,滋肝肾之效。该书称能"安神养血,滋阴壮阳,益智,强筋骨,泽肌肤,驻颜色"。似有抗衰美容之效。皆属药食两用平和滋补之品,凡心血不足、肝肾亏虚者可经常服用。

3. 首乌补血膏

何首乌 250 克,大枣、桑椹子、龙眼肉、黑芝麻各 500 克,煎煮,浓缩,炼蜜适量收膏。每日服 2~3 次,每次 15~30 克。

本方以养血为主，兼补气阴，益心脾，乌须发，润大肠。为平补阴血之品，宜于阴血不足，须发早白，心神不安，肠燥便秘者经常服用，亦可望发挥润肤泽肌、驻颜抗衰之效。

4. 当归补血膏

本药由武汉中联制药厂研制生产，方由当归、川芎、黄芪、甘草、党参、白芍、阿胶、茯苓、熟地组成。膏滋剂，服法见该药说明书。

本品能养血益气，适用于身体虚弱、面色萎黄、头痛眩晕、病后血虚、产后血亏等症。

2.4.3 滋阴膏滋

1. 二冬膏

天冬、麦冬各500克，煎煮，浓缩，酌加炼蜜收膏。每日服2～3次，每次15克。

此膏方载于《张氏医通》。有滋阴润肺清火之效。可治阴虚津亏，痰热咳嗽之症，亦宜于中老年阴虚肺燥者服用。

2. 二至膏

制女贞子、旱莲草各500克，煎煮，浓缩，加适量炼制砂糖收膏。每日服2～3次，每次服15克。

二至丸方见于《杨氏家藏方解》，改制为膏滋，仍有滋阴益肾养肝之效。可用于肝肾阴虚所致眩晕耳鸣，失眠多梦，须发早白，腰膝酸痛，遗精盗汗及阴虚出血之症。

3. 养阴膏

沙参、玉竹、麦冬、花粉、百合各250克，煎煮，浓缩，加适量炼蜜收膏，每日服2～3次，每次服15克。

本方滋阴生津，润养肺胃，宁心除烦。适用于肺胃阴亏津伤所致口燥咽干、干咳少痰，及心烦心悸等症。

2.4.4 助阳膏滋

1. 锁阳膏

锁阳 1500 克，煎煮，浓缩，酌加炼蜜约 250 克收膏。每日服 2 次，每次服 30 克。

本方见于《本草切要》。有补肾阳，益精血，润肠燥的功效。可用治肾阳不足、精血亏虚诸症及肠燥津亏便秘者。

2. 苁蓉二仙膏

肉苁蓉、淫羊藿各 500 克，仙茅 250 克，煎煮，浓缩，酌加经炼制之砂糖收膏。每日早、晚各服 15 克。

本方补肾阳，强筋骨，祛寒湿。适用于肾阳不足所致之阳痿、腰膝无力，筋骨不利，亦治风寒湿痹，肢体麻木等。药性燥热，若非阳衰之体，不宜久用。

3. 蛤蚧党参膏

蛤蚧党参膏由广西南宁中药厂研制生产，主要成分为蛤蚧、党参。膏滋剂，每瓶 250 克，每服 10 克，日二次，温开水冲服。

本药能益肾助阳，补肺健脾，止咳定喘，适用于各种原因引起的衰弱症，肾阳虚肺阴虚所致的慢性咳喘，贫血萎黄，消化不良等。

2.4.5 气血双补膏滋

1. 两仪膏

人参 120 克（或党参 250 克），熟地 500 克，煎煮，浓缩，酌加炼蜜或冰糖收膏。每日早、晚各服 15 克。

本方出自《景岳全书》。有补元气，养阴血之效，为平补气血之剂。凡精气内亏，阴血不足者宜常服之。

2. 十全大补膏

党参、蜜炙黄芪、炒白术、炒白芍、茯苓各 500 克，熟地黄、当归各 750 克，川芎、肉桂、蜜炙甘草各 250 克，煎煮，浓缩，依法制得清膏，取砂糖 530 克加水加热烊化，滤过，然后与上述清膏 1000 克混合，和匀即得。每日服 2 次，每次服 15 克，饭前用开水化服。

此方见于《江苏省药品标准》。为温补气血之方，凡有气虚血亏之证者均可服用。

3. 洋参双补膏

西洋参 30 克，山药、枸杞子各 500 克，桑椹子、大枣、龙眼肉各 750 克，煎煮，浓缩，加炼蜜或冰糖收膏。每日服 2 次，每次 30 克。

本方益气养血滋阴，平补心脾、肝肾，凡气虚血少阴亏者皆可服用。除西洋参外，其余各药均为药食两用之品。因西洋参较缺且昂贵，可用十倍量太子参代之。

2.4.6 补益五脏膏滋

1. 枸杞膏

枸杞子 500 克，煎煮，浓缩成膏，或兑适量炼蜜收膏。每日早、晚各服 15~30 克。

本方见于《寿世保元》。有补益肝肾，滋阴润肺明目之效。可治肝肾阴虚所致头晕目眩，视力减退，腰膝酸软及阴虚劳嗽等。

2. 苍术膏

苍术、茯苓各 500 克，煎煮，浓缩，兑适量炼蜜或砂糖收膏。每日服 2~3 次，每次服 15~30 克。

《卫生杂兴方》苍术膏即苍术、白茯苓、白蜜三味，现可改按前述膏滋常规制法配制。有健脾强胃益气之效。中老年劳伤心脾，脾胃虚弱，纳呆食少，精力衰减，健忘失眠及足胫浮肿、酸痛沉重者可以服用。

3. 茯苓膏

茯苓（蒸晒七遍）1000克，松脂（炼成者）500克，松子仁250克，柏子仁250克，上药捣筛为末，加蜜1000克拌和，置铜器内，微火煎一日夜成膏。每日服3次，每次服15～30克。

本方载于《太平圣惠方》，药味与《千金翼方》仙方凝灵膏相同。具有养心安神滋养强壮的功效。主治心气、心血不足而心神不安，心悸、失眠、健忘者。原书中注曰："顿食令饱，即可绝谷。久服轻身明目，不老复壮，发白更黑，齿落重生，延年益寿"。此皆补养心神之功。

4. 润肺膏

南沙参、麦冬、天冬、花粉、枇杷叶（去毛）、杏仁、核桃仁、冰糖各50克，川贝母120克，橘饼250克，诸药煎取浓汁去渣，再加入川贝末和冰糖末，以白蜜6000克收膏。每日服2次，每次服15克。

本方载于《江苏省药品标准》。有润养肺阴，止咳化痰之效。适用于阴虚肺燥，口燥咽干，干咳或痰少而粘者。

2.4.7 其他补益延寿膏滋

1. 琼玉膏

人参75克，生地800克，茯苓153克，白蜜500克。诸药为末，煎煮，浓缩，兑炼好之白蜜收膏。每日服2～3次，每次服15克。

此方源于宋代洪遵辑《洪氏集验方》，各药之比例亦按该书剂量推算。后世剂量有所改变，药味亦有增入沉香、琥珀者。有补气阴，生精血，滋肾益肺，健脾养心之效。不仅可以治疗虚劳干咳、咽燥咯血等症，中老年常服当有补虚扶正，固本祛痰，延缓衰老之效。本方配伍严谨，兼顾诸脏，气阴并补，滋而不腻，适于久服，故在清代宫廷医药中也甚受重视。近年的研究表明，服用本品可使老年人T淋巴细胞数明显增加，血清IgA含量明显降低，两者都已接近青年组水平。这种改善老年人免疫功能的作用,可视为琼玉膏扶正固本、祛病延寿的机理之一。

2. 益寿养真膏

生地黄 8000 克,人参末 750 克,茯苓末 1500 克,蜜 5000 克,天冬、麦冬、地骨皮各 250 克(均研末)。上 7 药和匀,入瓷缸内,密封,置于铜锅内煮 3 日夜,如水减则添暖水低于缸口,日满取出蜡纸封,浸井中 1 日夜,再入铜锅内煮 1 昼夜出水气。每日服 2~3 次,每次服 1~2 匙,温酒调服。

本方之剂量、制法均依《东医宝鉴·内景篇》所载。方中药物较琼玉膏增加天冬、麦冬和地骨皮,更加强了滋阴之力,适应症也类同。

3. 河车膏

党参、生地、枸杞子、当归各 60 克,紫河车一具,用水煎透,炼蜜收膏。每早用黄酒冲服 3~5 茶匙。

本方又名混元膏,见于《清太医院配方》。有补气养血,助阳滋阴,益精髓,补肝肾之效。据该书称:"治男妇诸虚百损,五劳七伤;或由先天秉受不足,元气虚弱,动转多病,不耐劳苦。男子肾虚阳痿,精乏无嗣;妇人子宫虚冷,屡经坠落,不成孕育,并皆治之。"并认为久服该膏可"返老还童"。凡中老年人因气血阴阳不足而体虚早衰者皆可服之,以图健身抗衰延年。该书指出,服此膏时当"戒气怒、房劳,忌食诸般血物、烧酒",亦当注意。

4. 龟鹿二仙膏

鹿角 500 克,龟板 250 克,枸杞子 100 克,人参 50 克,先将前两味锯截,刮净,水浸,桑火熬炼成胶,再将后两味熬膏,和入。每晨酒服 9 克。

此膏又名龟鹤二仙膏,载于明代《仙传四十九方》、《摄生秘剖》等书,以上剂量比例及制法、服法均照清代《医方集解》。本膏温阳益阴,滋补肝肾,峻补气血精髓,以"享龟鹿之年,故曰二仙"。"治虚损精极者,梦泄遗精,瘦削少气,目视不明等证","久服可以益寿"。

5. 红玉膏

玉竹、人参各90克，五味子、龟板胶、当归、大生地、茯苓、枸杞子各60克，川牛膝30克，白莲须15克，朱砂3克，煎煮，兑炼蜜收膏。每日服2～3次，每次15克。

此膏见于清代《集验良方》，称："此方填补精髓，固气养血，和五脏，利九窍，久服大益身心。"本方在琼玉膏基础上加味，加强了补肝肾，养阴血，安心神之效，宜于中老年虚损早衰者经常服用。以朱砂有毒性，宜去之，或易以其他镇养心神之品。

6. 加减扶元和中膏

党参45克，土炒白术、茯苓、土炒当归身、酒炒续断、生黄芪、炒谷芽、焙鸡内金各30克，炙半夏、生姜各24克，炙香附、炒大熟地各18克，砂仁、佩兰草各12克，红枣肉20枚，共以水熬透，去渣，再熬浓，兑冰糖为膏。每服9克，白开水冲服。

此为慈禧太后补益医方，载于《慈禧光绪医方选议》。有健脾益气养血，开胃消食化积，兼补肝肾之效。对久病体虚，脾胃虚弱，食少腹胀，干哕嘈杂，饮食不消者有效。

7. 加减扶元益阴膏

党参60克，炒白术、茯苓、山药、土炒当归身、女贞子各30克，醋炒白芍24克，丹皮、炙香附各18克，鹿角胶15克（溶化），砂仁12克，银柴胡9克，共以水熬透，去渣，再熬浓，加鹿角胶溶化，兑炼蜜为膏。每服12克，白开水冲服。

此亦为《慈禧光绪医方选议》所载慈禧太后补益医方。系逍遥散加减，并含四君子汤主要药，兼有健脾益气，调肝理脾行气，温肾益阴养血之效。本方兼顾气血阴阳和脾肝肾诸脏，是一个补通结合、较平和稳妥的膏方，尤宜于兼有肝郁气滞的虚损之证。

2.4.8 防治疾病保健膏滋

介绍几种有防病保健和辅助治疗康复作用较简易平妥的保健膏滋。

1. 菊花延龄膏

鲜菊花瓣适量，用水熬透，去渣再熬浓汁，少兑炼蜜收膏。每次服9～12克，白开水冲服。

此方为御医为慈禧太后所拟，载于《慈禧光绪医方选议》。有疏风清热、平肝明目之效。故本方宜于因肝阳、风热所致头晕目眩、头痛目赤症。结合现代药理及临床研究，亦可用治高血压病、冠心病等。古称"真菊延龄"，大约是通过防治这类中老年常见病，而获祛病延年之效。

2. 明目延龄膏

霜桑叶、菊花各30克，共以水熬透，去渣，再熬浓汁，少兑炼蜜收膏。每服9克，白开水冲服。

此方为《慈禧光绪医方选议》所载慈禧太后治眼病医方。功效应用与菊花延龄膏类似。

3. 加竹沥梨膏

黄梨100个，鲜竹叶100片，鲜芦根30支，老树橘红20片，荸荠50个（浓汁），竹沥适量依法制为膏滋。

此方出于《慈禧光绪医方选议》所载光绪皇帝治咳嗽医方。有养阴生津，润肺止嗽，清热化痰之效。宜于阴虚肺燥劳嗽者。

4. 利咽膏

麦冬、胖大海、天花粉各100克，黄梨1000克，鲜青果500克，桔梗、木蝴蝶各50克，甘草30克，双花75克，煎煮，浓缩，溶入柿霜30克，兑炼蜜收膏。每日服3次，每次9～15克，开水送服，或含口中噙化。

有清热滋阴，生津利咽之效。适用于咽喉肿痛，口干咽燥声哑等症，对教师、演员等亦有嗓音保健作用。

5. 首乌菊楂膏

何首乌、菊花、生山楂各500克,煎煮,浓缩,兑入适量炼蜜收膏。每日服3次,每次15~30克。

有滋补肝肾,平肝明目活血之效。用于高血压病、高脂血症、冠心病的预防、康复保健及患者的辅助治疗。

6. 益气活血膏

黄芪、丹参各500克,黄精、郁金、生山楂各250克,煎煮,浓缩,酌兑适量炼蜜收膏。每日服3次,每次服15克。

有益气活血之效。宜于气虚血瘀诸证,如冠心病、缺血性脑血管意外及后遗症、慢性阻塞性肺气肿及慢性肺心病的缓解期都常表现为气虚血瘀证候,可用本膏治疗。

7. 老鹳草膏

老鹳草500克,当归125克,白藓皮、川芎各62.5克,红花31克,用水煎透,浓缩,炼蜜成膏。每日服2~3次,每次9~15克。

该方载于《清太医院配方》。有祛风除湿,活血通络之效。主治风湿痹痛,筋骨不舒,拘挛麻木,跌打损伤,皮肤作痒等症。

2.5 保健药茶

药茶,即中药的茶剂剂型。传统的茶剂有两种类型:一种是含有茶叶或不含茶叶的药物经粉碎、混合而成的粗末制品,用开水沏后可象日常饮茶一样频频饮服,故也称代茶饮;另一种是将上述粗末加入面粉或神曲糊制成块状制品,如午时茶,亦用沸水泡服。后一种多属药厂的产品,前一种则制作服用方便,适合自我保健之用。故本节保健药茶即介绍代茶饮在养生保健中的应用。

我国是茶叶的故乡,种茶、饮茶已有几千年的历史。茶叶既是优良的保健饮料,也有药效,具有清头目、除烦渴、化痰、消食、利尿、解毒等作用。人们在饮茶过程中发现，若茶叶中加入适当药物，饮之有防治疾病之效，这就出现了中药代茶饮。早在1200多年前唐代王焘著《外台秘要》中就载有"代茶新饮方"。以后历代医著中都曾记载不少药茶方。在清代宫廷医药档案资料中，运用代茶饮法以治病和调理的记载甚多，应用范围颇广，形成清宫医药一大特色。近年来益寿茶、减肥茶、清宫仙药茶的应用，表明服饮药茶已成为现代中医自我保健的一种良好形式。

药茶有其独特的优点。药茶用药量较少，节约中药材；以开水沏后即可饮用，方便而节约能源；这种方式较之汤剂更宜于长期坚持服用；可兼作药疗、食疗，治疗和防病养生，因而应用广泛。由于这些特点，代茶饮可谓老少咸宜，广大群众乐于接受，用于自我保健尤佳。

代茶饮的应用范围很广，大体包括：轻症的治疗，慢性病的调理，重病的辅助治疗及康复善后，疾病的预防，养生抗老，以及防治口腔、咽喉、食道、胃肠等疾患。后者是因为频频饮入药茶液可较好地作用于各部的局部。

代茶饮的遣药组方也有特色。所用之药，性多平和，一般不用猛峻之药；味多甘淡，少用过苦药、动物药及质地坚硬、难以浸出之药；常选可食中药，多用瓜果蔬菜之类，多数药易得；还常适当应用蔗糖、蜂蜜等甘甜调味之品。代茶饮的组方有三少的原则，即选用药味精少，一般不超过5~7味，每味药用量少，一般不超过10克，每剂的总药量亦少。尽管用药少，代茶饮的组方也注重讲究辨证，配伍也是很严谨的。

代茶饮的加工制作很简单，但应注意选用优质清洁干净的中药饮片，必要时进行适当清洁处理，去除杂质和尘土，不得使用污染、变质的药物。宜将药物加工成粗末，细粉不宜过多，以免浸泡液混浊。如将药茶分装于滤纸袋中，成袋泡茶的方式，则更为方便。药茶制剂应干燥以便贮存，并应存于干燥处，注意防**虫、防霉**。

代茶饮的服用方法，一般可在茶杯、保温杯中，冲入开水，如普通饮茶一样饮用，并不断补加开水。也可使用平素饮茶的茶壶或保温瓶。也可将中药煎汤饮用，一般煎煮较短时间即可。亦有的药茶是以开水冲调饮服，如《仁寿录》观音面茶即是。

应用代茶饮防治疾病或养生抗衰也应注意辨证施用，根据不同个体的体质、病情、年龄以及用药时季节等，选用适当的、对症的代茶饮。代茶饮由于药量较轻，药性平缓，对某疾病只适合于辅助治疗，若遇急症重症，则应及时就医，以免延误病情。若以代茶饮摄生保健、延缓衰老，则应长期坚持，持之以恒，方易收效。

以下介绍各类保健药茶，凡注明出处者均系据有关文献，但有些叙述从简，剂量、制法、服法、功用分析等亦结合现代认识和经验而有所斟酌和调整。有的未注剂量者，可据一般用药规律酌情而确定，一般每味药用量 1.5~6 克为宜。未注明出处者系作者经验方。

2.5.1 补气、养血药茶

1. 参芪代茶饮

人参 3 克（或党参 9 克），黄芪 9 克，大枣 5 枚，陈皮 1.5 克，开水沏，代茶饮。

本方补益元气为主，兼以健脾开胃，使补而不滞，适合气虚体弱者常服，并有延缓衰老之效。

2. 五宝茶汤

黍米面、芝麻、牛乳、山药、牛骨髓各适量。将芝麻、山药研成末，用香油将牛骨髓化开，炒黍米面，再下牛乳，并药末和匀，每早用开水冲服。

此方载于《仁寿录》。有益气健脾，填补精血，滋养肝肾之效。宜于老衰体弱者食疗补益之用。

3. 观音面茶

炒黑芝麻、藕粉、粘黄米、白糖、炒山药各500克，上为细末，开水冲服适量。

亦为《仁寿录》方。有益气健脾，补精血，滋肝肾之效。适于体弱老衰者服用。

4. 五香奶茶

牛乳、白砂糖、蜂蜜、杏仁、芝麻各适量。将奶茶炖热，糖、蜜与芝麻、杏仁末和匀，每日食之，香甜异常。

《仁寿录》所载此方，有益气填精补血，滋补肝肾，润肺，及润肠通便之效。年老体衰而兼咳嗽、便秘者尤宜。

5. 术冬代茶汤

白术4.5克，麦冬（去心）3克，煎作汤，夏月服之代茶。

《串雅内外篇》此方，书中原名代茶汤，有益气健脾养阴，滋润心肺之效。适于脾气虚弱、心肺阴亏者服用。

6. 桑龙代茶饮

桑椹子、龙眼肉各15克，开水沏，代茶饮。

本方以补血为主，兼养阴益气，养心安神，生津润肠。适于阴血不足，眩晕耳鸣，失眠健忘，惊悸怔忡，食少体倦，须发早白及肠燥便秘者服用。

7. 益气生津代茶饮

人参、鲜石斛、麦冬、鲜青果、老米。

《清代宫廷医话》介绍慈禧太后曾用此方。有益气养阴生津，清热利咽之效。宜于气阴两虚，津液亏乏，口干咽燥，咽喉不利者。

8. 补血和胃代茶饮

当归身、川芎、白芍、生地、广木香、枳实、苍术、焦三仙。

据《清代宫廷医话》记载，光绪皇帝的珍妃曾用此方，方名原为和胃代茶饮，实为四物汤加健脾和胃、行气消导之品。脾胃健运，则饮食精微化生气血，故本方主要是补血。宜于脾胃不

· 565 ·

健、阴血亏虚者服用。

2.5.2 滋阴、助阳药茶

1. 玉石代茶饮

玉竹、石斛各6克，开水沏，代茶饮。

有滋阴润燥生津之效。宜于肺胃肾阴虚之证而见燥热咳嗽，阴虚劳嗽，津亏口干舌燥，腰膝软弱，视物昏花及阴虚消渴等症。

2. 二参二冬代茶饮

沙参、玄参、麦冬、天冬各6克，开水沏，代茶饮。

能滋阴生津，清热降火。用于肺胃阴伤，口咽干燥，干咳少痰，劳嗽咯血，食欲不振；热病伤阴，心烦失眠；虚火上炎，目赤咽痛及肠燥便秘等症。凡阴虚体质者，均可常服以上两种代茶饮。

3. 参苓代茶饮

沙参、茯苓、天冬。

据《清代宫廷医话》载，乾隆朝定贵人曾服此代茶饮方。有养阴兼扶脾之效。宜于肺胃肾阴虚而兼有脾虚者服用。

4. 仙灵脾茶

淫羊藿9克，肉苁蓉6克，开水沏，代茶饮。

有补肾助阳，壮筋骨，益精血之效。适用于肾阳不足，阳痿不孕，腰膝无力，冷痛等症。亦可用于肾阳虚型的高血压病、冠心病。

5. 复方杜仲茶

杜仲、桑寄生、怀牛膝各9克，开水沏，代茶饮。

有补肝肾、强筋骨之效。适用于肾虚腰痛，足膝痿弱之症，又可防治有肝肾不足见症的高血压病。

6. 新二仙代茶饮

仙茅4.5克，淫羊藿、杜仲、玄参、女贞子、枸杞子各6

克,开水沏,代茶饮。

此为仿二仙汤意而拟双调阴阳方,有补肝肾,温阳滋阴降火的功效。宜于阴损阳衰、肝肾不足,或兼有虚火上炎之症,有此见症之高血压病、冠心病患者用之尤宜。可根据阴阳虚衰的不同具体情况,适当调整助阳药与滋阴药的用量。

7. 复方枸杞茶

枸杞子、百合、何首乌、黄精、淫羊藿各6克,开水沏,代茶饮。

本方平补气血阴阳,兼顾五脏,适合身体虚弱者及中老年人经常服用,有抗衰强身、延年益寿之效。

2.5.3 调理脾胃、消食化积药茶

1. 和胃代茶饮

生白术、苍术、茯苓、陈皮、金石斛、谷芽、建曲、广砂仁。

此为《清代宫廷医话》介绍的光绪皇帝病后调补方之一。有健脾益胃,养阴消食的功效。宜于脾胃虚弱,胃纳减少,饮食不消,又兼胃阴不足者。

2. 二神代茶饮

茯神、神曲。

据《清代宫廷医话》载,嘉庆朝玉贵人病后调理曾用此方。有健脾安神、消食和胃之效。宜于脾虚纳少,饮食不消,心神不宁者。

3. 五仙代茶饮

神曲、炒山楂、**炒麦芽、炒谷芽**各6克,砂仁3克,开水沏,代茶饮。

此方重在消食导滞化积,佐以行气开胃,宜于饮食积滞,脘腹胀满,嗳腐食臭者。

4. 甘露茶

乌药、炒厚朴、炒枳壳、炒山楂各 24 克，陈皮 120 克，炒神曲 45 克，炒谷芽 30 克，红茶 90 克，共研成粗末，混合均匀，分装塑料袋，每袋 9 克。每次 1 袋，生姜 1 片煎服，或开水泡服。

此为《药剂学》所载。有理气、消食、化滞之效。用于食积气滞，脘腹胀闷，不思饮食，不服水土等症。

2.5.4 安神药茶

1. 安神代茶饮

煅龙齿 9 克，石菖蒲 3 克，水煎，代茶。

此为《慈禧光绪医方选议》所载治光绪皇帝心经病医方之一。有镇惊、开窍、安神之效。可用于心悸易惊者。

2. 圆肉二仙茶

龙眼肉、炒酸枣仁各 12 克，炒柏子仁 6 克，开水沏，代茶饮。

有养心安神之效，宜于心气、心血不足而心悸、失眠、健忘者。

3. 清心代茶饮

莲子心、灯心、竹叶各 3 克，炒酸枣仁 9 克，开水沏，代茶饮。

有清心火及养心安神作用，宜于心阴不足、心火亢盛而心悸、失眠者。有此见症的高血压病者用之更宜。

2.5.5 防治常见病症的药茶

1. 菊楂代茶饮

菊花、生山楂各 12 克，开水沏，代茶饮。

有降血压、降血脂、抗心肌缺血等作用。适用于高血压病、高脂血症、冠心病等。

2. 首乌决明茶

何首乌、决明子各12克，开水沏，代茶饮。

有降血脂、抗动脉粥样硬化和抗心肌缺血等作用。适用于高脂血症、动脉粥样硬化、冠心病等，兼有便秘者更宜。

3. 复方玉米须茶

玉米须30克，车前子15克，泽泻12克，开水沏，代茶饮。

有利尿、降压、降血糖、降血脂等作用。可用于肾炎水肿，肝硬化腹水，高血压病等。

4. 减肥代茶饮

乌龙茶6克，荷叶30克，泽泻、生山楂、薏苡仁各12克，陈皮3克，开水沏，代茶饮。

有降血脂，利尿，减肥等作用。单纯肥胖和高脂血症者可经常服用。

5. 消肥健身茶

消肥健身茶由广西百色地区制药厂生产，主要成分为田七、山茶、白皮根等。茶剂，每袋4～4.8克，每服1袋，日3次，白开水浸泡片刻，趁热饮服，每袋可连泡2～3次。

本品可调节机体代谢，促进脂肪分解，降低血脂，舒通血脉。适用于单纯性肥胖症，也可防治心、脑血管疾病，或作为老年人的一般保健品。

6. 复方罗布麻茶

罗布麻叶3克，钩藤15克，丹皮6克，开水沏，代茶饮。

有降血压作用。高血压病患者可服用，属于肝阳上亢者尤宜。

7. 黄玉石代茶饮

黄芪15克，玉米须30克，石韦21克，开水沏，代茶饮。

有补气、利水之效。肾炎蛋白尿者坚持服用，可有一定的消蛋白、消肿作用。

8. 荷佩防暑茶

鲜荷叶1张，佩兰、藿香、菊花、金银花各6克，开水沏，代茶饮。

有清暑热、祛暑湿之效。可用于预防中暑。

9. 温中茶

干姜6克，高良姜、陈皮各3克，吴茱萸、丁香各1.5克，开水沏，代茶饮。

有温中散寒止痛之效。可用于胃寒引起的脘腹疼痛，呃逆呕吐等症。

10. 健胃茶

徐长卿、麦冬各9克、生甘草6克，橘红4.5克，玫瑰花1.5克，开水沏，代茶饮。

据高树俊氏等发表于《新中医》杂志的报道，本方治浅表性与萎缩性胃窦炎，总有效率90.9%，显效44.26%。

11. 清解茶

金银花、菊花各12克，薄荷、生甘草各6克，黄连、竹叶各3克，开水沏，代茶饮。

有清热解毒之效。可用于防治热毒疮肿、目赤肿痛等症。

2.6 保健药粥

保健药粥即是将保健中药与米同煮而成的稀粥。药粥疗法则是在中医理论指导下，选择适当的中药，与米谷配伍，再加入一定的调味配料，同煮为粥，用以治疗疾病的一种食疗方法。

药粥疗法是一种重要的保健方法，"粥剂"是一种古老而独特的好剂型，它集中了药疗与食疗、药补与食补之优点，体现了米药协同作用的优越性，具有注重健脾养胃、补益后天、便于服食等特点。

食粥，是我国广大人民群众在长期的生活实践中形成的一种习惯，粥在我国已有数千年的历史。应用药物与米谷煮粥治疗疾病，最早见于汉·司马迁所著的《史记·扁鹊仓公列传》和马王堆汉墓中出土的十四种医学方剂书中。汉代名医张仲景对药粥的应用颇多阐发,追至唐、宋,药粥疗法有了很大发展,许多医者和人民群众都广泛采用药粥来防治疾病。元朝忽思慧的《饮膳正要》、邹铉的《寿亲养老新书》等书的问世,为药粥保健的发展作出了贡献。明、清以至近代,药粥疗法又有所发展,形成了一种系统的祛病强身、延年益寿的疗法。

药粥既可用于预防疾病,又可作为急性病的辅助疗法,或用于病后及妇女产后的调理,或用作慢性病人之自我调养,又不失为中老年人摄生自养的好方法。煮制药粥一般有中药直接同米谷煮粥、先将中药研为细末再与米谷煮粥、原汁同米煮粥、中药煎取浓汁去渣后与米谷煮粥等方法。服食药粥要注意辨证选粥、合理应用;注意应用药粥的季节性和地区性;注意药粥的配制煎煮方法;注意调味品和容器的选择以及忌口、疗程等问题。

保健药粥依选用药物之不同,而有偏于补气、养血、助阳、滋阴之差别,可据其功效灵活选用。

1. 人参粥

本粥选自《食鉴本草》,原料为人参末3克(或党参末15克)、冰糖少量、粳米100克。将人参末与粳米同入砂锅煮粥,将成时加入冰糖稍煮即可。本粥能益元气、补五脏、抗衰老,适用于年老体弱、五脏虚衰、久病羸瘦、食欲不振、慢性腹泻、心慌气短、失眠健忘、性机能减退等一切气血津液不足之病症。本粥适用于秋冬季节早晨空腹食用,忌食萝卜、茶叶,忌铁器,宜用砂锅。

2. 补虚正气粥

补虚正气粥方出自《圣济总录》,原料为炙黄芪30~60克、人参3~5克(或党参15~30克)、白糖少许、粳米100~150克。先将黄芪、人参切成薄片,冷水浸泡半小时,入砂锅煮沸后改用小火煎成浓汁,取汁后再如法煎取二汁。汁分两份,于每日早晚同粳米加适量水煮粥,粥将成时入白糖稍煮。人参亦可研成细粉入粥中煎煮。3～5日为一疗程，间隔2～3日再服。服粥期间忌食萝卜、茶叶。

本粥能补正气、疗虚损、健脾胃、抗衰老，适用于劳倦内伤、年老体弱、体虚自汗、食欲不振、气虚浮肿等气血亏虚之症。

3. 大枣粥

大枣粥方出自《圣济总录》，原料为大枣10～15个、粳米100克。两者共煮成粥。本粥可作点心或供早晚餐服食，痰湿较重的肥胖中老年人忌食。

本粥能补气血、健脾胃，适用于老年人胃虚食少、脾虚便溏、气血不足以及血小板减少、贫血、慢性肝炎、过敏性紫癜、营养不良、病后体虚等。

4. 参苓粥

参苓粥方出自《圣济总录》，原料为人参3～5克（或党参15克）、白茯苓15～20克、生姜3～5克、粳米100克。先将人参、生姜切片，茯苓捣碎，煎取药汁，再同粳米煮粥。本粥一年四季均可间断常服，每日早晚空腹温热食用。

本粥能益气补虚、健脾养胃，适用于气虚体弱、脾胃不足、倦怠乏力、面色㿠白、饮食减少、反胃呕吐、大便稀薄等症。

5. 山药粥

山药粥方出自《萨谦斋经验方》，原料为山药45～60克（鲜山药100～120克）、粳米100～150克。将山药洗净切片，与粳米同煮为粥。四季均可食用，早晚温热服。

本粥能补脾胃，滋肺肾，适用于脾胃虚弱、慢性久泻、虚劳喘嗽、食少体倦、糖尿病、慢性肾炎等。

6. 白扁豆粥

白扁豆粥方出自《延年秘旨》，原料为炒白扁豆60克（鲜白扁豆120克）、粳米100克。两者同煮为粥，煮时扁豆一定要烧至烂熟。宜于夏秋季早晚餐服食。

本粥能健脾养胃、清暑止泻，适用于脾胃虚弱、食少呕逆、慢性久泻、暑湿泻痢、夏季烦渴等。

7. 黄芪粥

黄芪粥方出自《冷庐医话》，原料为生黄芪 30～60 克、粳米 100 克、陈皮末 1 克、红糖少许。先将生黄芪浓煎取汁后，加入粳米、红糖同煮，粥将成时，调入陈皮末，稍沸即可。供早晚餐温热食用，阴虚体质者忌服。

本粥能补益元气、健脾养胃、利水消肿，适用于劳倦内伤、慢性腹泻、体虚自汗、老年性水肿、慢性肝炎、慢性肾炎、疮疡久溃不敛等气血不足之症。

8. 落花生粥

落花生粥方出自《粥谱》，原料为落花生（不去红衣）45 克、粳米 100 克、冰糖适量，怀山药 30 克或百合 15 克。花生洗净捣碎，加入粳米、山药片或百合片同煮，粥将成时放入冰糖稍煮即可。煮粥时花生红衣不宜去掉。本粥可长期食用，腹泻者不宜多食。

本粥能健脾开胃、润肺止咳、养血通乳，适用于肺燥干咳、脾虚反胃、贫血、产后乳汁不足等症。

9. 珠玉二宝粥

珠玉二宝粥方出自《医学衷中参西录》，原料为生山药 60 克、生薏苡仁 60 克、柿饼 30 克。本粥以山药代米，先将薏苡仁煮至烂熟，再将山药捣碎，柿饼切成小块同煮成粥。主要为慢性病调理之用，日食 2 次，5～7 日为 1 疗程。

本粥能补肺、健脾、养胃，适用于阴虚内热、劳嗽干咳、大便泄泻、食欲减退等一切脾肺气虚之病症。

10. 糯米阿胶粥

糯米阿胶粥方出自《食医心鉴》，原料为阿胶 30 克、糯米 100 克、红糖少许。先用糯米煮粥，将熟时放入捣碎的阿胶，边煮边搅匀，2～3 沸后，加入红糖即可。3 天为 1 疗程，可间断服用。脾胃虚弱者不宜多食。

本粥能滋阴补血、养血止血、安胎、益肺，适用于血虚、虚劳咳嗽、久咳咯血、吐血衄血、大便出血、妇女血虚经少、漏下不止、胎动不安、胎漏等。

11. 龙眼肉粥

龙眼肉粥方出自《老老恒言》，原料为龙眼肉15克、红枣3~5枚、粳米100克，共煮为粥。喜食甜者可加白糖少许。本粥须热服，每次用量不宜过大。风寒感冒、恶寒发热、舌苔厚腻者忌服。

本粥能养心安神、健脾补血，适用于心血不足之心悸、心慌、失眠健忘、贫血、脾虚腹泻、水肿、体质羸虚、神经衰弱等。

12. 仙人粥

仙人粥方出自《遵生八笺》，原料为制何首乌30~60克、粳米100克、红枣3~5枚、红糖适量。先煎取首乌浓汁，去渣后与粳米、红枣同入砂锅内煮粥，将成时入红糖再煮1~2沸即可。日服1~2次，7~10天为1疗程，间隔5天再服。大便溏泻者不宜食。食粥期间忌葱蒜，煮粥忌用铁锅。

本粥能补气血、益肝肾，适用于肝肾亏虚、须发早白、血虚头晕耳鸣、腰膝酸软、大便干结、高血压、冠心病、高血脂症、神经衰弱等。

13. 乳粥

乳粥方出自《臞仙神隐》，原料为牛乳或羊乳适量（幼儿也可用人乳）、大米100克、白糖少许。大米加水煮粥，至半熟时去米汤，加乳汁、白糖同煮成粥。供早晚餐空腹温热服食，夏季应注意乳汁保鲜。

本粥能补虚损、健脾胃，适用于一切虚弱劳损、气血不足、病后产后羸瘦、年老体弱、婴幼儿营养不良。

14. 海参粥

海参粥方出自《老老恒言》，原料为海参适量、粳米或糯米100克。先将海参发好，剖洗干净，切片煮烂后，与米共煮成稀粥。每晨空腹食用，疗程不限。

本粥能补肾、益精、养血，适用于精血亏损、体质虚弱、性机能减退、遗精尿频、神经衰弱等。

15. 桑仁粥

桑仁粥方出自《粥谱》，原料为桑椹20～30克（鲜者30～60克）、糯米100克、冰糖少许。先将桑椹浸泡片刻，洗净后与米同入砂锅煮粥，将熟时加冰糖稍煮即可。宜空腹服，可经常食用。忌用铁锅，便稀者不宜食。

本粥能补肝滋肾、养血明目，适用于肝肾阴虚、头晕目眩、视力减退、腰膝酸软、须发早白、肠燥便秘。

16. 鸡汁粥

鸡汁粥方出自《中国烹饪》，原料为1500～2000克母鸡1只，粳米100克。将母鸡剖洗干净后，浓煎鸡汁，以原汁鸡汤分次与粳米煮粥。宜温热服，发热者忌食。

本粥能滋养五脏、补益气血，适用于年老体弱、病后体虚、气血亏虚所致之一切衰弱病症。

17. 菟丝子粥

菟丝子粥方出自《粥谱》，原料为菟丝子30～60克（鲜者60～100克）、粳米100克、白糖适量。菟丝子洗净捣碎，水煎取汁后与米同煮，将成时加入白糖稍煮，每日早晚2次服用，须长期食用。

本粥能补肾益精、养肝明目，适用于肝肾不足、腰膝酸软、阳萎遗精、早泄、头晕耳鸣、小便频数等。

18. 苁蓉羊肉粥

苁蓉羊肉粥方出自《本草纲目》，原料为肉苁蓉10～15克、精羊肉100克、粳米100克、细盐少许、葱白2茎、生姜3片。将肉苁蓉、羊肉洗净后细切，先用砂锅煎取肉苁蓉汁，去渣后入羊肉、粳米同煮，沸后加入细盐、葱、姜煮至粥成。宜于冬季服食，5～7天为一疗程。夏季、便溏、性机能亢进者不宜食。忌铁器。

本粥能补肾助阳、健脾养胃、润肠通便，适用于肾阳虚衰、阳萎遗精、早泄、腰膝冷痛、宫冷不孕、素体羸弱、劳倦内伤、脾胃虚寒、老人阳虚便秘等。

19. 胡桃粥

胡桃粥方出自《海上集验方》，原料为胡桃仁10～15个、粳米100克。胡桃肉捣碎，与米同煮为粥。大便稀薄的老人不宜食用。

本粥能补肾、益肺、润肠，适用于肾亏腰痛腿软、肺虚久咳气短、慢性便秘、病后体弱、尿路结石等。

20. 荔枝粥

荔枝粥方出自《泉州本草》，原料为干荔枝5～7枚、粳米或糯米100克。荔枝去壳，与米同煮为粥。3～5日为1疗程，晚餐服食。阴虚火旺者忌食。

本粥能温阳益气、生津养血，适用于老人阳虚腹泻、五更泄泻、口臭等。

21. 栗子粥

栗子粥方出自《本草纲目》，原料为栗子10～15个（或栗粉30克）、粳米或糯米100克。栗子去壳（或栗粉）与米同煮为粥。早晚餐食，四季均可食用。

本粥能补肾强筋、健脾养胃，适用于老年体弱、肾虚腰痛、腿软无力、脾虚泄泻等。

22. 雀儿药粥

雀儿药粥方出自《太平圣惠方》，原料为麻雀5只、菟丝子30～45克、覆盆子10～15克、枸杞子20～30克、粳米100克、细盐少许、葱白2茎、生姜3片。先将菟丝子、覆盆子、枸杞子放入砂锅内煎取药汁，再将麻雀去毛及肠杂，洗净酒炒后与粳米、药汁加适量水煮粥,将熟时加入盐、葱、姜煮至粥成。宜冬季食用,3~5日为1疗程,发烧及性机能亢进者忌食。

本粥能壮阳气、补精血、益肝肾、暖腰膝,适用于肾气不足、腰膝酸冷而痛、阳萎早泄遗精、头晕耳鸣、小便清长、妇女带下等症。

23. 鹿角胶粥

鹿角胶粥方出自《本草纲目》,原料为鹿角胶15~20克、粳米100克、生姜3片。先煮粳米,待沸后加入鹿角胶、生姜同煮为粥。适用冬季服食,3~5日为1疗程。夏季、阴虚火旺或发烧者不宜食用。

本粥能补肾阳、益精血,适用于肾气不足、虚劳羸瘦、阳萎遗精早泄、宫冷不孕、崩漏、带下等。

24. 枸杞羊肾粥

枸杞羊肾粥方出自《饮膳正要》,原料为枸杞叶250克、新鲜羊肾一只、羊肉100克、粳米100~150克、葱白2茎、细盐少许。将羊肾剖洗干净,去内膜,细切,再把羊肉洗净切碎。煎取枸杞叶汁,同羊肾、羊肉、粳米、葱白一起煮粥,粥将成时加入盐稍煮即可。冬季食用为宜,无枸杞叶可用枸杞子代替,阳盛体质者不宜食用。

本粥能益肾阴、补肾气、壮元阳,适用于肾虚劳损、腰膝酸软、头晕耳鸣、性机能减退、老年阳虚等。

25. 山萸肉粥

山萸肉粥方出自《粥谱》,原料为山萸肉15~20克、粳米100克、白糖适量。山萸肉洗净去核,与粳米同入砂锅煮粥,将熟时加入白糖稍煮即可。3~5日为1疗程,病愈即可停服,发热或小便淋涩者不宜服用。

本粥能补益肝肾、涩精敛汗,适用于肝肾不足、头晕目眩、耳鸣腰酸、虚汗不止、遗精、遗尿等。

26. 玉竹粥

玉竹粥方出自《粥谱》，原料为玉竹15~20克（鲜者30~60克）、粳米100克、冰糖少许。煎取玉竹浓汁后入粳米，加水适量煮为稀粥，将成时加入冰糖1~2沸即可。早晚服食，5~7天为1疗程。胃有痰湿气滞、消化不良者忌食。

本粥能滋阴润肺、生津止咳，适用于肺阴不足、肺燥干咳少痰或无痰，或热病后烦渴、阴虚发热。服用本粥亦可作为各种心脏病、心功能不全的辅助疗法。

27. 天门冬粥

天门冬粥方出自《饮食辩录》，原料为天门冬15~20克、粳米50~100克、冰糖少许。煎取天门冬浓汁，与粳米煮粥，将成时加入冰糖稍煮即可。3~5日为1疗程，间隔3日再服。虚寒腹泻、外感风寒者不宜食。

本粥能滋阴润肺、生津止咳，适用于肾阴不足、阴虚内热、津少口干，或肺阴不足、干咳少痰、午后低热、夜间盗汗等。

28. 沙参粥

沙参粥方出自《粥谱》，原料为沙参15~30克、粳米50~100克、冰糖适量。先煎取沙参汁，然后与粳米同煮，粥熟后加冰糖稍煮即可。本粥宜稀薄，不宜稠厚。风寒咳嗽忌食。

本粥能润肺养胃、祛痰止咳，适用于肺燥干咳少痰，可肺气不足、肺胃阴虚之久咳无痰、咽干，或热病伤津口渴。

29. 百合粉粥

百合粉粥方出自《本草纲目》，原料为百合粉30克（鲜百合60克）、粳米100克、冰糖适量。将百合粉与粳米同煮，粥将成时加白糖稍煮即可。风寒咳嗽及脾胃虚寒者忌食。

本粥能润肺止咳、养心安神，适用于老年慢性支气管炎、肺热或肺燥咳嗽、热病后期余热未退、神经衰弱、更年期综合征等。

30. 莲子粉粥

莲子粉粥方出自《太平圣惠方》，原料为莲子粉15~20克、粳米或糯米 100 克。先将莲子煮熟后，切开去壳，晒干磨粉，与米同煮成粥。感冒发热、大便干燥者不宜食用。

本粥能养心安神、益肾补脾、抗衰老，适用于年老体弱、失眠多梦、慢性腹泻、夜间多尿等。

31. 酸枣仁粥

酸枣仁粥方出自《太平圣惠方》，原料为酸枣仁 30～45 克（生熟均可）、粳米 100 克。将酸枣仁捣碎，浓煎取汁，粳米加水适量煮粥，米半熟时，加入酸枣仁汁同煮为粥。宜于晚餐温热服食。

本粥能养肝宁心、安神、止汗，适用于神经衰弱、老年性失眠、心悸怔忡、自汗盗汗等。

32. 山楂粥

山楂粥方出自《粥谱》，原料为山楂 30～40 克（鲜山楂 60 克）、粳米 100 克、沙糖 10 克。先将山楂入砂锅煎取浓汁，去渣后入粳米、沙糖煮粥。可作三餐点心食用，7～10 天为 1 疗程。不宜空腹食，慢性脾胃虚弱者不宜食用。

本粥能健脾胃、消食积、散瘀血，适用于食积停滞、腹痛腹泻、产后瘀血疼痛、恶露不尽、痛经、小儿乳食不消、高血压、冠心病、高脂血症等，老年人常服有防病强身之作用。

33. 薏苡仁粥

薏苡仁粥方出自《广济方》，原料为薏苡仁粉 30～60 克、粳米 100 克。先将生薏苡仁洗净晒干，研成细粉，与米同煮为粥。供早晚餐，温热服食。

本粥能健脾胃、利水湿、抗癌肿，适用于老年性水肿、筋脉拘挛、风湿痹痛，服食本粥也可作为防治胃癌、肠癌、宫颈癌的辅助疗法。中老年人经常服食，有防病健体、抗老益寿之作用。

2.7 保健药糕

糕是用米粉、麦粉或豆粉等做成块状，经蒸制或烘制而成的食品，因其松软易消化，是我国人民喜用的食品品种之一。正如《本草纲目》对粳糕的评价："养脾胃，厚肠，益气和中"。若将具有保健作用的中药研为细粉，再与米粉、麦粉或豆粉相混合，或加适量白糖、食油，做成糕，蒸熟或烘制，即成保健药糕。

保健药糕既是味美可口的食品点心，因其中保健药物能发挥防治疾病、养生保健、抗老延年的作用，又是一种良好的食疗保健品种。

保健药糕多用于老年、小儿慢性脾胃疾病的调理和病后康复调养，也有些可防治各科疾病。据古代文献记载，某些药糕有补脾益肾，延缓衰老之效，尤宜于老人常服。由于药糕之药性多十分平和，在家庭中自制又很方便，是一种简便实用的自我保健方法。下面选介的各药糕，多出自有关文献，个别药物及方中剂量有所调整，有关叙述和分析亦结合现代认识和经验。未注出处者系作者经验方。

1. 阳春白雪糕

白茯苓（去皮）、怀山药、芡实仁、莲子肉（去心、皮）各150克，共研细末；与陈仓米、糯米各300克一起，蒸极熟取出，加入白砂糖900克同搅极匀，揉作一块，以印模作成饼状，晒干收贮。宜于男妇小儿任意取食。

明代太医院史目龚廷贤著《寿世保元》所载该药糕，有健脾养胃，益肾补心之效，宜于身体虚弱，脾胃不健，神疲倦怠，食欲不振者，不仅最益老人，而且"治虚劳百病……大有补益"。

2. 秘传二仙糕

人参、山药、白茯苓、芡实仁、莲子肉（去皮、心）各250克，糯米750克，粳米1750克，共为细末，和匀，将蜂蜜250克、白糖250克溶化，与药、米细末掺揉得宜，蒸熟成饭，取出作成棋子块，慢火上烘干，作点心食之。或为末，贮磁器，每早一大匙，白开水调下。

此药糕载于《扶寿精方》、《济阳纲目》，均为明代著作，称有"固齿黑发，壮阴阳，益肾水，养脾胃"之效。此方较阳春白雪糕多一味人参，则大大增强了培补元气的作用。两者适应范围相同，本方补益之力更佳。

3. 九仙王道糕

莲子肉、炒山药、白茯苓、苡仁各120克，炒麦芽、炒白扁豆、芡实各60克，柿霜30克；白糖600克，共为末，入糯米粉2500克，蒸熟为糕，切块，晒干。任意食，米汤下。

此方见于明·龚廷贤《万病回春》及清·赵学敏《串雅内外篇》，认为本药糕"养神扶元，健脾胃，进饮食，补虚损，生肌肉，除湿热"。本方药物比阳春白雪糕多苡仁、麦芽、白扁豆、柿霜，不仅增强健脾开胃之力，更以其消食祛湿、清热生津之效而使全方补消兼施，防止纯补易滞之弊。体弱或年老之人久服健身延寿，甚为适宜。

4. 八仙白云糕

干山药、莲子肉、白茯苓、芡实肉、薏苡仁各120克，白芍药、白术各60克，砂仁30克，共为细末，与上白米饭1500克、糯米750克和匀，再入白砂糖霜1250克，蒸糕，任意食之。

本方载于《明医选要济世奇方》，该书称之为"保养天和神品"。其药物比阳春白雪糕多4味：薏苡仁、白芍、白术、砂仁，既增强补脾健胃之力，复又能祛湿、行气、补血敛阴柔肝，故属平补脾胃，兼顾气血，滋而不腻的滋补药糕佳品。

5. 八仙早朝糕

炒白术、山药各120克，枳实、白茯苓、炒陈皮、莲子肉（去心、皮）、山楂（去核）各60克，人参30克（如气盛人以砂仁代之），共为细末，用白米2750克、糯米750克打粉，用蜂蜜

1500克（如无蜜可用糖2000克代之），入药末和匀，如做糕法，先划小块，笼中蒸熟，取出火烘干，瓦罐封，时取3～5片食之。

《济阳纲目》载本方，并云："主理脾胃，或泻泄不止者，最宜老人，服之神效"。其药物为秘传二仙糕去芡实，加白术、枳实、陈皮、山楂，重点是增强了行气开胃、消食化积作用，亦为一补通结合、补而不滞不腻的滋补药糕良方。适于脾虚气弱，纳呆食少的中老年人常服。

6. 八珍糕

薏米、芡实、扁豆、建莲、山药各90克，党参、茯苓各60克，白术30克，白糖240克，共研细末，同白米粉蒸糕。日进2～3次，随意取之。

此方出自《清太医院配方》，称之"不寒不热，平和温补之药，扶养脾胃为主，屡经奇效，百发百中，……此糕男妇小儿诸虚百损，无不神效。"此类药糕在清代宫廷中甚受推崇，乾隆、光绪、慈禧等皆喜食之。其药物较阳春白雪糕增加党参、白术、扁豆、薏米，更加强了益气健脾渗湿之力，诚为培补脾胃后天之佳品。适用于身体虚弱、脾气亏损者保健和有关病证的辅助治疗。该方之不足是缺乏行气消导之品，恐有滞胃气之弊。

山东中医学院在继承明、清以来药糕保健经验的基础上，结合现代科学研究成果，以药食两用之品组方，研制成功"八珍食品"，有山药、莲子肉、山楂等，体现了补消结合的原则，具有健脾养胃，和中消食，及补肾、养心、益肺、化滞、消积、渗湿、安神之效。经观察能促进儿童发育，增进食欲。实验研究表明，可促进幼小动物发育，提高血红蛋白，增强体力，调节消化功能，并使脾虚动物显著改善。这也提示保健药糕确有可靠滋补养生作用。

7. 健脾养心糕

茯神、莲子肉、山药、百合、龙眼肉各60克，共研细末，与白糖150克、糯米粉1000克和匀,蒸熟为糕,可随意食之。若切块,烘干,可贮存,平素常食。

本品健脾益气,养心安神,兼补肾养血,为双补心脾之食疗佳品。与前述各药糕相比,有较强的益心宁神作用是其主要特点。适于心脾气血亏虚,倦怠食少,健忘失眠,心悸气短,面色萎黄等症。

8. 和中消食糕

茯苓、白扁豆、莲子肉、山药、炒山楂、炒麦芽、炒谷芽各45克,砂仁9克,共研细末,与白糖150克、米粉1000克和匀,蒸熟为糕,可随意食之。或切成片,烘干,平素常食。

本品补脾健胃,益气和中,消食化积,理气行滞。为补消兼顾,补而不滞之补益药糕。最适于脾胃虚弱,食欲不振,食少腹胀,脘腹痞闷,饮食不消之症。

2.8 保健药饼

药饼也是一种传统中药剂型,有内服与外用两种。内服药饼是药膳食疗的一种常用形式,且常用于保健,本节即介绍此种保健药饼。

保健药饼是由具有保健作用的中药细末和麦粉、米粉或豆粉,或加枣肉,或白糖、食油等,做成饼状,经蒸、烙、烘烤或煎煿等法,制成的熟食。由于制法较简单,服食方便,比较可口,又确有效验,故服食此饼可为一种自我保健的好方法,尤宜于老幼及体弱者食用。保健药饼一般药性平和,收功亦较缓慢,常服久用,方能获良效。保健药饼中一般不用或少用药性较猛峻或有毒性之品。如方中有此类中药,应控制药的用量。按规定炮制,并严格限定药饼的服用量,以防发生毒副作用。

下面选介几种具有防病保健、养生抗老作用的保健药饼。出自有关文献者,对药物剂量及制法、功用分析等,结合现代认识和经验,有所斟酌调整。未注出处者系作者经验方。

1. 天门冬饼子

天冬 500 克,捣取汁 150 克,煎汁至 50 克,加入白蜜 100 克,胡麻末(微炒) 200 克,搅和,再加入适量黑豆黄末,捏成饼子,直径 9 cm,厚 1.5 cm,蒸、烙或烘成熟饼。每服 1 枚,嚼烂,可用温酒下,每日服 3 次。

本方载于《太平圣惠方》,有养阴精,补肺肾,坚齿黑发之效。该书称:"久服白发变黑,齿落重生,延年长生,气力百倍"。适用于虚劳绝伤,年老衰损,羸瘦,偏枯,及其他属于肺肾阴虚、精气衰少之症。天冬、胡麻属滋补抗衰老之品,久服此药饼可有抗衰延年之效。

2. 黄精饼

黄精适量,加水煎煮取汁,煎汁浓缩成膏,与适量炒黑豆黄末相和,作饼如钱大,蒸、烙或烘成熟饼。每服 2 枚,日渐加之。

本方亦见于《太平圣惠方》,原注曰:"百日知验,一年内即变老为少,气力倍增"。该药饼有填精益髓,养阴益气,强壮筋骨之效。宜于精髓不足,阴虚气弱,倦怠乏力,筋骨软弱,肺痨咯血等症。古认为黄精有益寿驻颜之效,现代研究表明,能增加冠状动脉血流量和心肌营养性血流量,预防动脉粥样硬化,降血压,降血糖,有益于抗老延寿。

3. 壮阳暖下药饼

炮附子 30 克(去皮),神曲 90 克,炮干姜 90 克,枣 30 枚(去皮、核),桂心、五味子、菟丝子(酒浸二宿,爆干为末)、肉苁蓉(酒浸一宿,刮去皱皮,炙干)各 30 克,蜀椒 15 克(微炒黄色),羊髓 90 克,酥 60 克,蜜 120 克,黄牛乳 1.5 升,白面 500 克。各药为细末,入面,用酥、髓、蜜、乳相合入枣,熟,搜于盆中盖严,令通风半日,顷即取出,再搜,令熟,摊作胡饼,入炉鏊中,上下以火煿熟。每日空腹食一枚。

此方见于明代徐春甫《老老余编》,以此"治五劳七伤,遗精数溺"。据其药物分析，主要功效为温肾助阳，散阴寒，填精髓。适用于肾阳亏虚，命门火衰、精髓不充的虚损劳伤，阳痿遗精，夜尿频数，腰膝酸软，畏寒肢冷等症。方中附子大热有毒，应经炮制，不得超量，所做药饼不宜大，服量不可多。

4. 期颐饼

生芡实 180 克，轧细，过罗；生鸡内金 90 克，轧细，过罗，置盆内浸以滚水，半日许；再入芡实、白面 250 克、白砂糖适量，用所浸原水，和作极薄小饼，烙成焦黄色，随意食之。

这是《医学衷中参西录》方。该书称此方"治老人气虚，不能行痰，致痰气郁结，胸次满闷，胁下作痛。凡气虚痰盛之人，服之皆效，兼治疝气。"本方有益肾固精，补脾消积，补消结合，脾肾双补之效，于中老年大有助益，可见"期颐"之名不虚。

5. 益脾饼

白术 120 克，鸡内金 60 克，各自轧细焙熟；干姜 60 克，轧细；与熟枣肉 250 克一起同捣如泥，作小饼，木炭火上炙干。空心时，当点心，细嚼咽之。

本方亦出自《医学衷中参西录》。该书以此方"治脾胃湿寒，饮食减少，长作泄泻，完谷不化"。该方有健脾温中，益气养血，消食化积之效，是一个平妥的温补中焦食疗方。宜于脾胃虚弱而有寒者，症如纳呆食少，脘腹冷痛，时作泄泻，完谷不化，受寒凉或劳累则加重。若无寒象，干姜酌减或不用。

6. 益寿饼

茯苓、山药、何首乌、莲子肉、枸杞子各 30 克，共为细末，与白面 500 克、白糖适量和匀，加水和面，作成饼干样小饼，烙、烤而成。若在烤箱内烘制更佳。制成之饼可供一周服食。

该方双补脾肾，益气充精。方中茯苓、首乌、枸杞等均为抗老益寿之佳品，故该饼适合于中老年常服，以抗衰防老。也适于身体虚弱，脾肾两虚者的日常滋补保健。

7. 九仙保健饼

茯苓、山药、薏米、芡实、百合、炒山楂、炒麦芽各 30 克,砂仁 9 克,共为细末,与炒黑芝麻 30 克、面粉 1000 克、白糖适量和匀,加水和面,作成饼干样小饼,烙、烤或烘制而成。平素可随意食之。

该药饼益心脾,补肝肾,固精安神,润养五脏,健胃行气,消食化积。9 味药都属药食两用之品,是一种作用平和,广泛适用的滋补保健食疗佳品,男妇老幼均可服用。

2.9 外用保健膏药

膏药,古称薄贴,是我国传统的外用中药制剂,属于膏剂的一种。以特殊的熬制法所制得的膏药,贴于皮肤,通过所含各种药物的作用,可以防治疾病,养生保健。我国运用膏药有悠久的历史。晋代葛洪《肘后备急方》中已有油、丹熬炼而成"膏"的记载,唐宋以来有广泛应用,明代龚廷贤《寿世保元》介绍常贴千金封脐膏有"还少"、"返童"之效,清代吴尚先的外治专著《理瀹骈文》所载各科膏药甚丰,清代宫廷御医也常用膏药为皇帝,太后等保健治病。

膏药的应用十分广泛,对内、妇、儿等科疾病可以"内病外治";对外科、骨伤科疾病可发挥消炎、止痛、活血、消肿、止血、生肌等作用。保健膏药一般贴于有关强壮穴位,能防病保健、抗衰延寿。由于其便于使用,药效缓和而持久,效果确实,是一种适合自我保健的好方法。

《理瀹骈文》指出:"外治之理即内治之理,外治之药亦即内治之药,所异者,法耳"。膏药外贴治病保健的作用,与药物的药性及内治的医理都是一致的。就保健膏药而言,药物多属温经散寒、助阳固元、补益脾肾、行气消瘀、通经活络之品,敷贴于神阙、气海、关元、肾俞等穴,则药性经皮肤,入腠理,通经络、归脏腑,从而温振阳气,固精培元,疏通经络,运行气血,故有强身健体、抗邪防病、延缓衰老之效。有人曾观察用丁香、肉桂等温肾助阳药贴神阙穴治疗慢性支气管炎病人，不仅改善症状，而且可改善机体的免疫状态，提高细胞免疫功能，并能预防感冒，增进食欲，可见确有保健作用。

膏药也有多种，用于保健的膏药一般是黑膏药。黑膏药系以食用植物油炸取药料，去渣后在高热下浓缩，再与铅丹反应而成的铅硬膏。植物油以芝麻油为最好。铅丹，一般称黄丹，为用铅加工制成的橙红色或橙黄色的粉末，主要成分为四氧化三铅。熬制黑膏药的基本方法步骤如下。

炸料　　将锅内适量芝麻油加热，放入药料，不断翻动，质地疏松的药宜在其他药料炸至枯黄后再下锅，并随时用漏勺把上浮的药物按入油中，此时宜文火，油温可达200°～220℃，不要超过240℃。待药料表面深褐色、内部焦黄色，停止加热，油温降至200℃以下时，把药渣捞去，所余油液为药油。

炼油　　武火熬炼药油，油温升至320°～330℃时，改用中火，并不断撩油，油温保持在这个温度范围，待油烟由黑而变为白色浓烟，油花由锅壁周边向中央集聚，并达到"滴水成珠"（沾取药油少许，滴于水中，油滴散开后又集聚时为度），药油即为炼好。

下丹成膏　　将炼好的药油连锅离火，置于平稳处，徐徐加入铅丹，均匀撒布，并不停地向一个方向搅拌，以防铅丹沉聚锅底。此时温度一般在320℃左右，可发生大量刺激性浓烟。待白烟冒尽，药油由棕褐色变为黑褐色时，取少量滴入冷水中，数秒后取出，若膏不粘手，稠度适当，即为膏药炼成。此为离火下丹法，为常用之法。另有火上下丹法，药油微炼即边加热边下丹，丹下完后，继续加热熬炼到成膏。关于铅丹的用量，一般为一斤油用150～210克丹，冬季可少些，夏季则略增。下丹前应炒干除去水分。

去"火毒"　　膏药制成后，徐徐倾入冷水中，用木棒不断搅动，使成带状，以利冷却。随时换冷水。凝结后取出，反复捏压，制成团块，浸于冷水中24小时至数日（每日换水），使火毒去净。不如此处理，贴后常对局部有刺激，出现红斑、瘙痒，甚至发泡溃烂。

摊涂　取膏药团块置适当容器中，在水浴上溶化，兑入细料（麝香、冰片细粉等），搅匀。以竹签沾取适量膏药，摊于布或纸上，即为膏药成品。

使用膏药时，可用火烘烤，或用盛开水的杯子热熨其布面，则膏药变软有粘性，即可贴于皮肤。贴前应将局部皮肤清洁洗净。

一般传统的膏药，药料中药味很多，常数十种，还常用麝香、虎骨等稀缺贵重药，自行配制不易，可购市售成品使用。下面介绍几种较为简便者，可按上面介绍的方法自行熬制。

1. 养心膏

党参、白术、云苓、甘草、生地、白芍、当归、川芎、黄连、瓜蒌、半夏、沉香、朱砂、栀子，麻油熬，黄丹收。

此方见于《理瀹骈文》。有养心活血，化痰清热之效。贴膻中。主治心虚有痰火。对气虚血瘀、痰阻热结的胸痹心痛症（冠心病心绞痛等）较为适宜。

2. 心肾双补膏

菟丝子90克，牛膝、熟地、肉苁蓉、附子、鹿茸、党参、远志、茯神、黄芪、山药、当归、龙骨、五味子各30克，麻油熬，黄丹收，朱砂30克搅匀。贴心口、丹田。

本方见于《理瀹骈文》。主要功效是温补心肾阳气。主治劳损心肾，虚而有寒。凡心气不足、肾阳虚衰者，可贴此膏，补虚强身。

3. 专益元气膏

牛肚一个，用麻油先熬去渣，入黄芪240克，党参、生白术、当归各180克，熟地、半夏、香附、麦冬各120克，五味子、茯苓、白芍、益智仁、补骨脂、胡桃肉、陈皮、肉桂、甘草各30克，砂仁、木香各21克，干姜15克，大枣10个，麻油熬，黄丹收。贴膻中或脐下。

此膏亦见于《理瀹骈文》。主治元气不足。元气为生命活动的动力源泉，乃先天之精所化生，赖后天摄入的营养精微不断滋生。本膏补肾助阳，健运脾胃，滋养精血，鼓舞五脏之气，所以适用于元气不足，精神衰减，五脏虚损之证。

4. 涌泉膏

海龙或海马1对，附子30克，零陵香、穿山甲、锁阳各9克，油熬，黄丹收，槐枝搅，下阳起石、冬虫夏草末、高丽参、川椒、丁香，搅匀。贴足心。少年勿用，徒起泡，无益也。

一方用海马、鹿茸、人参、大茴香、肉苁蓉、熟地、地龙、麻油熬，黄丹收，沉香、肉桂糁贴。用法同上。

上方均见于《理瀹骈文》多用助阳、温里之药，故有温肾补火、驱散阴寒之效。足心为涌泉穴，系足少阴肾经之井穴，贴于此穴更加强助火补阳之力。适用于因肾阳不足，命门火衰而有腰膝酸软，畏寒肢冷，阳痿遗精，耳鸣耳聋，发脱齿摇，面足浮肿，夜尿频多等症者。但年少体强或无阳虚者，忌此温燥助火之剂，以免相火妄动而出现头晕目眩，五心烦热，阳强遗精早泄等症。黄丹收膏之后所加各药，可研细粉在摊涂膏药之前投入溶化的膏药中混匀。原书未列用量者，酌用适量即可。

5. 四淫百病膏

川乌、草乌、羌活、独活、南星、半夏、麻黄、桂枝、苍术、大黄、细辛、当归、白芷、豨莶草、海风藤各30克，姜、葱、蒜、槐枝各500克，麻油熬，黄丹收，松香60克，木香、乳香、没药、轻粉、川椒末各15克搅匀。贴肾俞处。

以上处方见于《理瀹骈文》。方中诸药多为祛风胜湿散寒及活血行瘀之品，故可防治风寒暑湿四淫邪所致诸病。贴肾俞穴更能固肾益元强身，使外邪难以侵袭，有防病保健之效。

6. 保元固本膏

党参、炒白术、鹿角、当归、香附各45克,川芎、炙附子、独活、干姜、川椒、杜仲、鳖甲、荜拨、草果仁、白芍各30克,生黄芪45克,用麻油1500克,将药炸枯,去渣,再熬至滴水成滴,入飞净黄丹560克,再加入肉桂、沉香、丁香各9克共研之细末,候油冷,加入搅匀成坨,重120~150克,候去火气,3日后方可摊贴。

此方载于《慈禧光绪医方选议》,为光绪7年5月21日几位御医为慈禧太后所拟方,系摊贴脐部以治脾肾不足肠胃功能失调之用。诸药健脾补肾,助阳滋阴,益气养血,兼散寒行气活血,故有固本保元之效,可作为中老年体虚者保健良方。

7. 毓麟固本膏

杜仲、熟地、附子、苁蓉、牛膝、补骨脂、续断、官桂、甘草各120克,生地、大茴香、小茴香、菟丝子、蛇床子、天麻子、紫梢花、鹿角各45克,羊腰子1对,赤石脂、龙骨各30克,用香油4000克,熬枯去渣,用黄丹1500克收,再入雄黄、丁香、沉香、木香、乳香、没药各30克,麝香0.9克,阳起石1.5克。此膏妇人贴脐上,男子贴左右肾俞穴各一张,丹田穴一张,用汗巾缚住,勿令走动,半月一换。

此方载于《清太医院配方》及《慈禧光绪医方选议》,后者将此方列于光绪皇帝种子医方。前者称此膏"能固玉池,真精不泄,……气血流畅,精髓充满,保固下元,固本全形,……强阳健力",可治"下元虚冷,诸虚百损,五劳七伤,阳痿不举,举不坚固,久无子嗣,下淋白浊,小肠疝气,遗精盗汗,手足顽麻,半身不遂,单腹胀满,腰腿疼痛,……妇人脾胃虚弱,经水不调,赤白带下,气血亏虚,久不孕育,干血劳瘵,或系屡经小产,……兼崩漏不止,症瘕血块等症。"该书还认为此膏能助孕种子:"此膏充实血海,能暖子宫,易得孕育,……固精种子"。光绪皇帝无子嗣,又久患遗精,贴此膏药是指望补其肾,固其精,以种子承祧。此膏的保健功效也很值得重视,《清太医院配方》称:"男妇如能常贴此膏者,气血充足,容颜光彩,诸疾不生,乌须黑发,……此膏终身永贴者,体健身轻,返老还童,虽八十老人,阴阳强健,目能远视,行不困乏,……如系衰老之人,贴至百日之后,其效可验"。虽难免有言过之嫌,但对于体弱和老衰之人,不妨将贴敷此膏作为一种值得试用的简便自我保健之法。

8. 益寿比天膏

牛膝、杜仲、制虎骨、木鳖子、蛇床子、肉豆蔻、菟丝子、紫稍花、续断、穿山甲、远志、天麻子、鹿茸、苁蓉、生地、熟地、官桂、川楝子、山萸肉、巴戟天、补骨脂各 30 克、海蛆 15 克、甘草 60 克,桑枝、槐枝各 22 cm,香油 3000 克,浸一夜,慢火炸至黑色,每净油 500 克,入黄丹 195 克,用柳棍不住手搅,再下黄丹、雄黄、龙骨、赤石脂各 6 克,母丁香、沉香、木香、乳香、没药、阳起石、麝香各 12 克,黄蜡 15 克。每用两张,贴两腰眼上,或贴脐一张亦可。每贴 1 次半月 1 换。

此方载于《清太医院配方》。谓"最能添精补髓,保固肾精不泻,善助元阳,润滑皮肤,壮筋骨,理腰膝,……能通二十四道血脉,坚固身体,返老还童。"主治"下元虚冷、五劳七伤、半身不遂;或下部痿软,脚膝酸麻,阳事不举,夜梦遗精"及妇女赤白带下,砂淋血崩等。清代宫廷之中以此类外贴膏药之法保健延寿用之颇多,慈禧太后所用者就有益寿膏两方、培元益寿膏等,药味甚多,其法相似,故只选录 1 则,可供参考。个别稀缺昂贵之品可免,或易以代用品。

2.10 保健药枕

药枕是以适当中药填充枕芯,用于睡眠枕头,从而发挥防治疾病或保健作用。这是我国中医传统外治法之一,历来受到重视。湖南长沙马王堆一号汉墓出土有绢质绣花枕 1 个,内装有佩兰。河北满城县陵山汉代中山靖王刘胜墓中也有内装花椒的鎏金镶玉铜枕。说明在 2100 多年前已使用药枕。其后,在宋代《圣济总录》、《保生要录》,元代《御药院方》,明代《审视瑶函》、《本草纲目》,清代《理瀹骈文》等众多古代医著方书中,都记载有各种药枕。近年来,各地相继研制的药枕,不仅在国内很受欢迎,而且已有多种销往国外,为国内外人民保健作出了贡献。

药枕保健治病独具特点。首先是简便易行,在正常的睡眠中接受治疗,无需煎药、服药。其次,节省药材,一个药枕中只用不到 1 公斤中药,可以使用数月,平均每日耗药只几克,大大低于汤剂用药量。使用药枕最容易长期坚持,尤便于慢性病的防治和养生保健。大量临床观察证明,药枕疗效可靠,而且具有长效特点。作者等曾观察特制保健药枕对高血压病的降压作用,1 个月、2 个月与半年的观察,降血压作用都很显著。还发现药枕具有良好的调节作用,上述能使高血压者降血压的药枕,血压正常者使用后血压并不下降,而稳定在原来正常的水平。药枕的应用十分广泛,可治疗高血压、颈椎病、神经性头痛、神经衰弱、冠心病、呼吸系统疾病等多种疾病,还可预防感冒等疾病,有适于儿童用的保健药枕,也有中老年人适用的祛病保健或抗衰延年的药枕,加之药枕的制作比较简单,因而成为中老年自我保健的佳品。

药枕的中药组方也十分讲究辨证施治的原则,要求注意药物配伍。药枕所用中药以各类芳香性中药为多,含有各种挥发油,所以也有人称为"香枕"。药枕的作用在一定程度上与所含的挥发油有关,所以在选药组方时应不仅要考虑药物的性味、归经、功效,还要了解所含挥发油的情况及其药理作用等。药枕处方中药味的多寡悬殊很大,有单味药者,如菊花枕、决明枕,也有数十味药者,如《圣济总录》神枕方 32 味药。目前常用的药枕一般 10 味药左右。

自行制作药枕,首先要把按处方备齐的中药作适当加工,一般粉碎为粗末即可。不加破碎则影响药性的挥发,粉碎过细则药效散失过快，使用期缩短，细的粉末也容易从枕袋中漏出。药物粉碎前应注意去除杂质、尘土，不能使用污染、霉变的药物。枕袋以纯棉布质为宜，内袋装以加工好的药物成为枕芯，外套以外袋以便经常洗涤。枕袋的大小，一般长35～45 cm，宽20～30 cm，可视药物的多少及使用者的习惯而定，儿童使用的可再小些。每个药枕的中药总量一般500～1000克。

使用药枕时，应平整地置放于一个普通枕头上，调整该枕的高度，使加药枕后总高度适中，枕之舒适为度。使药物均匀平整。每使用数日后，可适当翻整枕内药物。枕巾与外套应适时洗涤，保持清洁。药枕应保持干燥，防潮湿、防霉、防虫蛀，避免曝晒。连续使用半年到1年之后，可更换其中药物。为保证使用效果，应坚持长期使用，每日使用时间不少于6小时。

应用药枕保健，应注意根据不同的病情、体质、年龄等，辨证施用药枕。最好在中医师的指导下使用。危、急病症一般不单独用药枕治疗，病情较重者一般只用药枕作辅助治疗或病后康复之用。

药枕防治疾病，在祖国医学是按照传统的"闻香治病"的理论来解释，是一种气味疗法，或称香味疗法之一种。就现代认识来说，药枕中的药物散发出各种挥发油或其他生物活性物质，这些物质在枕头附近形成一个药香淡雅的小气候，人体通过呼吸道粘膜、皮肤吸收，既可作用于局部，又能进入体液，也可以通过反射性起作用，因而对机体心、脑血管功能以及其他方面的机能可以发挥良好的调节作用。这样就能够防治疾病，抗衰延寿。至于药枕保健的具体机理，尚需深入研究探讨。

下面介绍若干种保健药枕，可供选购或自制者参考。古代药枕均按原剂量单位作换算，其比例可供自制时参考。

1. 歧黄牌高效保健药枕

由菊花、薄荷、川芎、细辛、柏子仁、藁本、白芷等10余种中药组成。

系山东中医学院综合借鉴宋代《圣济总录》"神枕方"、《保生要录》"药枕方"、元代《御药药方》"神枕法"、明代《审视瑶函》"药枕方"及清代《理瀹骈文》"丁公仙枕"等及现代药枕的用药特点,参考中药化学成分、药理作用、临床疗效等,反复筛选有效药物,而研制成功。现由山东中医学院实验药厂生产。该药枕有平肝潜阳,清热凉血,养心安神,开窍通脉,活血祛风,通痹止痛等功效。适用于高血压病、脑动脉硬化、颈椎病、冠心病、高脂血症、神经衰弱及神经性头痛等病的防治和中老年养生保健。经临床观察,对缓解头痛、头晕、颈项强痛、耳鸣、失眠等症状有显著效果;高血压病患者使用,有显著的降血压效果,使用1个月及2个月其收缩压下降率为14.86%及12.92%,舒张压下降率为16.11%及11.88%;非高血压病患者使用该药枕,血压无显著变化。还观察到使用药枕1.5月后脑血流图上升时间显著缩短,表明颅内血管弹性改善,或血管紧张度降低、外周阻力减小、流入道通畅,即反映了脑循环可能得到一定程度的改善。心阻抗微分图法测定表明,用药枕1.5月后左心功能似有改善,高血压患者总外周血管阻力降低。这些客观指标的改善,对中老年保健有重要意义,也表明药枕的疗效是肯定的。

2. **神枕方**

当归、川芎、白芷、辛夷、杜仲(去粗皮)、藁本(去苗土)、肉苁蓉、柏子仁、薏苡仁、蘼芜、秦椒、木兰皮、蜀椒、肉桂(去粗皮)、干姜、飞廉、防风(去叉)、款冬花、人参、桔梗、白薇、蔓荆子、白术、白藓皮、乌头(去皮)、附子(去皮尖)、藜芦(去芦头)、皂荚、莽草、半夏、矾石、细辛(去苗叶),共32味,各18.65克。

以上为《圣济总录》所载方,药物置于柏木枕内,盖上钻孔120个,以绛纱三重裹之。据称:"枕及一百日,筋骨强壮,身面光泽,即去一重纱;二百日,血气充实,百疾皆愈,又去一重;三百日又去一重,一年一易……三年后,齿发益壮,容色还童矣。"相传西汉时泰山下有一老人，85岁时已头白齿落，得一道士传授"绝谷，但服术饮水，并作神枕枕之"，以后"白发更黑，齿落更生，日行三百里"，老人180岁时将此神枕方给了来到泰山狩猎的汉武帝。传说虽有夸张，但其养生延年之效还是值得重视的。现代应用时，药物可适当加减出入。

3. 《保生要录》药枕方

蔓荆子3.0克，甘菊花3.0克，细辛2.2克，香白芷2.2克，白术1.5克，芎䓖2.2克，通草3.0克，防风3.0克，藁本3.0克，羚羊角3.0克，犀角3.0克，石菖蒲3.0克，黑豆0.33升，拣择拣令净。上药细锉去碎末，相拌令匀，以生绢囊盛之欲达其气，次用碧罗袋重盛，缝之如枕样。纳药直令紧实，置于盒子中，其盒形亦如枕。纳药囊令出盒子唇一寸半。欲枕时，揭去盒盖，不枕即盖之，使药气不散。枕之日久渐低，更入药以实之，或添黑豆，令如初。三、五月后，药气歇则换之。

该书指出，久枕此药枕，"治头风目眩，脑重冷痛，眼暗鼻塞，兼辟邪。"从药物组成来看，主治病症是可信的。所述制枕、用枕方法，亦很有借鉴价值。唯羚角、犀角均稀缺、贵重，可易为磁石之类，或据病情而作加减。

4. 丁公仙枕

川椒、桔梗、蔓荆子、柏子仁、姜黄、吴萸、白术、薄荷、肉桂、川芎、益智仁、枳实、当归、川乌、千年健、五加皮、藜芦、羌活、防风、辛夷、白芷、附子、白芍、藁本、苁蓉、细辛、牙皂、芫荑、甘草、荆芥、菊花、杜仲、乌药、半夏等分各37.3克，咀片研末，绢袋盛，装枕睡。

《理瀹骈文》所载此方，较前述神枕方药物有些增减，据称："能除百病，寿高，多子"。可供研制现代保健药枕参考。

5. 高血压病药枕

滁菊花500克，晚蚕砂500克，国槐花500克，正川芎200克，香白芷300克，将后2者研成粗末，与前3种共拌匀，同装入小麻布袋中,外套细夏布做成的枕套。睡时即以此药枕作枕头。

此方见于《中草药外治验方选》,有平肝凉血、祛风、活血、止痛之功效,宜于高血压病人使用。

6. 保健药枕

野菊花 500 克,艾绒 200 克,夜交藤粗末 100 克;牡丹皮、枸杞子、山海螺、虎杖、白芷各 20 克,樟脑 5 克,均为细末;香精少许,箬壳丝 500 克。先将菊、艾、夜交藤平摊于箬壳丝上,其他各药和匀分装于 5 只棉毛针织布小袋中,缝好,枕芯四角与中心各放 1 只。用纱布做枕芯袋,以利药物气味透出;用浅蓝色棉布做枕套,有利于安定情绪,消除疲劳。

此为金亚城氏等研制,报道于浙江中医杂志 1986 年第 8 期。该药枕对老年慢性支气管炎、高脂血症、神经衰弱的临床有效率 73~87%,对健康老年人亦有抗衰老效果,可使衰老见症积分显著下降。有上述疾病者或中老年人可酌情使用。

7. 健康长寿药枕

杭菊花、冬桑叶、野菊花、辛夷各 500 克,薄荷 200 克,红花 100 克,冰片 50 克。混合粉碎后(冰片另拌)装入布袋,作枕头使用。

此为王健生氏所介绍的基础方,见于浙江中医学院学报 1986 年第 1 期。有平肝潜阳、疏风散热、消肿解毒、活血祛风、通经止痛之效。适于高血压、动脉硬化、脑震荡、脑血栓后遗症引起的头部不适和正偏头痛、眩晕症、神经衰弱、斑秃及目赤肿痛、急慢性鼻炎、咽喉炎、后颈部毛囊炎等患者应用。

8. 颈椎病药枕

通草 300 克,菊花 200 克,白芷、红花、佩兰、川芎、厚朴各 100 克,石菖蒲 80 克,桂枝 60 克,加工并掺合为软硬适度的枕芯。颈项酸困不适加苍术 60 克、豨莶草 100 克;头晕、鼻塞者加葛根 60 克、辛夷花 60 克;肢体麻木加麻黄 50 克、桑枝、防风、羌活各100克。

姚昌晔氏在中国康复医学杂志1986年第1期介绍的此药枕,有芳香利窍、清头疏风、活血理气通痹之效,适于颈椎病患者使用。

9. 小儿鼻渊药枕

1号方:苏叶、白芷、荆芥、防风、陈皮、藿香各60克,桂枝、川椒、川芎、菊花各30克,檀香20克,细辛15克。

2号方:藿香100克,菊花、薄荷、荆芥、防风、白芷各60克,川芎、陈皮各30克,辛夷花、檀香各20克,细辛15克。

江苏中医杂志1985年第6期赵孝明氏介绍上述1、2号方,分别用治外感风寒、风热或风寒化热之鼻渊。鼻渊又称脑漏,主要症状为鼻塞、经常流带恶臭味的脓浊鼻涕,并可出现头痛、头晕、目眩等症状,相当于副鼻窦炎。成人此类病症也可以上述药枕防治。

10. 李时珍药枕

由薄荷、野菊花、青木香、淡竹叶、生石膏、白芍、川芎、冬桑叶、蔓荆子、磁石、晚蚕砂等药物组成。

葛火普氏等在中医杂志1984年第12期介绍该药枕,治疗高血压病有显著的降血压效果,总有效率88.5%,有关症状亦明显改善。该药枕由上饶市中医院、上饶市卫生保健品服务公司研制生产。

11. 神农牌保健药枕

其中有适于老年人用的长寿保健药枕,适于中青年用的逍遥保健药枕,适于小儿用的健儿益智保健药枕。由成都市新都县保健用品厂生产的这几种药枕,特别适合头痛、头昏、头晕、失眠和神经衰弱患者使用。

12. 益寿药枕

由杭菊、竹茹、夏枯草、灯芯等30余种中药制成。

陕西省蒲城县益寿药枕厂生产的该药枕,有滋阴降火,明目清心，安神醒脑，清心解毒，防暑驱邪等功效，主治高血压病、神经衰弱、神经官能症、美尼尔氏综合症等，对有头痛、目眩、耳鸣、失眠等症的老年人有一定的疗效。

3 非药物保健方法

3.1 针灸保健

针灸是中华民族发明的一种独具特色的医疗保健术,不仅对保障我国人民的健康作出重大贡献,而且在 1400 多年前就开始流传到朝鲜、日本,4 个多世纪前开始传到欧洲,受到各国人民的重视与欢迎。

针灸学是由针刺和灸疗两种治疗方法组成。针灸疗法是在人类与疾病斗争过程中,逐渐形成和发展的。早在一万多年以前的旧石器时代,我国人民就懂得使用打制石器刺病解痛。到新石器时代,已把磨制的石针作为专门的医疗工具,古称这种原始的针刺工具为砭石。此后,随着社会生产力和科学技术的发展,不断改进针刺工具,又出现竹针、骨针、铜针、铁针、金针、银针、不锈钢针。灸法也大约起源于旧石器时代,人们知道用火后,发现用火熏烤、烧灼身体某些部位可以减轻病痛,开始萌发灸法。后来发展为艾灸及其它灸法。我国古代对针灸防治疾病总结了丰富的实践经验,形成了一整套完整科学的理论。近年来在理论、临床和现代科学研究方面获得更迅速发展。

针法和灸法均可应用于保健防病,灸法更适于自我保健,称保健灸法。

3.1.1 针灸的保健作用

针灸是通过针刺、艾灸调整机体的经络脏腑气血的功能,而防治疾病,增进健康。健康的机体,应该阴阳协调,气血充盛,脏腑功能正常,经络畅通,营卫调和,这样才不致发生疾病,也不容易过早衰老。否则,阴阳失调,气血虚弱,脏腑亏损,经络气血不畅，营卫失调，则易生百病，早衰损寿。针灸通过作用于穴位和经络，并通过经络与脏腑组织的密切关系，而发挥疏通经络、调畅气血、协调阴阳、调整脏腑、调和营卫，及祛除病邪等作用。这种整体调节作用，能使机体保持生命力旺盛的健康状态，而防治疾病，预防早衰，延年益寿。

方便易行、效果显著的保健灸法，是我国古今备受推崇的保健方法，对于保健延寿发挥的作用可以归纳为以下几个方面。

1. 温通经络，祛除阴寒

灸法是一种温热性刺激，加以艾的温散寒邪的作用，故能温通经络、经脉，祛除风湿、风寒阴邪，预防风寒湿邪的侵袭，防治痹证，促进康复。

2. 补火助阳，延缓衰老

中年之后，命门之火日渐不足，阳气衰退，故老衰之象接踵而来。保健灸法以艾之性温芳香和燃艾之温热作用于神阙、关元、气海、命门、肾俞等穴，长于补命门之火，温振阳气，从而增强中老年生命的活力，延缓衰老。

3. 扶助正气，预防疾病

体质虚弱者或老年人，由于正气不足，腠理不密，脏气亏虚，往往难以抵御外邪的侵袭，六淫之邪容易乘虚而入，使人患病，甚至危及寿命。保健灸法可以扶正补气益元，密固腠理肌表，改善脏腑功能，从而增强抗御外邪，预防疾病的能力。身体素虚，经常患病者，特别是中年以后，应坚持保健灸，以祛病延年。

4. 健运脾胃，培补后天

常灸足三里、中脘等穴，可以温运脾阳，健胃消食，补益中气。脾胃为后天之本。脾胃健运，受纳运化功能正常，水谷精微化生精血充盛，后天培养得力，则身强体健。如《景岳全书》所说："人自有生以来，惟赖后天以为立命之本，……其有先天所禀原不甚厚者，但知自珍而培以后天，则无不获寿"。

5. 调畅气血，散结消肿

正常的机体应当气血和畅。气血凝滞，经络不通，则生瘀血痰浊。痰瘀结聚，则导致症瘕、肿结、中风、诸痛等症。常施保健灸，能调畅气机，行气活血，疏通经络，可预防上述诸证，或起辅助治疗、促进康复的作用。

3.1.2 针灸保健的机理

经过用现代科学的方法所进行的大量临床和实验研究，发现针灸可从多个方面发挥整体调节作用，从而达到保健抗老的目的。

1. 改善免疫功能

针灸对外周血液中淋巴细胞计数、活性及其相关指标有调节作用，对外周血流中白细胞总数、吞噬功能有调整作用，可增强网状内皮系统的功能；还能调节血清免疫球蛋白含量，增加血清补体含量，增加某些特异性补体的含量。表明针灸增强细胞免疫功能，调整体液免疫功能，因此能够防病保健，抗衰防老。

2. 调整心血管功能，改善微循环

针灸对心血管功能有良好的调节作用，可调节血管舒缩，调节血压，改善心脏功能，改善冠脉循环和微循环，保护缺血的心肌，对实验性心肌梗塞也有防治作用。因而可以预防心、脑血管疾病，并能促进已患病者及早康复。

3. 改善消化吸收功能

针灸足三里等保健穴位，可以调节胃肠的运动功能，改善消化吸收，促进整个消化系统的协调，从而增强体质和抗病能力。

4. 改善其他多系统功能

针灸还能调节神经系统功能、调节垂体、肾上腺等内分泌腺功能，调节呼吸、泌尿、生殖等方面的功能，都有利于发挥保健养生作用。

3.1.3 常用保健穴位

针灸的理论基础是经络学说。经络是人体气血运行的通路，内属于脏腑，外布于全身，将各部组织、器官联结成为一个有机的整体。经络系统包括十二经脉，奇经八脉，等等。

腧穴，一般称穴位，又称输穴、俞穴，是针灸施术的特定部位。腧穴具有输主气血、反应病痛、扶正祛邪的作用。在腧穴上施以针刺、艾灸等刺激，就能通过经络系统有效地发挥调整机能，从而防治疾病和保健。

腧穴包括十四经（十二经脉和督脉、任脉）的腧穴361个，以及经外奇穴、阿是穴。腧穴的定位，又称取穴，直接影响施术的效果。常用的取穴方法有以下3种。骨度分寸折量法，即将人体的各个部分分别规定其折量长度，作为量取穴位的标准。例如，腹部脐中上至歧骨（胸剑联合）为8寸，下至横骨上廉（耻骨联合上缘）为5寸。手指同身寸法，即以患者的手指为标准进行测量取穴，有3种具体方法。中指同身寸，以患者的中指中节屈曲时内侧两端纹头之间作为1寸。拇指同身寸，以患者拇指指间关节的横度作为1寸。横指同身寸，是令患者将食指、中指、无名指和小指并拢，以中指中节横纹处为准，4指横量作为3寸。体表标志法，以人体各种解剖标志（固定标志及采取某动作姿势时出现的动作标志）作为取穴的依据。下面重点介绍常用的保健穴位，至于其他大多数穴位和经络的具体情况请参看有关针灸学专著。

1. 足三里

屈膝，从髌骨下缘外侧凹陷处向下3寸，胫骨前嵴外一横指处，胫骨前肌中。可直刺0.5~1.2寸。可灸。主治脾、胃、肾、肝、心、肺、脑等脏腑病证，特别是消化系统疾病，如胃痛、呕吐、呃逆、腹胀、肠鸣、泄泻、痢疾、便秘、肠痈、完谷不化等，及中风、瘫痪、头晕、失眠、癫狂、咳嗽、气喘、水肿、乳痈、脚气、膝胫酸痛等。为强壮保健要穴，治虚劳赢瘦、痞积等。对该穴常施以保健针灸，可增强脾胃功能，强壮身体，提高免疫抗病能力。据传一老人每月初 8 天连续灸足三里穴，始终不渝，寿 174 岁以上。

2. 神阙

在脐窝正中，即脐中，禁针。可灸。主治腹痛、肠鸣，中风脱证，脱肛，泄泻不止等。是常用的保健灸穴位。古籍记载一老人"每岁灸脐中"，"年逾百岁而甚健壮"。灸此穴有补阳益气，温肾健脾作用。

3. 中极

在腹正中线，脐下 4 寸。可直刺 0.5~1.0 寸。可灸。主治阳痿，遗尿，遗精，小便频数，小便不通，崩漏，月经不调，痛经，带下，阴痒，阴挺，小腹痛，疝气等。

4. 关元

在腹正中线，脐下 3 寸。可直刺 0.8~1.2 寸。可灸。主治阳痿，遗尿，遗精，小便频数，小便不通，崩漏，月经不调，痛经带下，产后出血，小腹痛，疝气，完谷不化，泄泻，脱肛，中风脱证等。为强壮保健要穴。

5. 气海

在腹正中线上，脐下 1.5 寸。可直刺 0.8~1.2 寸。可灸。主治阳痿，遗尿，遗精，崩漏，月经不调，痛经，闭经，带下，产后出血，腹痛，疝气，泄泻，痢疾，便秘，水肿，中风脱症，气喘等。为强壮保健要穴。为诸气之海，施之针灸有补肾助阳，益气固精等作用。

6. 肾俞

在第 2 腰椎棘突下，旁开 1.5 寸。可直刺 0.8~1.2 寸。可灸。主治阳痿，遗精，遗尿，月经不调，白带等及腰痛，腰膝酸软，头昏目眩，耳鸣，耳聋，水肿，气喘，泄泻等。施之针灸有补肾壮阳益精作用。

7. 命门

在第 2 腰椎棘突下。可直刺 0.5～1.0 寸。可灸。主治脊强，腰痛，阳痿，遗精，月经不调，带下，泄泻，完谷不化，水肿，头昏耳鸣等。施之针灸，有补肾壮阳，健脾益胃的作用。

8. 三阴交

在内踝高点直上 3 寸，胫骨内侧面后缘。可直刺 0.5～1.0 寸。可灸。孕妇禁针。主治阳痿，遗精，遗尿，小便不利，崩漏，月经不调，痛经，带下，阴挺，不孕，腹痛，肠鸣，腹胀，泄泻，水肿，疝气，阴部痛，下肢痿痹，头痛，眩晕，失眠等。

常灸以上 6 穴，可补元阳，助命火，健肾脾，益精气，填骨髓，壮筋骨，养血，坚齿，乌发，对中老年保健尤有助益。《扁鹊心书》指出："常灸关元、气海、命关、中脘"，"可保百余年寿"。

9. 中脘

在腹正中线上，脐上 4 寸。可直刺 0.5～1.2 寸。可灸。主治胃痛，吞酸，翻胃，呕吐，饮食不化，腹胀肠鸣，泄泻，痢疾，黄疸及失眠等。常灸本穴与足三里穴可健脾益胃，培补后天。

10. 天枢

在脐中旁开 2 寸。可直刺 0.7～1.2 寸。可灸。主治消化系统诸病，如腹痛，腹胀，肠鸣，绕脐痛，泄泻，痢疾，便秘及月经不调，水肿等。

11. 曲池

屈肘，当肘横纹外端凹陷处。可直刺 1.0～1.5 寸。可灸。主治咽喉肿痛，齿痛，目赤肿痛，瘰疬，风疹，上肢不遂，腹痛，吐泻及热病等。常灸本穴与足三里，可调整血压，预防中风，提高抗病能力。

12. 内关

腕横纹上 2 寸，掌长肌腱与桡侧腕屈肌腱之间。可直刺 0.5

~0.8寸。可灸。主治心痛，心悸，胸闷，癫狂，痫症，失眠，胁痛，胃痛，恶心，呕吐，呃逆，热病，烦躁，疟疾，肘臂挛痛等。针灸本穴对心血管系统有良好的调节和保健作用。

13. 神门

在腕横纹尺侧端，尺侧腕屈肌腱的桡侧凹陷中。可直刺0.3~0.5寸。可灸。主治心痛，心烦，怔忡，惊悸健忘，不寐，癫狂，痫症，痴呆，胁痛，目黄等。

14. 大椎

在第7颈椎棘突下，约与肩相平。可向上斜刺0.5~1.0寸。可灸。主治头项强痛，疟疾，热病，癫痫，骨蒸潮热，咳嗽，气喘，感冒，脊背强急等。为调整诸阳经之要穴，针灸本穴有助阳，调经络之气的作用。

15. 肺俞

在第3胸椎棘突下，旁开1.5寸。可斜刺0.5~0.7寸。可灸。主治咳嗽，气喘，胸闷，胸痛，咯血，骨蒸潮热，盗汗等。

常灸以上两穴，可益气助阳，补肺固表，增强抗御外邪的能力，尤宜于体质虚弱常易患感冒者。

16. 心俞

在第5胸椎棘突下，旁开1.5寸。可斜刺0.5~0.7寸。可灸。主治心痛，健忘，惊悸，心烦，癫狂，痫证，咳嗽，咯血，梦遗，盗汗等。针灸本穴有益于心肺保健。

17. 肝俞

在第9胸椎棘突下，旁开1.5寸。可斜刺0.5~0.7寸。可灸。主治胁痛，黄疸，目赤，目眩，雀目，癫狂，痫症，及脊背痛，吐血，鼻衄等。针灸本穴有益于肝胆保健。

18. 脾俞

在第11胸椎棘突下，旁开1.5寸。可斜刺0.5~0.7寸。可灸。主治胃脘痛，腹胀，纳呆，呕吐，泄泻，痢疾，便血，黄疸，月经过多，水肿，背痛等。

19. 胃俞

在第12胸椎棘突下，旁开1.5寸。可斜刺0.5~0.7寸。可灸。主治胃脘痛，纳呆，腹胀，翻胃，呕吐，肠鸣，泄泻，胸胁痛等。

针灸以上2穴有益于脾胃保健。

20. 环跳

侧卧屈股取穴，在股骨大转子与骶管裂孔的连线上，中1/3与外1/3交界处。可直刺1.5~2.5寸。可灸。主治腰腿痛，下肢痿痹，半身不遂等。

21. 涌泉

在足底，足趾跖屈时呈凹陷处，约当足底（去趾）前1/3与后2/3交点。可直刺0.3~0.5寸。可灸。主治头痛，头昏，目眩，咽喉痛，舌干，失音，大便难，小便不利，小儿惊风，昏厥，足心热等。常灸本穴可补肾壮阳，有强壮作用。

22. 百会

在头部正中线上，前发际直上4.5寸，约当两侧耳廓尖连线之中点取之。可横刺0.3~0.5寸。可灸。主治头痛，眩晕，耳鸣，鼻塞，昏厥，中风失语，癫狂，脱肛，阴挺等。

23. 膻中

在前胸正中线，平第4肋间隙处，两乳头连线之中点，可横刺0.3~0.5寸。可灸。主治胸痛，胸闷，心痛，心悸，气喘，呃逆，噎膈，乳汁少等。

3.1.4 针灸保健方法

1. 针刺保健方法

（1）毫针刺法

应选用针柄无松动，针身挺直、圆滑、坚韧而富有弹性，针尖无钩的毫针。患者应取适当体位。针具和所取穴位处应严格消毒。根据穴位部位和针的长短，采取适当进针手法。如指切进针，骈指进针，舒张进针及挟持进针等。正确掌握针刺的角度和深度。进针后要施行一定的行针手法，以使患者产生针刺感应。若患者有酸、麻、胀、重等感觉，医者的指下同时也常有沉紧感，即得气，达到得气，才能取得较好的效果。得气后留针15～20分钟，亦可适当延长。留针过程中可酌情间歇行针。出针时，先以左手拇、食两指按住针孔周围的皮肤，右手持针轻微捻转并慢慢退至皮下，然后将针起出并以无菌棉球轻揉针孔，防止出血。针刺有补、泻不同手法。毫针刺法自我保健常选足三里穴，及三阴交，曲池等穴，一般不用其他穴位。保健常用补法，一般进针达到一定深度后，轻微捻转针柄，捻转的幅度较小，速度较慢。提时用力较轻，速度较慢，插时用力较重，速度较快为补法。

(2) 皮肤针刺法

梅花针和七星针均称为皮肤针，用于在皮肤表面经络、穴位处叩击浅刺，可以疏通经络气血，调节脏腑功能，是一种自我保健的好方法。

七星针，针柄长17～20cm，一端固定有莲蓬状的针盘，上嵌不锈钢短针7支。

梅花针，针柄长约33cm，一端固定捆扎在一起的5～7支不锈钢针。可以用竹筷和小号的缝衣针自行制作。这两种针具都要针锋平齐，针尖不要太锐，不能带钩。

操作时针具及叩刺的局部皮肤均应注意严格消毒。手握持针柄的后段，用手腕之力进行弹刺，使针尖垂直叩打在皮肤上，并迅速提起，反复快速操作。轻叩时用力较小，使局部皮肤潮红充血即可；重叩用力较重，以皮肤微出血为度。叩完后再消毒局部皮肤。

皮肤针叩打的部位，一般沿有关的经络循行路线，及有关穴位，也可在病痛局部。用于强壮保健时常叩腰背部正中线（督脉）及其两侧各旁开1.5寸、3寸的共4条经络线（足太阳膀胱经)。皮肤针既可用于保健，又可用于头痛、眩晕、失眠、胃肠病、妇科病、皮肤病及痿症、痹症等的防治及病后康复调理。

(3) 皮内针刺法

皮内针是一种专用于皮内埋藏的短针，一般用30～32号不锈钢丝制成。有两种形状：图钉形，形如图钉，针身长约0.3cm，适用于耳廓部埋藏；麦粒形，针柄形如麦粒，针身长约1cm，适用于人体各部的腧穴或压痛点上。皮内针刺法又称埋针，由于将针身刺入皮内，固定留置一定时间，可有持续的刺激作用。既可用于保健，又可用于防治某些需要久留针的慢性或疼痛性疾病，如头痛、胃脘痛、失眠、哮喘、遗尿、痛经、月经不调等。

操作时应首先对针身及局部皮肤严格消毒，用消毒镊子将针身刺入皮内，以胶布固定针柄。一般夏季留针不宜超过两天，以免因多汗而易发生感染；秋冬季则可视病情适当延长留针时间。埋针期间应注意清洁，不宜洗澡，以避免感染。皮肤若有破溃或化脓性炎症时不宜埋针，亦不宜在关节处埋针。

2. 保健灸法

灸法有多种，这里主要介绍保健灸常用的艾灸法。艾灸包括艾炷灸、艾条灸和温针灸，后者系与针刺相配合治疗疾病，这里从略。艾叶为菊科植物家艾的叶，性温，气味芳香辛烈，能振扶阳气，温经散寒，通行诸经，调理气血。艾叶捣烂为艾绒，则易燃烧，且其火力温和，又易透热于皮肤、肌肉深处，故作为施灸的材料。将艾绒少许置于平板上，以拇、食、中指捏为圆锥体形，即为艾炷。艾炷小者如麦粒至半个枣核大，用于直接灸；大者如拇指大，高约1cm，底部直径约0.8cm，用于间隔灸。以桑皮纸把艾绒卷成一定大小的烟卷状，为艾条，用于艾条灸，简便易行。艾条一般可作成直径约1.5cm，长约20cm。

(1) 艾炷灸

艾炷灸又分直接灸和间接灸。每燃烧一个艾炷称为一壮。

A. 直接灸　　是把艾炷直接放置在穴位上燃烧，古时此法应用最广。若待艾炷烧到1/2或2/3，患者感到灼痛时，则除掉未燃尽的部分，另换一壮艾炷再灸，皮肤不致成泡、化脓，称为无瘢痕灸。若施灸前用葱液或蒜汁涂于穴位处以增加艾炷的粘附性，整个艾柱燃尽，再加一壮继续燃点，一般灸5~10壮，使局部皮肤烧伤、起泡，以后局部化脓，愈合后留有瘢痕，称瘢痕灸。此法有一定痛苦，又不宜施于影响容颜之处，故不如无瘢痕灸应用广。两法均用于慢性虚寒性疾病和保健强壮。

B. 间接灸　　又称间隔灸，是于艾炷下加垫适当药物。这样既不直接烧及皮肤，又能发挥所垫药物的作用。据所垫药物的不同，有隔姜灸、隔蒜灸、隔盐灸、附子饼灸等多种。隔姜灸用于阳虚病症，脾胃虚弱、泄泻、腹痛及痹症等。隔蒜灸用于毒虫咬伤，疮疡初起及肺痨、瘰疬等。附子饼灸用于肾阳虚衰的阳痿、早泄及顽固性的阴寒证、虚证。隔盐灸施于神阙穴，有回阳救逆之效，可救治虚脱病症，又治腹痛、疝痛、泄泻、久痢等。古籍记载，隔盐灸神阙，灸至三五百壮，有愈疾延年之效。明代李梴《医学入门》以"炼脐法"为题介绍"彭祖固阳固蒂长生延寿丹"也是有于灸脐的。此方药料为：人参、附子、胡椒各21克，麝香、夜明砂、没药、虎骨、蛇骨、龙骨、硃砂、白附子、五灵脂各15克，青盐、小茴香各12克，丁香9克，乳香、木香各6克，雄黄3克，用白面作条，圈于脐上，将前药一料为末，分为三份，内取一份，先填麝香末1.5克入脐眼内，又将前药一份，入面圈内，按药令紧，中插数孔，外用槐皮一片盖于药上，艾火灸之，无时损易，壮其热气。灸时慎风寒，戒油腻生冷。若妇人灸脐，去麝香，加韶脑3克。该书称："凡一年四季各熏一次，元气坚固，百病不生，及久嗽久喘，吐血寒痨，遗精白浊，阳事不举，下元极弱，精神失常，痰膈等疾，妇人赤白带下，久无生育，子宫极冷，凡用此灸，则百疾顿除，益气延年。"上法可供借鉴，但药物可作调整。如《针灸大成》"蒸脐治病法"所用药物有五灵脂、青盐、乳香、没药、夜明砂、地鼠粪、葱头、木通、麝香。《明医选要济世奇方》"灸脐固基法"则以夜明砂30克,五灵脂30克,枯矾60克,麝香6克为春分、秋分、夏至、冬至计4次灸脐的用量。

(2) 艾条灸

艾条灸是近代常用灸法,尤以保健灸多用此法。本法是将艾条的一端点燃,熏灼穴位局部,又分温和灸和雀啄灸两类。

A. 温和灸 是使艾条点燃的一端与穴位保持一定的距离,使穴位局部受到适宜的熏灼,有温热感,以局部皮肤发红为度。连续熏灸时间一般以5~10分钟为宜。

B. 雀啄灸 是将艾条燃着的一端,对准皮肤穴位处,如麻雀啄食般地一上一下移动施灸,也可均匀地左右移动或反复旋转施灸。

施用任何一种灸法,都应掌握好施灸的量。一般根据患者的体质、病情、年龄和施灸的部位,来决定艾柱的大小多小,或艾条灸的时间长短。除瘢痕灸外,要避免因施灸过量而使局部皮肤出现水泡。如出现水泡,注意不要擦破,保持局部清洁,可自然吸收结痂而愈。如水泡较大,可局部消毒后用消毒毫针刺破,放出水液,以消毒敷料复盖。瘢痕灸局部化脓者,要作好局部清洁、消毒,用消毒敷料保护灸疮,使之顺利愈合。

3. 针灸保健的穴位选配

(1) 强壮身体和延年益寿主要穴位

足三里 神阙 关元 气海 大椎 涌泉

(2) 补肾助阳固精主要穴位

命门 肾俞 中极 关元 气海 三阴交 涌泉

(3) 健脾益胃补气及消化系统保健、防病和康复主要穴位

足三里 中脘 天枢 脾俞 胃俞 神阙

(4) 心血管系统保健、防病和康复主要穴位

心俞 内关 膻中 神门

(5) 呼吸系统保健、防病和康复主要穴位
肺俞　大椎　心俞　膻中
(6) 泌尿生殖系统保健、防病和康复主要穴位
肾俞　命门　三阴交　中极　关元　气海
(7) 调摄精神情志的主要穴位
神门　内关　心俞　三阴交
(8) 中风病的预防和康复主要穴位
足三里　曲池　百会　环跳
(9) 肝胆病的预防和康复主要穴位
肝俞　脾俞　足三里
(10) 预防感冒主要穴位
大椎　肺俞　足三里
(11) 虚脱症辅助治疗和康复保健主要穴位
神阙　关元　中极
(12) 头部疾病的预防和康复主要穴位
百会　涌泉
(13) 腰腿疾病的预防和康复主要穴位
肾俞　命门　环跳　三阴交
(14) 癫、狂、痫症的预防和康复主要穴位
内关　神门　大椎　心俞　肝俞　百会

在具体实施针灸保健时，上述穴位不必全部选用，一般每次选1~3个穴位即可。可选1~2个最重要的穴位，长期坚持，并随时视具体情况选加1~2个穴位。

4. 针灸保健注意事项

(1) 针灸保健多用灸法，对体质虚弱和年老者更是如此。身体过度虚弱或过饥、过饱、过度劳累、醉酒时忌用针刺法，施灸也宜慎重。

(2) 施行针灸保健时应采取较舒适而能持久的姿势，常取卧位或坐位。

(3) 针刺时要注意有些穴位（如少腹部、腰骶部的穴位）孕妇禁针，有些穴位（腹背胸部的穴位）施针时应防止刺伤重要脏器，施针时还要避开血管及局部炎症、溃疡或外伤处。还要严格注意针具和局部皮肤的消毒。

(4) 施灸时要避免灼伤皮肤，施瘢痕灸时要防止感染扩散。患实证、热证或阴虚发热者一般不要施灸。老年或行动不便者施灸时应防止烧坏衣物，甚至发生火灾。孕妇的腹部或腰骶部都不宜施灸。颜面五官和有大血管的部位不宜施瘢痕灸。

(5) 注意针灸保健后的调摄。按照有关文献对施灸后调摄的要求，可归纳为以下几点：灸后不可就饮茶及进食；灸后宜入室静卧，远人事，远色欲，平心定气，百事俱要宽解；尤忌大怒、大劳、大饥、大饱、受热、冒寒；宜忌生冷瓜果，宜食茹淡养胃之物；忌酗醉；忌房劳。这些调摄宜忌，利于养生保健，可供针灸保健者参考。

(6) 针灸保健要持之以恒，疗程之间可有适当间歇。一般可每日或隔日1次，10次为1疗程，疗程间可休息数日，坚持几个疗程就逐渐见效。古代文献中亦有每月、每季或每年按一定时间施灸的，可供参考，有待在实践中探索验证。

3.1.5 穴位磁疗保健

据一些临床观察和实验研究，磁疗有通调气血，防治疾病，保健延寿的作用。在保健方面的应用，一般是用适当的恒磁体，贴敷在保健穴位上，可获健身防病抗衰老之效。此种方法可称为穴位磁疗保健。其中应用较广的是"三里磁"，即足三里穴位贴敷恒磁体。有报道约有90%的患者或正常人，用此法后饮食、睡眠、肌力、血压均有不同程度的改善。具体运用时要注意掌握好磁感应强度和敷磁的时间。选用直径1cm左右适当磁感应强度的恒磁体，缝在单层条形布带中，使磁体对准足三里穴，把布带绑敷固定。无严重疾病者，磁感应强度宜0.01~0.03T（特斯拉），每日绑敷 2~4 小时。如血压及白细胞低者，无其他疾病，磁感应强度宜减至 0.005~0.02T。如患胃肠病、高血压及关节炎等病，磁感应强度可增至 0.04~0.1T，并可延长绑敷时间，甚至长期使用。借鉴此法，也可探索和观察在其他重要保健穴位贴敷适当磁感应强度恒磁片对人体的保健效果，并宜从较小的磁感应强度开始试用。

3.2 气功保健

气功是我国劳动人民创造出来的一种传统养生方法，适宜于各种人群，尤其是中老年人。气功为现代通俗名称，包括古代"导引"、"吐纳"、"术数"、"行气"、"坐禅"、"按跻"、"静坐"等。它以阴阳五行、脏腑、经络、气血学说为基础，以"气"为动力，在入静和放松的状态下，经过三调（调身、调心、调息）进行自我控制、自我调整、自我修复和自我建设，达到防治疾病、健身延年之目的。

气功起源于（传说）唐尧时期，奠基于春秋战国，以后历代有所发展。气功流派甚多，从形式上分，有动功与静功；从练法上分，文练称为气功，武练称为硬气功；从呼吸方式分，有气息内功与声息气功；从功用上分，有健身的内壮功和治病的保健功；从性能上分，有内气功与外气功，等等。不同的功法既有区别，又有联系。其共同特征谓之内练"精、气、神"，外练"筋、骨、皮"。气功锻炼有两个基本特点：强调自我锻炼，强调内因与整体的关系。通过气功锻炼，可以养精守神、调和气血、平衡阴阳、活血化瘀，从而达到防病治病、益寿延年之目的。由于气功功法、流派甚多，本节只作简略介绍，详见有关专著。

3.2.1 气功的功法

功法，即练气功的方法，气功功法不胜枚举，汇历代各派之精华，可概括为"调"（调阴阳、调气血、调营卫）、"练"（练姿势求轻、松、静,练呼吸求细、深、长,练意守求归丹田),然后达到"功"。通过练功者发挥主观能动作用,对身心进行自我锻炼,达到养生却病之目的。

每种气功大致都包括互相联系、互相影响、互相促进、同时进行的3个基本环节,即调身、调心、调息。其中调心和调息是关键环节。

1. 调身

调身又称姿势或体势,通常分为站、坐、卧、行4种基本类型,多以坐式为主。具体选用则要因人因时因地而异。

(1) 站式 站式一般为健康者锻炼的方式,以健身为目的。站式又可分为三圆式、自然站式、随意站式等,以三圆式最为常用。其做法是:两脚分开,宽与肩齐,脚尖稍向内,膝微屈,含胸;两臂抬起,与肩同高,然后缓缓下降,手与乳头平,两手相距约30cm,两臂如抱大球,两手指屈曲作握球状;眼口微闭,面带笑容。

(2) 坐式 坐式既适于健康人练习,又适于恢复期病人之康复训练。常用的有平坐式、自由盘膝式和单盘膝式。

平坐式要求端坐在方凳上,足着地,两腿分开,躯干与大腿、大腿与小腿均为90°角;双手放于膝盖上或握拳放小腹前;下颏回收,垂肩含胸,口眼微闭,舌抵上腭,面带微笑。

自由盘膝式要求端坐在木板床上,两腿叉成八字型,自然盘坐,两手放小腹前或两膝盖上。

单盘膝式则应端坐在木板床上,右小腿放于左小腿上面,或左放右上。其他要求同自由盘膝式及平坐式。

(3) 卧式 卧式适于久病体弱、阳气虚衰的患者,以及各种慢性病人。分为仰卧式和侧卧式。

仰卧式要求仰卧于木板床上,上半身垫高,呈斜坡状;腿伸直,手放于两侧。头面部要求同平坐式。

侧卧式是侧卧于木板床上,头枕平,上身直;上腿弯曲放下腿上，上面的手放于臀部，下面的手放于枕上，手心向上。头面部要求同平坐式。左右侧卧均可，心脏病人以右侧卧为宜。

(4) 行式　行式为气功与武术相结合的姿势，不同派别有不同的动作。一般静站 2～3 分钟，先左脚向前迈出一步，脚跟先着地，上身和两手向右摆动，鼻吸气，口呼气；当左脚落实后，再将右脚向前迈出一步，脚跟先着地，身子和两手向左摆动，鼻吸气，口呼气。如此一步步向前走，20～30 分钟后收功。

2. 调心

调心又称意守或练意，是练功者在练功时通过意念活动的锻炼以调整生理功能的一种方法。调整精神状态使之入静，是气功最基本的功夫。练功效果取决于入静的程度，越静效果越好，反之则差。入静是指一种稳定的安静状态，无杂念，集中意念于一点，即意守丹田或留意呼吸。这时对外界刺激（如声、光等）的感觉减弱，甚至连位置感和重量感也消失，亦即大脑皮层进入了保护性抑制状态。常用的入静方法有 5 种。

(1) 意守法　意念高度集中于身体某一点，常用的是意守丹田或气海（脐下一寸三分）。意守时，要排除杂念，但不必过分用意。要似守非守，不即不离，松静自然，恰到好处。

(2) 随息法　意念集中在呼吸上，只留意于腹式呼吸的起伏，但不可加意指挥。要意气和一，达到入静。

(3) 数息法　1 呼 1 吸谓 1 息。练功时，默数呼吸次数，从 1 到 10，10 到 100，数到耳无所闻，目无所见，心无所虑，便可自然入静。

(4) 默念法　默念的字句要单纯，其目的是用 1 念代万念，用正念代邪念，以帮助入静。

(5) 听息法　用耳朵听自己的呼吸，以听不到为好，在听不到的情况下去听，以助入静。

初练时，可从意守法开始，逐渐过渡到随息法或听息法，或始终练1种。

3. 调息

调息又称为气息或练气,是气功锻炼的重要环节。通过锻炼,改胸式呼吸为腹式呼吸,改浅呼吸为深呼吸,最后练成自发的丹田呼吸,以扩大肺活量,促进气体代谢和血液循环,"按摩"内脏,帮助消化吸收,达到保健强身、防治疾病之目的。常用的呼吸方法有8种。

(1) 自然呼吸法　这是生理呼吸,丝毫不加意念支配,呼吸自然、柔和、均匀,缺点是不够深长。

(2) 顺呼吸法　吸气时膈肌下降,腹部外凸;呼气时膈肌上升,腹部内凹。这种呼吸法膈肌上下移动幅度大,腹肌前后运动量大,可逐渐练成腹式呼吸。

(3) 逆呼吸法　与顺呼吸法相反,吸气时膈肌上升,腹部内凹;呼气时膈肌下降,腹部外凸。较顺呼吸法之运动幅度和强度为大。

(4) 停闭呼吸法　有两种。一是在1呼1吸之间将呼气时间拉长,另是在1呼1吸之间将吸气时间拉长。

(5) 鼻吸口呼法　呼吸道有病变,内腔狭窄,呼吸不畅时可用此法。

(6) 气通任督脉法　采用逆呼吸法,用鼻吸气,同时以意领气,意想气到了丹田,然后下至会阴;呼气时以意领气,意想气由会阴循脊柱至百会(头顶),由鼻呼出。因气循体内1周,故又名小周天呼吸法。

(7) 潜呼吸法　这是在练顺呼吸法或逆呼吸法后,自然出现的一种呼吸法。其特点是:吸气绵绵,呼气微微,息息均匀。呼吸时手置于鼻,没有明显的感觉,故又称潜息法。

(8) 真息法　即古人所云"盖凡息即停,而真息自动"的状态。息停,不是强闭不出,而是虚极静笃,神凝气结,止此一息。此时从外表看好象呼吸停止,实际上仍在用肚脐呼吸,腹中在旋转跳动,故又称"胎息"。这是功夫的较高阶段。

练呼吸要与养呼吸相结合,不论选练哪种呼吸法,每练10～20分钟后,都要改为自然呼吸法,以免呼吸肌过于疲劳。练呼吸要在柔和自然的基本原则指导下,逐步做到深长、细匀、缓慢,切不可急于求成。

3.2.2 气功的功种

气功的功种甚多,常用于保健、防病、益寿的有松静功、内养功、强壮功等。

1. 松静功

松静功侧重于练放松。

准备工作　练功的环境应尽可能选在安静、空气新鲜之处。室内练功要通风换气,但不要迎着风向,以防感冒。要宽衣松带,解除束缚,使身体舒适,血液循环畅通。练功前20分钟左右应休息一下,安定情绪,精神愉快。

姿势　不论采取哪种姿势,都要端正,合乎自然。姿势端正易于入静。端正姿势后,两眼微闭,注视鼻尖;口微闭,舌抵上腭。

放松法　放松可采取坐、站、卧、行等不同姿势,要求自头上向脚下放松。做到虚灵顶颈(头轻轻顶起之意),垂肩坠肘,胸部不外挺,腹部回收,腰部正直,全身无紧张不适之处。精神放松,面带微笑。

呼吸法　松静功采用顺呼吸法。吸气时默念"静",呼气时默念"松"。放松的越好入静越快。要求呼吸自然柔和,舒适自得,使气沉丹田(气海)。呼吸是练气功的主要环节之一,要循序渐进,每次练20～30分钟即可。

静坐法　练完呼吸法后,接练静坐法。要求意守肚脐或气海,进入无杂念的境界。但静是相对的,入静的程度因人而异,特别是练功初期,不可勉强追求,急于求成。必要时可用一念代万念，也可收到一定效果。

收功法　练完气功后，不要急于起来，用1只手掌心按在肚脐上，另1手掌心贴在此手背上，两手同时以肚脐为中心，由内向外、由小到大缓缓划圈，左转30圈，稍停，再由外向内、由大到小右转30圈，到肚脐处停止。而后活动身体。如加练太极拳、八段锦或慢跑步等，则收效更大。

本功适于健康者、中老年、体弱者以及患有心血管、呼吸、消化系统慢性疾病者锻炼。

2. 内养功

内养功侧重于练调息。准备工作、姿势、放松法的要求同松静功。

呼吸法　内养功采用停闭式呼吸法。可以在吸→停→呼→吸……或吸→呼→停→吸……两种呼吸方式中任选1种。每次练功必须注意呼吸深长、轻细、均匀，努力建立鼻呼鼻吸、气沉丹田的条件反射。要求在练呼吸时，通过意念诱导气体下降到小腹（气海穴）。气贯丹田，则小腹膨大，然膨大之程度因人而异，在练功的各个阶段也不一样。不宜故意用力鼓肚子，或以为越高越好。

静坐时可采用1种或2种调息法，尤以随意法、止息法、静息法为优。静坐及收功要求同松静功。

本功最宜于年老体弱及慢性消化系统病患者。

3. 强壮功

强壮功侧重于练入静。一般在松静功的基础上容易练成。练本功的要领是姿势正确、调节呼吸、意守入静。准备工作、姿势、放松法要求同松静功。

呼吸法　一般男子用顺呼吸法，女子用逆呼吸法。本功要求：平时顺呼吸者练腹式逆呼吸法，平时逆呼吸者练腹式顺呼吸法，每练10～20分钟后改为自然呼吸。练呼吸时不要注意吸气，而要注意呼气的柔和自然。

静坐法　本功意在练入静，也可不练呼吸而径练静坐法。静坐时可以采取意守丹田法或听息法、数息法、默念法等诱导入静，使之进入似睡非睡、似醒非醒、忘我的状态。静坐30～40分钟。

练完静坐法，以意领气从肚脐开始划圈，先自左而右划24圈，再自右而左划24圈，而后离坐。或加练动功。

强壮功对增强体力、保健益寿、防病却病有独到效果，对神经衰弱、神经官能症、植物神经功能紊乱等有良好疗效。

3.2.3　气功锻炼的要领

进行气功锻炼，必须掌握要领，方能取得效果。

1. 要有信心、决心、恒心。要求长期锻炼，深信气功具有防病治病、健身延年的作用。
2. 生活要有规律，避免"七情"干扰，保持精神愉快，戒烟忌酒。
3. 练功前要排除大小便，松解衣带，全身放松，安下心来，消除杂念。
4. 姿势因人而异，每次可练30～60分钟，每天练1～2次。练功地点宜安静，空气新鲜。
5. 练功初应做准备功，练功末应当收功，练功过程中则要求松静自然，不可急于求成。
6. 对于自发动功，决不可强求，一般应在老师指导下进行。动作要有柔有刚，有缓有急，经常变化。只有练出一定的动作规律来，才能减少偏差。

3.3　推拿保健

推拿，又称按摩，是我们的祖先在长期的生活实践中创造出来的一种有效的摄生保健方法，推拿疗法是指运用手和手指的技巧，在自身或他人皮肤、肌肉组织上连续动作，用来保健或治病的方法。它勿需药物和器械，经济、简便、安全、疗效可靠，尤其适于某些老年性慢性疾病，又是老年保健和健康人养生的理想方法。

推拿疗法有着悠久的历史，远在两千多年前的春秋战国时期，按摩就被广泛应用于医疗中。以后历代都有发展，至今已形成了一套完整的理论体系和切实有效的方法。

推拿可导致局部和全身反应，从而调整人体功能，消除病因，达到治病、健身之目的。现代则认为，推拿手法的物理刺激，使作用区产生生物物理、生物化学变化，局部组织发生生理反应。这种反应通过神经反射与体液循环的调节，一方面得到加强，另一方面又引起整体的继发性反应，从而产生一系列病理生理过程的改变，起到治疗或保健效果。推拿手法作用于人体，可以平衡阴阳、调节功能、调节经络、扶正祛邪、活血散瘀、强筋壮骨、镇痛、移痛、消痛、止痛。

推拿疗法的总原则是治病求本，具体施行手法时应根据体质、年龄、疾病种类、时间等情况灵活掌握。

推拿疗法的内容甚多，本节仅以自我保健为主，进行简略介绍，详见推拿专书。

3.3.1 推拿的种类与常用手法

1. 推拿的种类

推拿疗法有主动、被动之分。自我操作，即自己对自身进行推拿的保健方法，称为主动推拿，亦谓自我按摩，主要用于预防保健；他人操作，即医师对病人进行推拿的治疗方法，称为被动推拿，主要用于医治疾病。

2. 推拿的手法

推拿手法复杂多变，因流派不同操作各异。大抵有推、拿、按、摩、揉、捏、擀、擦、运、搓、摇、捻、刮、拍、叠、点、压、押、弹、分、合等手法，其中以前8种最为常用，自我按摩又常用拍、点、压等法。

(1) 推法

用指、掌或肘部着力于一定部位上,进行单方向的直线推动,称为推法。推时用力要稳,速度要缓慢,着力部分要紧贴皮肤。推法适用于人体各部位。本法能增强肌肉的兴奋性、促进血液循环、舒筋活络。

(2) 拿法

用大拇指和食、中两指,或用大拇指和其余四指对称地用力,提拿一定部位和穴位,进行一紧一松的拿捏,称为拿法。拿法动作要缓和而有连贯性,不要断断续续;用劲要由轻到重,不要突然用力。拿法刺激较强,常配合其他手法使用于颈项、肩部和四肢等穴位。本法具有祛风散寒、开窍止痛、缓解肌腱肌肉痉挛等作用。

(3) 按法

用拇指或掌根等部按压一定部位或穴位,逐渐用力深压捻动,按而留之,称为按法。分为拇指按、掌根按、4指按、2指按等。按法是一种较强刺激的手法,常与揉法结合使用,组成"按揉"复合手法。拇指按法适用于全身各部穴位,掌根按法常用于腰背及下肢部,4指按法适于颈部或肋间部位,2指按法适用于手指或细柔肌肉处。本法具有诱导止痛、开通闭塞、放松肌肉、矫正脊柱畸形的功能。

(4) 摩法

用手掌掌面或食、中、环指指面附着于一定部位上,以腕关节连同前臂作环形有节律的抚摩,称为摩法。操作时,肘关节微屈,腕部放松,指掌自然伸直;指掌着力部分要随着腕关节连同前臂作盘旋活动,用劲要自然;摩动时要缓和协调,每分钟120次左右。本法刺激轻柔缓和,是胸腹、胸胁部常用手法。具有和中理气、消积导滞、调节肠胃蠕动的功能。

(5) 揉法

用手掌大鱼际、掌根部分或手指罗纹面部分,吸定于一定部位或穴位上,作轻柔缓和的回旋揉动,称为揉法,分为掌揉和指揉法。操作时手腕应放松,以腕关节连动前臂一起作回旋活动,腕部活动幅度可逐步扩大,压力要轻柔。一般每分钟120~160次。本法轻柔缓和,刺激量小,适用于全身各部,具有宽胸理气、消积导滞、活血祛瘀、消肿止痛之作用。

(6) 捏法

用拇指与其他指相对捏住肌肉或肌腱,沿其走向辗转挤捏推进,称为捏法。分为2指捏、3指捏和5指捏。适用于大腿、小腿、肩背等部位。具有舒筋通络、行气活血之作用。

(7) 擦法

用手背近小指侧部分或小指、环指、中指的掌指关节部分,附着于一定部位上,通过腕关节屈伸外旋的连续活动,使产生的力持续作用于治疗部位上,称为擦法。操作时,肩臂不要过分紧张,肘关节微屈(约120°角),手腕放松。擦动时小鱼际部分要紧贴体表,不要跳动或使手背拖来拖去摩擦。运用压力要均匀,动作协调而有节律。每分钟120~160次。本法压力较大,接触面较广,适用于肩背、腰臀及4肢等肌肉较丰厚的部位。具有舒筋活血、滑利关节、缓解痉挛、促进血液循环、消除疲劳等作用。

(8) 擦法

用手掌面、大鱼际或小鱼际部分着力于一定部位上,进行直线来回摩擦,称为擦法。擦时应直线往返,不可歪斜,往返距离要拉得长;着力部分要紧贴皮肤,但不可过压,以免擦破皮肤;用力要稳,动作要均匀连续。每分钟100~120次。本法是一种柔和温热的刺激,具有温经通络、行气活血、消肿止痛、健脾和胃、提高局部体温、加速血液和淋巴循环之作用。掌擦法多用于胸胁及腹部,小鱼际擦法多用于肩背、腰臀及下肢部,大鱼际擦法适于胸腹、腰背、4肢等部位。使用擦法时,治疗部位应暴露,并涂适量的润滑油或药膏。

(9) 拍法

用虚掌拍打体表,称为拍法。拍时手指自然并拢,掌指关节微屈,平稳而有节奏地拍打患部。拍法适用于肩背、腰臀及下肢部位。具有舒筋通络、行气活血、消除疲劳、缓解痉挛之作用。

(10) 点法

根据不同的施治部位,用1指或2指向应点部位的上下左右或周围进行点压,称为点法。本法刺激很强,常用在肌肉较薄的骨缝处。具有开通闭塞、活血止痛、调整脏腑功能之作用。

(11) 压法

用手压患处的方法称为压法。用中指或其他指的正面压称为指压,适于头面部;用单掌或双掌压为掌压,适用于躯干各部。本法能放松肌肉、活血止痛。

3.3.2 自我推拿保健方法

自我推拿是常用的推拿保健方法,通常分为局部推拿与全身推拿两种。前者指小面积推拿,侧重于局部治疗;后者指头部、躯干、4肢等处的大面积推拿,多用于预防保健。全身自我推拿是一种较理想的保健方法,尤其适用于老年体弱者。

1. 自我推拿的适用范围

局部推拿　　适用于患病的局部。凡是感受风寒引起局部肌肉疼痛、酸麻、萎缩、功能减退者,皆可采用局部推拿法。局部神经痛、消化不良等也可应用。

全身推拿　　主要用作预防保健、强身壮体、延年益寿,也可用于疾病的治疗。

2. 自我推拿的方法

这里重点介绍一种强身防病的全身推拿方法,此法尤宜于老年、体弱者。本法包括20个相连续的动作。

(1) 叩齿

口唇轻闭,有节律地叩击上、下齿 30~40 次。

(2) 净口

口唇轻闭,用舌在齿唇之间用力卷抹,左、右各转 30 次。

(3) 搓手

两手掌相对,用力搓动,由慢而快,约 30~40 次,搓激为止。

(4) 摩脸

搓热手掌后摩脸。手指微屈,5 指并拢,两手轻作遮面状,由额向下拂,如同洗脸。20~30 次。

(5) 梳头

10 指微屈,以指尖接触头皮,从额前到枕后、从颞颥到头顶进行"梳头"。20~30 次。

(6) 揉太阳

用两手中指端按压两侧太阳穴,旋转揉动,先顺时针,后逆时针,各转 7~8 次。

(7) 揉眼

用两手食、中、环三指指节,沿两眼眶旋转揉动,先由内向外,再由外向内,各转 7~8 次。

(8) 点睛明

用两手食指指端分别点压双睛明穴(在目内眦外约一分凹陷中)15~30 次。

(9) 按太阳

用两手食指指端分别压在双侧太阳穴上,旋压转动。顺、逆时针方向各 10~15 次。

(10) 鸣天鼓

两手掌心紧按两耳孔,两手食、中、环三指轻击头后枕骨 15 次。然后掌心掩按耳孔,手指紧按头后枕骨部不动,再骤然抬离,连续开闭放响 15 次。最后两中指或食指插入耳孔内旋转三次,再骤然拔开,如此反复 3~5 次。

(11) 揉胸脯

两手掌按在两乳外上方,旋转揉动,顺、逆时针各揉 10 次。揉胸脯宜用力,不宜滑动。

(12) 抓肩井

以右手拇指与食、中指配合捏提左肩肌(肩井穴周围);再以左手拇、食、中指配合捏提右肩肌。如此左右手交叉进行,各捏提 10~15 次。抓肩肌要有力度。

(13) 豁胸廓

两手微张 5 指,分别置于胸骨两旁的胸壁上,手指端沿肋间隙从内向外滑动,各侧重复推 10~15 次。

(14) 揉腹

以 1 手 5 指张开,指端向下,从胃脘部起,经脐左侧揉到下腹部,然后向右、向上、向左、向下,沿着大肠走向擦揉。反复擦 10~15 次。

(15) 搓腰

两手搓热,紧按腰部,用力向下搓到尾尖部,左右手一上一下,两侧同时进行。共搓 30 次。

(16) 点环跳

先以左手拇指端点压左侧环跳穴(右侧卧位,右腿伸直,左腿弯曲,在大转子最高点后上方约 2 寸凹陷中),再用右手点压右侧环跳穴,交叉进行。每侧 10 次。

(17) 擦大腿

两手抱紧一侧大腿部,用力下擦到膝盖,然后擦回大腿根。来回擦 20 次。擦大腿要用力均匀,不可忽轻忽重。

(18) 揉小腿

用两手撑挟紧一侧小腿腿肚,旋转揉动,每侧揉动 20~30 次。揉小腿要有力。

(19) 擦涌泉

两手搓热,搓涌泉穴(在足心陷中,前三分之一交界处),

快速用力,约30～40次,至脚心发热为止。先左后右。

(20) 呼吸

站立,两腿分开如肩宽,两手由腹部向上抬至喉头,同时抬头、伸腰、吸气;然后两手由喉头下引到腹部,同时低头、弯腰、呼气,呼气时顺序发出"哈、呵、唏、嘘"4音。重复3遍。

上述动作应依次完成。体质差者,可先选择部分动作,逐渐至全部完成。

3. 自我推拿的注意事项

(1) 过饱或过饥不宜推拿。

(2) 应保持推拿地点的空气新鲜。

(3) 一般每天早晚各推1次,每次20分钟左右。可根据个人情况增减。

(4) 推拿量应因人而异,以感舒适愉快、精神振奋为最佳。

(5) 推拿时应思想集中,情绪稳定,全身放松。

(6) 推拿期间应适当补充营养,避免劳累,节制性生活。

(7) 应保持全身皮肤清洁。推拿前应洗净双手,剪短指甲并使之圆滑,4肢及多毛部位可涂少许滑石粉,以防损伤皮肤。

(8) 推拿应直接接触皮肤,不宜隔衣操作。

3.3.3 推拿的适应症和禁忌症

1. 推拿的适应症

推拿疗法的应用范围较广,内、外、儿、骨(外)、伤、保健等科都可应用,或作为辅助疗法。推拿较适于内伤性疾病,尤其是慢性病、功能性疾病,对某些疾病的急性期也有较好疗效,如腰椎间盘突出症、急性扭伤、急性乳腺炎、小儿发热、小儿消化不良、小儿腹泻等。防病强身、延年益寿亦为推拿之一大适应范围。

2. 推拿的禁忌症

各种急性传染病、恶性肿瘤的局部、溃疡性皮肤病、烧伤、烫伤，各种传染性、化脓性疾病和结核性关节炎、严重的心脏病、肝病，严重的精神病，胃及12指肠等急性穿孔，各种危重症患者以及出血性疾病等，均为推拿的禁忌症。妇女月经期、妊娠期不宜推拿腹部和腰骶部。

THE ENGLISH–CHINESE ENCYCLOPEDIA OF PRACTICAL TCM
(Booklist)

英汉实用中医药大全

(书目)

VOLUME	TITLE	书名
1	ESSENTIALS OF TRADITIONAL CHINESE MEDICINE	中医学基础
2	THE CHINESE MATERIA MEDICA	中药学
3	PHARMACOLOGY OF TRADITIONAL CHINESE MEDICAL FORMULAE	方剂学
4	SIMPLE AND PROVEN PRESCRIPTION	单验方
5	COMMONLY USED CHINESE PATENTMEDICINES	常用中成药
6	THERAPY OF ACUPUNCTURE AND MOXIBUSTION	针灸疗法
7	*TUINA* THERAPY	推拿疗法
8	MEDICAL *QIGONG*	医学气功
9	MAINTAINING YOUR HEALTH	自我保健
10	INTERNAL MEDICINE	内科学

11	SURGERY	外科学
12	GYNECOLOGY	妇科学
13	PEDIATRICS	儿科学
14	ORTHOPEDICS	骨伤科学
15	PROCTOLOGY	肛门直肠病学
16	DERMATOLOGY	皮肤病学
17	OPHTHALMOLOGY	眼科学
18	OTORHINOLARYNGOLOGY	耳鼻喉科学
19	EMERGENTOLOGY	急症学
20	NURSING	护理
21	CLINICAL DIALOGUE	临床会话

(京)112号

The English—Chinese
Encyclopedia of Practical TCM
Chief Editor   Xu Xiangcai

9

MAINTAINING
YOUR HEALTH

Chief Editors   Xu Xiangcai
                 Zhang Wengao

英汉实用中医药大全
主编 徐象才
9
自我保键
主编 张文高
      徐象才

*

高等教育出版社出版
高等教育出版社照排技术部照排
新华书店总店北京科技发行所发行
高等教育出版社印刷厂印装

*

开本 850×1168 1/32 印张 20.625 字数 530 000
1992年12月第1版 1992年12月第1次印刷
印数 0 001—5 273
ISBN7—04—003868—4/R·17
定价